Surgical
Techniques in
Obstetrics
and
Gynaecology

To
Jack and Evelyn (Sissy) who gave so much to their sons
and
Cheryl, Charlotte and Sophie for every single day

Commissioning Editor: Ellen Green
Project Development Manager: Duncan Fraser
Project Manager: Frances Affleck
Designer: Sarah Russell
Illustration Manager: Bruce Hogarth

Surgical Techniques in
Obstetrics and Gynaecology

Edited by

DARRYL J MAXWELL FRCOG MRANZCOG

Consultant Obstetrician and Gynaecologist,
Honorary Senior Lecturer,
Women's Services Directorate
Guy's and St Thomas' Hospital Trust,
London, UK

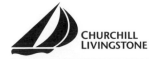

CHURCHILL
LIVINGSTONE

EDINBURGH   LONDON   NEW YORK   OXFORD   PHILADELPHIA   ST LOUIS   SYDNEY   TORONTO   2004

CHURCHILL LIVINGSTONE
An imprint of Elsevier Limited

First published 2004

ISBN 0443071497

British Library Cataloguing in Publication Data
A catalogue record for this book is available from the British
Library

Library of Congress Cataloging in Publication Data
A catalog record for this book is available from the Library
of Congress

Notice
Medical knowledge is constantly changing. Standard safety
precautions must be followed, but as new research and
clinical experience broaden our knowledge, changes in
treatment and drug therapy may become necessary or
appropriate. Readers are advised to check the most current
product information provided by the manufacturer of each
drug to be administered to verify the recommended dose,
the method and duration of administration, and
contraindications. It is the responsibility of the practitioner,
relying on experience and knowledge of the patient, to
determine dosages and the best treatment for each
individual patient. Neither the Publisher, the editor nor the
contributors assume any liability for any injury and/or
damage to persons or property arising from this
publication.

Printed in Spain

Contents

1 General principles

2 Obstetric techniques

Contents

List of contributors

Mr Vincent Argent
Consultant Obstetrician and Gynaecologist,
Eastbourne District Hospital, King's Drive,
Eastbourne, East Sussex BN21 2UD, UK

Mr Simon Atkinson
Consultant Gastrointestinal Surgeon,
Department of Surgery, 1st Floor North Wing,
St Thomas' Hospital, London SE1 7EH, UK

Miss Helena Baxter
Tissue Viability Specialist, Hinchingbrook
Healthcare NHS Trust, Huntingdon,
Cambridgeshire PE29 6NT, UK

Dr Catherine Elliott
Senior Medical Claims Handler, Medical
Defence Union, 230 Blackfriars Rd, London
SE1 8BJ, UK

Mr David J. Gerrard
Consultant Vascular Surgeon, Department of
Surgery, Frimley Park Hospital, Portsmouth
Road, Frimley, Surrey GU16 7UJ, UK

Mr Donald Gibb
Independent Consultant Obstetrician and
Gynaecologist, 137 Harley St, London
W1G 6BG, UK

Dr Kate Harding
Consultant Obstetrician and Gynaecologist,
Women's Services Directorate, 10th Floor North
Wing, St Thomas' Hospital, London SE1 7EH,
UK

Mr Patrick Hogston
Consultant Obstetrician and Gynaecologist,
St Mary's Hospital, Milton Road, Portsmouth
PO3 6AD, UK

Mr Frank Loeffler
Consultant Obstetrician and Gynaecologist,
86 Harley St, London W1N 1AE, UK

Mr Derek Mercer
Consultant Plastic Surgeon, Department of
Plastic Surgery, 3rd Floor Lambeth Wing,
St Thomas' Hospital, London SE1 7EH, UK

Mr David Oram
Consultant Obstetrician and Gynaecologist,
Department of Gynaecological Oncology,
St. Bartholomew's Hospital, West Smithfield,
London EC1A 7BE, UK

Mr John Pereira
Consultant Plastic Surgeon, Queen Victoria
Hospital, Holtye Rd, East Grinstead, West Sussex
RH19 3DZ, UK

Mr Rick Popert
Consultant Urologist, Department of Urology,
1st Floor Thomas Guy House, Guy's Hospital
SE1 9RT, UK

Miss Janice Rymer
Consultant Obstetrician and Gynaecologist,
Department of Obstetrics and Gynaecology,
10th Floor North Wing, St Thomas' Hospital,
London SE1 7EH, UK

Dr Michael Scott
Consultant Anaesthetist, Royal Surrey County
Hospital, Egerton Rd, Guildford
Surrey GU2 7XX, UK

Professor Phillip Steer
Academic Department of Obstetrics and
Gynaecology, Chelsea and Westminister
Hospital, Fulham Rd, London SW10 9NH, UK

Mr Christopher Sutton
Consultant Obstetrician and Gynaecologist,
Guildford Nuffield Hospital, Stirling Rd,
Guildford Surrey GU2 7RF, UK

Mr Peter R. Taylor
Consultant Vascular Surgeon, Department of
Surgery, 1st Floor North Wing, St Thomas'
Hospital, London SE1 7EH, UK

Foreword

Training in all branches of surgery has undergone progressive change during my professional lifetime. In years gone by it was usual for a trainee to have no more than alternate evenings off duty and to spend many more hours than now in the operating theatre assisting and carrying out both elective and emergency surgery. As a consequence, by the time an appointment as consultant was obtained a trainee was very widely experienced in operative surgery. Indeed, in many instances, full consultant responsibility could have been assumed much earlier. Today, with the length of training better defined and the working week being so much shorter (and to be shorter still in the future), a trainee needs to have the very best study aids readily available to amplify their lessened practical experience.

Twenty-five years ago the majority of trainees entering a career in obstetrics and gynaecology gained wide experience in general surgery, culminating in the completion of the FRCS diploma, before embarking on experience in obstetrics and gynaecology leading to the MRCOG. Today, a comprehensive preliminary general training is less common and most trainees progress far more quickly, after pre-registration jobs, into their chosen specialty. This has many advantages but it can also cause difficulties when faced with an unexpectedly tricky situation in the operating theatre.

This book takes into account these changes in training, each of which has impinged on the safe learning of operative obstetrics and gynaecology. As such, it is a valuable addition to the surgical literature. Throughout the text there is particular emphasis on the general principles of operative surgery as applied to obstetrics and gynaecology including wound healing, complications and peri-operative care. There are individual chapters relating to techniques used in general surgery, vascular surgery, urology and plastic surgery that will be of particular use to the gynaecologist. These sections will be of special value to those trainees who have not had clinical exposure in these disciplines. New areas that have gained great importance in the past few years are also well covered, including clinical governance, risk management, clinical negligence, the meaning of informed consent and the importance of patient choice. One hardly need add that detailed descriptions and illustrations of the standard operative repertoire in obstetrics and gynaecology occupy many pages and that minimal access surgery as it relates to the specialty is also fully covered.

All in all, I believe this book will prove of great value to the obstetrics and gynaecology trainee, and I suspect that some of their Chiefs may find parts of value as well. As a colorectal surgeon, who has long recognized the close interface that exists within the pelvis between gynaecological surgery and the various branches of general surgery, I can only say how much I wish that there had been a volume such as this available when I was at an early stage of my own career.

Sir Barry Jackson MS FRCS FRCP
President, The Royal Society of Medicine
Past-president, The Royal College of Surgeons of England

Preface

My first thoughts that this book should be written were about four years ago. I have always felt that it would have been advantageous if my own core surgical skills had been acquired earlier in my career. From discussions with colleagues I knew I was not alone in this view. Another issue consistently regretted by us all was the fact that as we became more senior there were less and less opportunities to operate with colleagues, thereby reducing the chance to reappraise one's own techniques by observing others.

My trigger to action was the considerable revision that training in obstetrics and gynaecology has undergone in recent years. Teaching how to operate safely has changed with the traditional 'consultant firm' and apprenticed surgical training being replaced by a more fragmented approach. I noted that trainees seemed to read less often the definitive textbooks on gynaecological surgery or operative obstetrics; their place being supplanted by an increasing number of courses on the varied surgical modalities. I strongly felt that teaching of sound, core surgical principles should be maintained. A series of one-day seminars were initiated. They were well received and have evolved to become this text.

The objective has been to develop a manual that:

- is useful from the start of an individual's surgical career;
- continues to be of assistance as more experience is gained; and
- assists the more established practitioners wishing to review their basic approach.

This book is aimed primarily at the trainee, but is also intended for a wider readership encompassing all obstetricians and gynaecologists of any seniority. It was never intended to be an exhaustive surgical text but to be read in conjunction with them. It outlines sensible practical principles for operating in the pelvis but deliberately does not deal with assisted vaginal delivery. Core methods and the avoidance of surgical pitfalls using safe techniques have been emphasised plus the essential measures to take when encountering problems. Unique features are the inclusion of relevant tips from allied surgical disciplines and an appendix dealing with common instrumentation in obstetric and gynaecological surgery.

Because the contributions deal with core concepts and practical tips pertaining to sound surgical technique, there is overlap, repetition and sometimes conflict between the chapters. However, in surgery there is frequently more than one way to deal with technical issues and a rich diversity of opinion should always be welcomed. The mission for contributors was to critically evaluate their personal experience and to convey their advice and tips in a way that they felt would have been helpful if presented to them at the outset of their own careers. I asked for a reasonably didactic style explaining why each contributor had chosen their preferred surgical method over alternative approaches.

I thank and congratulate the chapter authors for what they have achieved in turning my initial thoughts and 'directions' into a most readable and informative text. The pleasures and pains of planning and editing this sort of project have, at times, been keenly felt. Nevertheless, I can honestly say I have enjoyed it thoroughly—in large part because of the quality of each contributor's submission. I sincerely hope that readers will find their text as thought provoking and helpful as I have.

D. J. Maxwell
2003

Acknowledgements

It is so difficult to adequately record my appreciation to all those who supported and guided me in the aspects of my career that have culminated in this volume. John Malvern, David (EDM) Morris and Tim Coltart at Queen Charlotte's Maternity Hospital, Chelsea Hospital for Women and Guy's Hospital gave me fine examples to follow as well as support and wise counsel. Special thanks always to Professors Jack Dewhurst and Richard Lilford who gave me my chance for which I will always be grateful. Professor Bert Brant, Humphrey Ward and Anthony Silverstone at University College Hospital are all people I am proud to have known and been taught by. To Michael Chapman and David (DGM) Morris for being such staunch friends over the years.

My gratitude for assistance received in preparing the book itself extends to Tristan Murray and colleagues at instrument makers S. Murray and Co. and Suzy Herridge and colleagues at New Splint plc. Both groups were very helpful in preparing the appendix. Thanks also to my colleague Kate Langford with whom it is always good to bounce ideas around and who invariably gives a straight answer! And finally at Elsevier, sincere thanks to Ellen Green who did seem to believe in this venture from the start and Duncan Fraser who provided help and support when things looked wobbly from time to time.

Figure acknowledgements

Figure 1.1 adapted, with permission from The Royal College of Obstericians and Gynaecologists from, Hogston, P., 2001. Suture choice in general gynaecology. *The Obstetrician & Gynaecologist* 3, 127–31

Figure 6.7 redrawn, with permission, from F. G. Cunningham, P. C. MacDonald and N. F. Ganr. *Williams' Obstetrics*, 18th edition. 1989, Appleton and Lange

Figure 6.8 redrawn, with permission from, T. F. Baskett. *Surgical Management of Obstetric Emergencies*. 1985, Wiley

Figure 6.9 redrawn, with permission, from Hankins, Clark, Cunningham and Gilstrap. *Operative Obstetrics*. 1995, Appleton and Lange

Figures 6.10 and 6.11 redrawn, with permission, from C. B-Lynch, A. Coker, A. H. Lawal, J. Abu, and M. J. Cowen. 1997. The B-Lynch surgical technique for the control of massive postpartum haemorrhage: an alternative to hysterectomy? Five cases reported. *British Journal of Obstetrics and Gynaecology*. 3, 372–5

Figures 6.12, 6.13, 6.14 and 6.15 redrawn, with permission, from the American College of Obstericians and Gynaecologists. Hayman *et al*. *Obsterics and Gynaecology* 99, 502–6

Figure 6.16 redrawn, with permission from, C. Pauerstein. Clinical Obstetrics. 1995, Wiley

Figure 10.5 redrawn, with permission from, M. S. Baggish, J. Barbot and R. F. Valle. *Diagnostic and Operative Obstetrics: A Text and Atlas*. 1989, Year Book Medical Publishers Inc.

General principles

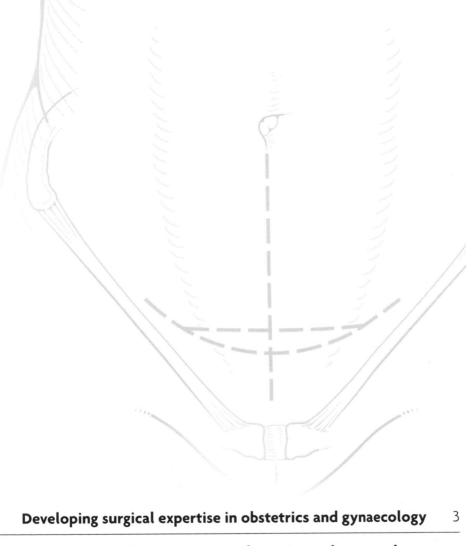

Developing surgical expertise in obstetrics and gynaecology

Frank Loeffler

CHAPTER

1

Acquiring surgical expertise—the changing picture

Surgical practice in obstetrics and gynaecology

All branches of surgery have changed radically in the past 150 years or so. In the 19th century it was the introduction of inhalation general anaesthesia (ether and then chloroform in the 1840s) and the Listerian principles of antisepsis (1865) that gave surgery its kick start. The 20th century brought with it antibiotics, the recognition of blood groups, blood transfusion, muscle relaxants, intravenous anaesthetic agents, a much better understanding of the biochemistry and physiology of surgery, the laser, fibreoptics and, finally, endoscopic and minimal-access surgery. Gynaecological surgery, like all other surgical specialties, is now more technical, more sophisticated and more demanding than ever before.

The growing sophistication of surgery in general has greatly enhanced the safety of caesarean section. Resort to abdominal delivery now solves the problems that were once dealt with by complicated interventions (like destructive operations, internal versions and breech extractions, difficult forceps deliveries) aimed at achieving a vaginal delivery in days when opening the abdomen was shunned because of subsequent sepsis. This explains why, unlike gynaecological surgeons, the obstetricians of today require, if anything, less practical skills in the labour ward than their forbears. That is not to say that obstetrics has been without its technological advances, but their focus has been on imaging and on surveillance of the fetus and using sophisticated ultrasound-guided techniques to obtain detailed haematological, biochemical and genetic information about the unborn child. The latter skills are outside the remit of this book.

The consumer, litigation and the trainee

Paternalism is rapidly becoming obsolete in obstetric and gynaecological practice. Many patients now have access to medical articles or texts, not to mention the internet. They arrive in the doctor's surgery very well briefed and therefore require very full information and counselling. Having obtained this, decisions about the treatment options open to them are usually made by the patients themselves and expectations of outcome are higher than they ever were. While this is not a bad thing, it does put new pressures on those involved in surgical care, as does the growing demand that hospital practice should be consultant-led.

The more developed a country is, the steeper is the rise in the incidence of medical litigation; some of the claims are justified, some not. Small wonder, then, that in the UK the annual professional indemnity insurance premium for an active obstetrician and gynaecologist has risen more than a hundredfold over the past 30 years.[1] Again, this puts pressures on those involved in operative procedures.

The increasing complexity of surgery, the demands made by the consumer, the growing threat of litigation, all referred to already, mean that trainee doctors are obliged, more so than previously, to attain the highest possible levels of expertise before they embark on independent practice. Under the 'New Deal' governing junior doctors' hours in the UK and in Europe, and as a result of the demands of the streamlined 'structured training' programme introduced to the UK by Calman, it has been calculated that the time available for trainees to gain experience in the clinical setting has been reduced, in recent times, by as much as 50%.[2,3] If one adds to the disappearance of the 80-hour week the increasing demands by patients that surgery should not be delegated to junior doctors, it is easy to see why

both trainees and trainers have worries about being able to prepare young doctors adequately for the demands facing the surgeons of today.[4,5] These considerations constitute the background for comments on the basic steps that need to be followed by those seeking to develop surgical expertise in obstetrics and gynaecology.

Acquiring expertise in 'open' gynaecological surgery

The theory

A general understanding of anatomy and detailed knowledge of abdominal and pelvic anatomy are non-negotiable prerequisites for a surgical trainee in gynaecology and obstetrics. Equally important are an understanding of relevant biochemistry, physiology and pathology. These subjects are usually studied in the first 2 years of the medical curriculum, but they need to be revisited by any surgical trainee and the MRCS and Part I of the UK MRCOG reflect this need.

There are many manuals of operative surgery, and trainees are well advised to find and to study one that suits them. Not everything can be described by written words, pictures and diagrams. Gaps in information are usually plugged by competent surgical teachers who will explain what they are doing as they operate, or answer questions about matters not covered in standard texts. The greater this sort of exposure, the better.

Knots

The heading of this section seems banal enough to insult the average trainee. But trainees in gynaecological surgery can make no headway without learning how to tie basic knots with their eyes shut. All that trainees need for this vital portion of their training is a piece (or two) of string, something to loop it round (the handle of a locker in the surgeon's room is ideal!), a pair of hands, an artery (or similar) forceps and illustrated instructions. It should not take them more than an hour to learn a one-handed reef

Fig. 1.1 Commonly used suture materials

Type of suture	Chemical name	Trade names	Advantages	Disadvantages	Absorption rate
Polyfilament	Polyglycolic acid	Dexon	Good knot security Predictable resorption	Rapidly absorbed	Complete absorption by 60–90 days
	Polyglactin	Vicryl	As above		Complete absorption by 60–90 days
	Nylon	Neurolon	Strong	Knots slip	Degrades at 15–20% per year
	Polyester	Ethibond, Ti-cron	Very strong	Needs to be removed if infected	Non-absorbable
Monofilament	Nylon	Dermalon, Ethilon	Strong	Knots slip, many throws needed	Degrades at 15–20% per year
	Polydioxane	PDS	Intermediate strength	May last longer than Maxon	Complete absorption by 180 days
	Polyglyconate	Maxon	Intermediate strength	May be easier to handle	Complete absorption by 180 days
	Polybutester	Novafil	Strong, can stretch under tension	Potential for sinus formation	Non-absorbable
Natural	Silk		Easy to handle	Provokes inflammatory response	Absorbed slowly over 1–2 years

knot, an instrument tied reef knot, a slip knot and a surgeon's knot (a reef knot with a double throw for its second half). It is not acceptable for trainees to ask to be taken through any surgical procedure without being armed with the basic 'knotty' skills that are the very foundations of open surgery.

Needles and sutures

Surgeons must know their needles and their suture materials. Needles can be round-bodied or cutting, and the latter may be tapercuts (most usual for the pelvic surgeon) or cutting throughout. The shape of the needle may be straight, 1/4, 3/8, 1/2 or 5/8 circle, J-shaped or with a compound curve, and needles come in varying sizes. Most needles nowadays are eyeless, being swaged to the suture material so that the tissues are not damaged unnecessarily by the redundant strand of a threaded needle. As for the suture materials, they come in varying thicknesses and strengths and may be absorbable or non-absorbable, monofilament or polyfilament and from man-made or natural fibres.

The features of the commonly used suture materials are shown in Fig. 1.1 which is adapted from a recent article by Hogston (2001).[6]

Instruments and other materials

An exact knowledge of operating theatre paraphernalia and how it works is a huge advantage: good workmen know their tools. Fig. 1.2 lists

Fig. 1.2 Basic types of equipment used in non-endoscopic gynaecological surgery

- Scalpels and knives
- Scissors
- Dissecting forceps
- Haemostats
- Pedicle clamps
- Needle holders
- Retractors
- Diathermy/coagulation apparatus
- Vaginal speculums
- Cervical dilators
- Uterine sounds
- Vulsellum and other cervix grasping forceps
- Sponge and polyp forceps

the main types of instruments used in major gynaecological surgery. Time spent with Theatre Nurses or Operating Department Assistants (ODAs) going over, naming and understanding instruments (and sutures) is worth more than three encyclopaedias of operative surgery. The gowns, gloves, operating tables, drapes, skin preparations and swabs used and the methods of checking swabs and instrument numbers might also be reviewed. Time so spent sets the scene for good understanding and team work between surgeons and all the operating theatre staff. These are as essential to achieving high standards as is the individual surgeon's expertise.

Learning by assisting

It is difficult to think of a more productive way of learning than by assisting a competent surgeon. Variety is the spice of life, and assisting a number of different surgeons gives trainees an opportunity to study a variety of techniques and viewpoints and to choose those that most appeal to them. Because of the limit on hours worked by trainees in the UK, assisting at operations has become more difficult to organize and one can only recommend that clock-watching should not be allowed to interfere with the benefits of learning by assisting and apprenticeship. Watching televised operations is of some value, but nothing can beat the impact of actually being there to observe technique at first hand and to receive explanations, or the opportunity to handle tissues and get the feel of anatomical structures and tissue planes.

'Solo' performances

There comes a time when trainees embark on their first 'solo'—an unforgettable learning experience. In the ideal world, trainees who start doing procedures on their own should either be assisted by a teacher, or should know exactly where to get hold of an experienced colleague in the event of difficulties, should they arise. Twin theatre lists, with the trainee operating on one side and the mentor on the other, is the ideal arrangement.

The amount of operating time that trainees appeared to need was investigated by sending out a questionnaire to all 53 Specialist Registrars (SpRs) in post in Wales during January 2000.[7] There were 48 replies, from which it seemed that SpRs feel that they must be able to get their hands on at least one major procedure a week to develop sufficient confidence to feel comfortable with independent practice at the end of their 5 years in training. Even at these levels of experience, one out of three SpRs in the first 3 years of training, and one out of six in their final 2 years, felt that the amount of operating they were getting was insufficient to prepare them for independence. While this study gives only a snapshot of SpR opinion, there can be little doubt that the more operating experience that trainees get, the better, even if it does mean working more than the prescribed number of hours.

Achieving expertise in obstetric procedures

Most of what has so far been said about gynaecological surgery applies to gaining expertise in obstetric procedures. But obstetric emergencies cannot be scheduled, and familiarity with the indications for, and the methods of carrying out, obstetric procedures can only be obtained by spending time in the labour ward. So training programmes must provide this time, regardless of other teaching demands, and the range of experience gained should be carefully recorded in log-books, which should be reviewed regularly by both trainees and trainers, so that gaps in experience can be identified and plugged.

Gaining experience in endoscopic surgery

General comments

It is generally accepted that a training in 'traditional' surgery (i.e. open abdominal surgery, vaginal surgery and minor procedures) must precede, or at least accompany, training in endoscopic surgery. Endoscopic procedures sometimes turn into open procedures or result in complications requiring open surgery, and if this happens, endoscopic surgeons should be able to handle the situation even if they decide, in the end, to seek the help of a surgical colleague in dealing with the problem that has arisen.

The equipment

The basic equipment required in well-organized endoscopic surgery is listed in Fig. 1.3. Endoscopic surgeons should be thoroughly conversant with the handling, maintenance and repair of this equipment, because suitably trained theatre staff are not always on hand (particularly 'out of hours') to provide the technical support that forms so large a part of endoscopic surgery.

Early training

Assisting at minimal-access procedures is an essential part of early training in endoscopic surgery. Assistants usually start by working the camera, and that can be very instructive. After that, assistants may be given certain steps of the procedure to complete and the final stage is a solo performance.

The surgical training laboratory

In recent years, numerous surgical training laboratories have been established, which are

Fig. 1.3 Basic equipment used in endoscopic surgery

- Colour television monitor
- Camera system
- Light source
- Insufflator
- Monopolar and bipolar electrosurgery
- Laser
- Endoscope
- Veress needle
- Trocars
- Tissue dissectors
- Graspers
- Scissors
- Needle holders
- Suture and knot-tying devices
- Stapling/clipping devices
- Irrigation and suction apparatus

used for the training of gynaecological and other minimal access surgeons, minimal access procedures having spread to nearly all branches of surgery. Most laboratories have simulators on which the steps and tricks involved in hysteroscopic or laparoscopic surgery can be rehearsed and learnt. In some laboratories, three-dimensional 'virtual reality' can be produced from computer programs somewhat similar to those used for training pilots in flight simulators. Trainees can use these 'clinical simulators' to practise procedures for which there are computer-generated responses that mimic the real-life situation.[8] Some European laboratories are equipped for opportunities to practise minimal access surgery on animals, e.g. pigs. Where such opportunities do not exist, apples, bananas, tomatoes and slices of liver must suffice.

It is most important that minimal access surgeons spend time in training laboratories because minimal access surgery inevitably has a steeper learning curve than 'open' surgery, and the training laboratory can be used to get trainees through the steep part of the learning curve away from the clinical setting and thus without putting patients at any risk.

Much recent research has been directed towards objective computerized methods of assessing operative skills, and there is convincing evidence of the efficacy of surgical training laboratories.[9] It is also believed that computerized assessment is capable of identifying that very small group of people who just have not got the basic 'hand–eye co-ordination' that is required for endoscopic surgery. If such people can be identified, there is benefit in spotting them early enough to divert their training into appropriate alternative channels.

The levels of endoscopic surgery

Four levels of laparoscopic surgery and three levels of hysteroscopic surgery were identified by an RCOG (Royal College of Obstetricians and Gynaecologists) Working Party in 1994.[10] These levels are shown in Fig. 1.4. Most generalist gynaecological surgeons reach Level 2 in laparoscopic surgery and Level 1 in hysteroscopic procedures. To perform endoscopic surgery above

Fig. 1.4 Levels of endoscopic surgery[10]

Level	Laparoscopic procedures	Hysteroscopic procedures
1	Diagnostic laparoscopy	Diagnostic hysteroscopy and biopsy Removal of simple polyps Removal of intrauterine devices
2	Laparoscopic sterilization Needle aspiration of simple cysts Ovarian biopsy Minor adhesiolysis (not involving bowel) Ventrosuspension Diathermy to endometriosis AFS Stage I	Proximal Fallopian tube cannulation Minor intrauterine adhesions Removal of pedunculated fibroid or large polyp
3	Laser/diathermy to polycystic ovaries Laser/diathermy to endometriosis—AFS Stages II and III Linear salpingostomy and/or salpingectomy for ectopic pregnancy Salpingostomy for infertility Salpingectomy/salpingo-oophorectomy Adhesiolysis for severe adhesions or adhesions involving bowel Laparoscopic ovarian cystectomy Removal of ovarian or other endometrioma Laparoscopically assisted hysterectomy	Division/resection of uterine septum Endoscopic surgery for Asherman's syndrome Endometrial resection or ablation (primary or repeat) Resection of submucous leiomyoma
4	Myomectomy Lymphadenectomy Presacral neurectomy Dissection of obliterated Pouch of Douglas Incontinence surgery	

AFS, American Fertility Society

these levels requires special training, and many hospitals insist on certification that such training has been received and that people doing the more complicated procedures have an adequate backing of training and experience.

The 'proctoring' or 'mentor' system

Anyone doing an endoscopic procedure for the first time should always be assisted by someone experienced in that procedure. After that, supervision should be provided until an adequate level of experience is achieved. It is most desirable that a proctor or mentor is identified who has the responsibility of fashioning a trainee's skill to the level of competence necessary for independent practice. These mentors will be in the best position to judge when their trainees have completed their training and are ready for a certificate of competence. There is no room for 'dabblers' or 'cowboys' in this branch of surgery. It requires strict regulation if disastrous

complications leading to litigation are to be avoided.

The continuum of care

A surgical procedure is but a single episode in a continuum of care. No one would deny that an operation needs to be done with appropriate skill. But the success of the procedure depends on more than that. The operation chosen must be the right one for the clinical circumstances. The patient needs to be fully informed and sign consent willingly to what is being done. Appropriate preoperative investigations and assessment are important, anaesthetists must be fully involved in planning procedures, the co-operation of a theatre team is vital. Postoperative care must be of a high standard, with the aim of administering reassurance, relieving pain and recognizing complications with a minimum of delay. And when the patient is discharged from hospital, appropriate follow-up arrangements must be made. The operating surgeon has a duty to ensure that provisions are made for each step in the continuum. To concentrate solely on the technicalities of any surgical procedure does not ensure the best results.

Limitations and continuing education

Much has been said about acquiring expertise. It is of equal importance for surgeons to know their limitations and to seek help without any hesitation when they cross the boundaries of their capabilities. Most surgeons do not consider the attainment of specialist status as the end of the road of training. They are usually well aware of their duty to keep up to date by spending a significant amount of time on continuing education and keeping abreast of new developments in their area of expertise. Continuing medical education, and the move towards introducing revalidation systems, are testimony to this need and make the practice of surgery the intensely absorbing vocation that it is.

REFERENCES

1. Symonds E M 2000 The impact of the courts on obstetric and gynaecological practice. In: O'Brien P M S (ed.) Yearbook of obstetrics and gynaecology. RCOG Press, London, p 33
2. Calman K 1995 Hospital doctors: training for the future. British Journal of Obstetrics and Gynaecology 102:354–356
3. NHS Executive Guidance 1998 The working time regulations (Series Number HSC 1998/160). NHS Executive, London
4. Wright, C S W 1999 Specialist registrar training in obstetrics and gynaecology: have we got it wrong? Hospital Medicine 60:291–293
5. RCOG National Training Committee 1997 Survey of training. RCOG, London
6. Hogston P 2001 Suture choices in general gynaecological surgery. The Obstetrician and Gynaecologist 3(3):127–131
7. Myerson N A, Pugh D H O 2001 Surgical training of specialist registrars in obstetrics and gynaecology in Wales. The Obstetrician and Gynaecologist 3(3):152–156
8. McCloy R, Stone R 2001 Virtual reality in surgery. British Medical Journal 323:912–915
9. Vossen C, van Ballaer P, Shaw R W, Koninckx P R 1997 Effects of training on endoscopic intracorporeal knot tying. Human Reproduction 12(12):2658–2663
10. RCOG 1994 Report of the RCOG Working Party on Training in Gynaecological Endoscopic Surgery. RCOG Press, London

Clinical governance in obstetrics and gynaecology: risk management and consent

Vincent Argent and Catherine Elliott

Clinical governance

Introduction

The concept of clinical governance in the NHS was introduced by the incoming government through a White Paper in 1998.[1] Clinical governance is now being implemented at local level. To many doctors in training it may seem an exercise that is more relevant at management level. It does, however, provide a framework for many activities that will have profound effects on the way obstetrics and gynaecology are practised, and so it is in every doctor's interest to understand the basic concepts.

Clinical governance has been defined by Scally and Donaldson (1998) as:

A framework through which NHS organisations are accountable for continually improving the quality of their services and safeguarding high standards of care by creating an environment in which excellence in clinical care will flourish.[2]

The key areas therefore are:

- increased accountability
- being able to set and monitor standards of care
- provision of a working environment in which these standards can be achieved.

A statutory duty to ensure quality of care was placed on all NHS organizations by the 1999 Health Act.[3] Clinical governance is a means of providing this quality at a local level. On a national level, clinical governance is overseen by the Commission for Health Improvement (CHI), soon to become the Commission for Health

Audit and Inspection, and supported by the NHS modernization agency, which includes the Clinical Governance Support Team established in September 1999.[4] Their website (http://www.cgsupport.org) provides a useful overview of clinical governance and its implementation for those with an interest or an interview looming!

The Clinical Governance Support Team

The NHS Clinical Governance Support Team (CGST) includes consideration of consent issues within its development programmes. Its three main aims are, first, to support the development of clinical governance in the NHS; second, to raise the profile and provide information about clinical governance; and, finally, to create, capture and spread ideas and good practice in clinical governance. The team is multidisciplinary and includes members from primary care, nursing and midwifery, communications, health management, clinical medicine and education. Clinical governance support is provided through a range of multi-level development programmes, by the provision of information and by providing a forum for discussion.

The general Clinical Governance Development Programme gives support to teams of multi-disciplinary delegates—these have included clinical teams from obstetrics and gynaecology—as they explore the use of the 'RAID' strategy to help implement clinical governance locally (this is: Review their local service, Agree changes, Implement changes and Demonstrate improvements).[5]

Implementing clinical governance

Clinical governance, risk management and consent are closely linked to accountability, professional regulation, clinical audit, standards and education and evidence-based practice; all having the ultimate aim of providing high-quality and safe health care.

The implementation of clinical governance includes:

1. Setting and maintaining standards:
   (a) setting clear standards;
   (b) measures to ensure quality-assured practice by all staff;
   (c) a robust system of inspection to ensure that standards are being met and proper quality improvement systems are in place at every level;
   (d) accountability for service quality in every NHS organization.

Many of these activities fall within the performance of effective audit and link with professional regulation.

2. Risk-management activities:
   (a) effective systems of adverse event recognition and analysis with positive action on potential failings of systems or personnel.

3. Education and training:
   (a) strong mechanisms to spread and learn from good practice and research evidence; this applies to local training and education and national training and regulation programmes;
   (b) active participation of and information for patients.

It has been said that the values behind clinical governance—accountability, transparency and openness—are not new. The aim of clinical governance is to formalize these laudable values and place them into a patient-centred framework, which can then be applied to the many different areas of the NHS. This framework also reflects the changing relationship between those receiving and those providing health care, which is discussed further below.

Risk management and patients as 'consumers'

Risk management is a process used widely in commercial and industrial areas outwith the NHS, and the procedures developed there are now being adapted to clinical risk management. The four phases of any risk management strategy are:[6]

1. Risk identification: this is often done by adverse event reporting but could be achieved by other methods.
2. Risk analysis.
3. Risk control.

4. Risk funding: this describes how the NHS should fund the potential costs of risks and is covered under the Clinical Negligence Scheme for Trusts.

The Royal College of Obstetricians and Gynaecologists (RCOG) definition of clinical risk management is: 'Methods for the early identification of adverse events, using either staff reports or systematic screening of records. This should be followed by creation of a database to identify common patterns and develop a system of accountability to prevent future incidents'.[6] Risk management aims to identify potential risk and to reduce the occurrence of untoward outcomes that harm patients, staff and corporate organizations. These untoward outcomes include harm to the health or lifestyle of a patient, damage to the professional reputations of staff and loss of reputation and public confidence in the employing authority. It is important that risk management is not viewed as a purely defensive process attempting to contain the impact of litigation, but rather as a positive process leading to improved patient and staff welfare. Patients are now undeniably viewed by themselves and by the government as consumers of health care services, and this fact has had a fundamental role in the development and application of clinical governance and risk management. Modern health care consumers are often well informed; they expect to know about their conditions, any proposed treatments, and to receive safe and high-quality care with positive outcomes. Valid consent enables the consumer to be a partner in deciding on treatment and care. Such an approach is particularly relevant to obstetrics and gynaecology, where many patients are young and in tune with the modern consumerist approach to medical practice. They are unlikely to tolerate unexpected events and may assume that the health care delivery system is at fault. In addition, obstetrics and gynaecology patients are often healthy individuals requiring care for natural events such as childbirth or for other procedures such as abortion and sterilization, and this leads to greater expectations. The many consumer groups and self-help organizations provide patients with a wealth of information and knowledge about health care. There is a high risk of litigation and 50% of all claims involve obstetrics and gynaecology, accounting for 80% of the value of claims. The most common reason for litigation in gynaecology is failed female sterilization.[7]

Adverse incident reporting and the National Patient Safety Agency

Adverse incident reporting is an integral part of clinical governance and risk management and is crucial to the success of a high-quality service.[8] Such reporting must be undertaken in a no-blame environment to allow openness and support in identifying suboptimal outcomes. Adverse incident reporting is now being overseen by the National Patient Safety Agency (http://www.npsa.org.uk).[9] The NHS Incident Record Form IRI (Safecode) or local variations of this are commonly used.

The RCOG publications, *Maintaining good medical practice in obstetrics and gynaecology*[10] and the *Clinical Governance Advice* guideline,[6] provide a list of reportable untoward events in obstetrics and gynaecology. Adverse events reported then need to be looked at by a departmental review group, and any factors contributing to them identified. This will include looking at whether guidelines or protocols were available and, if so, whether they were appropriate for the situation, whether they were correctly followed and whether correct decisions were made. If necessary, a plan must then be formulated and applied to try to prevent the recurrence of such errors.

Used correctly, the system of risk identification, analysis and control should provide a positive way in which a unit can identify and move forward upon potential areas of weakness in its systems and staff. It should also provide an opportunity to identify areas where training and education of all staff can be improved, and ultimately should benefit doctors in training.

Provision of quality care in obstetrics

The previously mentioned publication *Maintaining good medical practice in obstetrics and gynaecology*[10] provides suggested areas in which good quality of care should be ensured:

1. The need for clear arrangements concerning which professional is responsible for the care at all times, and equally for a clear definition of the professional responsible for intrapartum care.
2. Guidance on the transfer of care in the intrapartum period should also be transparent.
3. There should be an agreed mechanism for direct referral to a consultant from a midwife and for personal handover of care when medical and nursing shifts change.
4. Any handover to obstetric locums should be done personally, either by the post holder or senior member of the team, and vice versa.
5. A named consultant should have designated responsibility for labour ward matters, while a doctor with at least 12 months of obstetric experience should be resident on the labour ward at all times, or available within 5 min. A doctor with at least 3 years of experience in obstetrics should be available within 30 min.

It is good medical practice to subject the delivery interval in caesarean section for fetal distress to an annual audited standard.[10]

Clinical Negligence Scheme for Trusts

The Clinical Negligence Scheme for Trusts (CNST) was established in 1995 to aid NHS Trusts in the management and payment of claims for medical negligence. The CNST has a Risk Management Scheme that defines main standards, and three levels of accreditation with attached financial incentives for their achievement.

Consent

Valid consent must be obtained prior to health care interventions. It is the agreement by the patient that permits the health care team to carry out any investigation, procedure or treatment. It provides the doctor with a defence against a criminal accusation of assault. For consent to be deemed valid, three general consent principles must be adhered to: the patient must have the mental capacity to give consent to the particular procedure; adequate provision of information must be given prior to consent; and consent must be freely given.

Legal theory and informed consent

Although this phrase is widely used within the medical profession, it has a narrow legal meaning and does not simply mean the provision of adequate information to obtain valid consent.[11] In legal usage, it refers to the amount of information that a patient needs in order to give valid consent. There are three ways in which this can be assessed. The first is a 'doctor standard', whereby the doctor is expected to give the information that another competent doctor in the field would provide; thus an individual doctor's actions are judged against the actions of his peers. Secondly, there is a 'prudent patient standard' whereby the doctor's information is judged against what it is felt that a 'reasonable' patient in that situation would wish to know. This is the standard that appears now to be accepted by the English courts. Thirdly, there is the individual patient standard in which a doctor would be judged by what that particular patient in his or her own circumstances would wish to know about that particular procedure. It is this latter, exacting standard which is known as 'informed consent' and which has been used as a standard in some North American court judgements. It has been clearly stated that there is no doctrine of informed consent in English law.[12] It has been said that the expression 'informed consent' begs the question, 'How informed is informed?'[13] Informed consent has been described as a euphemism and a form of ritual deception that is never completely possible except when the patient is another doctor.[14] It is, therefore, unfortunate that many documents use the term 'informed consent'.

The legal basis of consent in English law serves to illustrate what is required of the practitioner who seeks the permission of the patient to carry out an intervention. The original, and often quoted, Bolam principle[15] was formulated as a rule that a doctor is not negligent if he acts in accordance with a practice accepted at the time as proper by a responsible body of medical opinion. Although the courts still often uphold this general principle, it has been modified by subsequent rulings, for example those in the cases of Sidaway[11] and Bolitho.[16] In Sidaway, the issue of consent was dealt with and Lord Scarman compared the patient standard as opposed to the medical standard and the increasing tendency to make consent patient-focused. There can be little doubt that, in the ruling on this case, there was a move towards the North American principle of informed consent, although it was agreed that there is no doctrine of informed consent in English law. The English case of Bolitho[16] did not deal specifically with consent, but demonstrated a willingness of the courts to question the rationality of medical opinion rather than accepting it as given, and demonstrated a move towards a 'patient oriented' rather than 'doctor oriented' standard of care.

Valid consent

Four prerequisites to ensure valid consent were given in the case of Canterbury v. Spence:[17]

1. The root premise is the concept that every human being of adult years and of sound mind has a right to determine what shall be done with his own body (this enshrines the ethical principle of autonomy).
2. Consent is the informed exercise of choice, and that entails an opportunity to evaluate knowledgeably the options available and the risks attendant on each.
3. The doctor must, therefore, disclose all 'material risks'; what risks are 'material' is determined by the 'prudent patient' test. A risk is material when a reasonable person, in what the physician knows, or should know, to be the patient's position, would be likely to attach significance to the risk in deciding whether or not to forgo the proposed therapy.

However, the doctor has what the court called 'therapeutic privilege'. This exception means that if a reasonable medical assessment of the patient indicates to the doctor that disclosure of infor-

mation would pose a serious threat of psychological detriment to the patient, the doctor can reasonably withhold that information.

The General Medical Council (GMC) has published recommended professional standards for the disclosure of information during the consent process. The first principle, published in the GMC document, *Seeking patients' consent: The ethical considerations*, is that successful relationships between doctors and patients depend on trust.[18] To establish that trust you must respect patients' autonomy; their right to decide whether or not to undergo any medical intervention, even where a refusal may result in harm to themselves or their own death. Patients must be given sufficient information, in a way that they can understand, in order to enable them to exercise their right to make informed decisions about their care. This GMC document provides clear guidance on providing information and obtaining consent and should be read by all doctors.

In addition to providing information, doctors must adjudge that an adult is competent to consent to treatment in order for the consent to be valid. Competence to consent must always be assumed unless otherwise proven. In order to consent, an adult must be able to retain and understand information given and apply it to their condition. Refusal to consent, for example, to caesarean or any other operation does not demonstrate a lack of competence.

The philosophical and ethical principles of self-determination and autonomy are now enshrined in the Human Rights Act 1998. Article 3 of the Act states that 'No one shall be subjected to … degrading treatment'. This article is considered to be fundamental to the question of valid consent.[19]

The Patient's Charter stated that all patients have a National Health Service right: 'to be given a clear explanation of any proposed treatment, including any risks involved and available alternatives, before you decide whether to agree to the treatment'.[20,21] There may be a tendency to interpret 'any' risk as every or all the risks, and, if this is so, movement is towards a patient standard of consent. The more recent publications on consent from the NHS Executive and the Department of Health (DoH) build on this initial work and are similar to the GMC guidelines (http://www.gmc-uk.org/standards/default.htm). *12 Key points on consent 2001*[22] provides guidance for health professionals on the following issues:

- when health professionals need consent from patients
- whether children can consent for themselves
- who is the right person to seek consent?
- what information should be provided?
- whether the patient's consent is voluntary
- whether it matters how the patient gives consent
- refusals of treatment
- adults who are not competent to give consent.

The NHS Executive has also published *Good practice in consent*,[23] which discusses the Department of Health's Reference guide to consent for examination or treatment (March 2001) and has published an implementation guide containing model consent forms and a new model consent-to-treatment policy.[24] Consent-to-treatment forms, accompanying information for patients and the adoption of the new policy commenced use in April 2002.

The new model consent forms, with guides for patients and health professionals, are available online,[25] and the expectation is that they will become recognisably the same across the NHS. The consent forms and the consent policy indicate the importance of making written information available to patients on their treatment options, to back up what they have been told face to face. Asking patients what they understand and how much they want to be involved in decisions regarding treatment is a good start for doctors, to ensure that they are adopting good practice. Not all patients want to make their own decisions; however, the ability to make any decisions is impaired if they are not given adequate information.

Standard information

There is a perceived lack of national standards for information about procedures in obstetrics and gynaecology. It is reasonable to assume that there should be a national standard to ensure consistency, although it is recognized that individual patients will have different requirements. Many Trusts are currently designing information leaflets, but there has been little networking to ensure that the information given is similar. Without consistency, patients may become confused and health care professionals may be vulnerable to litigation. A legal approach consistent with the Bolam case would suggest that the level of information would be tested by reference to professional standards.

Existing national information standards are likely to carry far more weight than individual publications by NHS Trusts and other local organizations. Some of the RCOG's evidence-based guidelines do contain standard recommendations on information that should be given to patients prior to certain procedures. The *Care of women requesting induced abortion* guideline gives an evidence-based list; it is somewhat technical and the practitioner should go through it with the woman. *Male and female sterilisation* contains three adjuncts to the provision of information and the consent process: there is a patient record standard, which includes the outpatient counselling to be recorded in the preoperative notes; a recommended standard information leaflet *Choosing and using male and female sterilisation*, published by the Family Planning Association; and special consent forms for female sterilization and vasectomy, which should be used in addition to the new Department of Health forms. The Royal College has also endorsed two books that provide comprehensive health information to women; they are *Complete women's health*[26] and *Everywoman's lifeguide*.[27] The use of such national publications should provide some consistency. Good-quality information for people seeking fertility treatment, to donors and the general public, has been produced by the Human Fertilisation and Embryology Authority, and patients can be given copies of national guidelines or useful information downloaded from a website; for example, the patient information site concerning microwave endometrial ablation.[28]

Obstetrics and gynaecology is a specialty where the patients expect to be well informed. It is worthwhile giving an overview of the risk management and provision of information in the most contentious areas of the specialty.

High-risk areas in obstetrics

Antenatal screening

Antenatal screening problems are an increasing source of patient dissatisfaction, complaints and litigation. Much of this stems from poor information and communication, and the difficulty of understanding the limitations of screening and testing. Better co-ordination of the currently available national standards in screening, testing, training and experience would be helpful in removing present variations, together with a robust quality assurance programme.[29]

In legal cases, claims that it would have been better not to have been born (wrongful birth and wrongful life) are unlikely to succeed as they are not favoured in English law, and to bring a claim successfully a plaintiff will usually allege negligence in that the health care team failed to offer a test or failed to detect an abnormality.[30]

Antenatal screening is a voluntary, opt-in service and patients must be provided with comprehensive, accurate literature before they make their choice. They should be fully informed about the implications of high-risk and low-risk results, detection rates, local figures and the limitations.[31] When screening tests indicate a high risk of a problem, the parents require careful counselling; it is important that they are not told that a screening test is positive as this implies a definite result. Obviously, the situation is complex, as the screening tests may then be followed by invasive tests with a risk of fetal loss and the option of termination of pregnancy.[32]

No assumptions should be made about a patient's wishes. Particular care must be taken with age and religious beliefs. Successful legal actions have occurred where a test or a termination of pregnancy has not been offered because of the patient's religion. Younger women, with a low risk of chromosomal abnormality, may still occasionally request invasive testing, and it would be prudent to grant their wishes after a full and frank discussion.

Antenatal care

The current trend is to divide pregnant women into low-risk and high-risk categories, with obstetricians concentrating their efforts on the latter. Women should be aware of the practitioner who is managing their care. This practitioner is likely to be fully responsible for clinical decisions, but will be working as part of a team according to protocols agreed by the service provider. Risk prediction and evaluation is a fundamental part of modern antenatal care, tempered by the knowledge of the sudden occurrence of minor and major unpredictable events. *Changing childbirth*[33] emphasized the importance of choice, and pregnant women should still be managed as individuals with their own personal views and needs. Among the most challenging risk management areas are:

- detection of intrauterine growth retardation
- early detection of pre-eclampsia and avoidance of eclampsia
- detection of thromboembolic disease
- prediction of shoulder dystocia
- detection of breech presentation, external cephalic version (ECV) and caesarean delivery
- caesarean section at the patient's request
- mode of delivery following previous perineal damage
- induction for post-maturity
- sterilization consent obtained during pregnancy.

An interesting example of provision of information and risk management is the recent result of the Term Breech Trial Collaborative Group.[34] This suggests that elective caesarean section is safer than planned vaginal delivery for the fetus in a breech presentation at term. Some units have, therefore, adopted a policy of caesarean section. It is important to ensure that women are made fully aware of such information.

Intrapartum care and operative obstetrics

Complaints and claims about intrapartum care involve acts of omission as well as commission.   17

Failure to act on the occurrence of a high-risk event is difficult to defend. While the 2001 National Institute for Clinical Excellence (NICE) guidelines on electronic fetal monitoring (based on the RCOG guidelines) should be followed, there must also be adequate training, with regular updates using skill station exercises, and cardiotocograph (CTG) review meetings.

Often, there are problems in communication between staff, and allocation of responsibility: inappropriate delegation to less-experienced staff and failure to alert senior staff are common.[35] Even in times of emergency, a dialogue with the patient and the partner must be maintained so that they are fully informed of the problems and intended action. The newer concepts of triage and prioritization are well taught on the Advanced Life Support in Obstetrics (ALSO®) and Managing Obstetrics Emergencies and Trauma (MOET) life support courses.[36]

It is now accepted that trained, experienced practitioners should undertake operative obstetrics and there is no place for the unsupervised trainee. Competency levels must be determined. It is particularly important that locums are supervised; nearly 50% of claims for intrapartum problems involve locum staff. It is desirable that senior or consultant obstetricians should be physically present for the following:

- anticipated shoulder dystocia
- change of instruments, e.g. Ventouse to forceps
- rotational forceps
- vaginal breech delivery
- twin delivery
- difficult caesarean section, e.g. previous caesarean section, placenta praevia, at full cervical dilatation and after unsuccessful instrumental delivery
- any major problem!

Undiagnosed breech in labour is a major problem. The Term Breech Trial has led to more caesareans, and few obstetricians maintain their expertise at vaginal delivery, leading to minimal opportunity for training junior staff. It is advisable to have a strict shoulder dystocia protocol. All midwives and obstetricians should undertake regular skills drill locally, as well as attending the ALSO/MOET courses. Logical progression through the management protocol avoids panic and ineffective measures.

There is still significant discussion and debate around the delivery interval for emergency caesarean section. The classification of urgent-emergency, urgent-scheduled and elective[37] is helpful, but no timings have been attached. Several national publications still describe a 30-minute interval, although recent publications have pointed out that there is little clinical evidence for this and that it is not an achievable audit standard.[38,39] The so-called '30-minute rule' does cause medico-legal problems, but courts usually have the wisdom to judge each case individually.

Fetal damage following instrumental delivery is usually ascribed to the obstetrician pulling too hard. One of the most important medico-legal cases concerning instrumental delivery served to distinguish the difference between an acceptable error of judgement and negligence.[40] Many units no longer use rotational forceps, and thus practitioners have problems maintaining their expertise.

Further complaints and medico-legal problems arise from perineal damage. It has been suggested that women should be educated and informed about the prospects of perineal and pelvic floor damage prior to the construction of their birth plan. Al-Mufti et al (1996)[41] showed that just over 30% of female obstetricians would prefer an elective caesarean to reduce later stress incontinence. A later study by Keighley et al (2000)[42] suggested that women should be informed of the risks of anal sphincter damage before childbirth. The repair of third-degree tears must be undertaken by senior staff, ideally those who have attended a special training course. Perineal problems and dyspareunia are best dealt with in specialist pelvic pain clinics.[43]

Cerebral palsy

Cerebral palsy claims, if successful, can lead to damages of several million pounds. In order to bring a successful claim it must be shown not only that actions were negligent but also that this negligence was causative of the damage. It has been said that proving that observed associations are causally related is an infamously difficult problem in philosophy and science.[44] There is no widespread agreement about the contribution of birth asphyxia and perinatal hypoxic events to neurodisability.[45] Courts will listen to the opposing views of experts and largely resist the temptation to be sympathetic to such terrible suffering in the absence of negligence. The NHS Litigation Authority continues to record an increasing number of claims for cerebral palsy, as well as alleged deafness, intellectual deficit and behavioural problems, related to birth asphyxia. The difficulties of establishing a causal link are:

1. Cerebral palsy can occur without intrapartum asphyxia, so the concurrence of intrapartum asphyxia and cerebral palsy is not of itself proof of causation.
2. It is impossible to be certain that the brain was normal before the onset of labour, using the investigations commonly available.
3. Fetuses with abnormal brains may withstand the stresses of birth poorly and show outward signs of having suffered intrapartum asphyxia, when in fact they have not.
4. It is difficult to define and quantify intrapartum asphyxia using current methods, and therefore difficult to establish when asphyxia has been severe enough to cause brain injury.
5. Intrapartum asphyxia does not necessarily lead to permanent brain injury, and fetuses vary in their susceptibility to brain injury as a result of other factors, such as their genetic make-up and prior environmental influences.

Cerebral palsy claims are best defended by careful analysis of antenatal and intrapartum events, meticulous record keeping, careful attention to signs of fetal stress, intervention by senior staff where necessary, and the measuring of cord blood gases after delivery. Impartial advice from an expert who understands the difficulty of causation is invaluable.

High-risk areas in gynaecology

Clinical examination

Allegations of unprofessional practice during clinical examination can have grave consequences, including suspension, professional conduct hearings and criminal prosecution for sexual assault. In the first place, gynaecologists should be careful with the language they use and should avoid patronizing or talking down to women. Plain and sensitive English is always preferable.

It may be prudent to offer a chaperone or third party for all parts of the consultation, including the history and discussion as well as the examination; this should apply whatever the sex of the practitioner. The use of audio or video recording can be offered and is helpful in reducing allegations of inappropriate behaviour, as well as acting as a source of information about the consultation for the patient and the doctor. If a patient declines a chaperone, then this should be recorded in the patient's notes. The RCOG guidelines on intimate examination should be followed.[46]

Female sterilization

This social operation attracts litigation for failure.[7] Currently damages are available for the pain and suffering of further pregnancy and other procedures, but only for the upkeep of a disadvantaged child, not a normal healthy child.

Preoperative counselling and records

The word 'sterilization' suggests a permanent state of affairs, and the patient should be told that sterilization is the intent of the procedure. It is essential to discuss other methods of contraception, including the levonorgestrel intrauterine system and vasectomy. Special care should be taken with the nulliparous and those under 25 years of age. Information should be given according to the recommendation of the RCOG guidelines on male and female sterilization.[47] The patient should be told that reversal operations are difficult, with a limited success rate, and that they may not be available on the NHS. In the case of a failed procedure, an experienced consultant, who can give a full explanation of the problem, must see the patient.

Consent form

The RCOG recommended consent form should be used in conjunction with the new Department of Health general form. Special consent forms are favoured by the defence societies.

Timing of the operation

Ideally the operation should be performed in the first half of the cycle but it is recognized that this may be impractical. A full menstrual and sexual history must be taken on the day of admission. It is wise to postpone the operation if the patient has had unprotected sex at mid-cycle. If she wishes to proceed, then she should be fully counselled about the risk of existing early pregnancy and this must be recorded in the notes. Many units now carry out routine pregnancy testing on all patients.[48]

Methods, equipment and training

Mechanical occlusive devices, clips or rings, should be used. Diathermy can be taught as a back-up method, but the patient should be advised that there is a small risk of undiagnosed bowel burns with unipolar diathermy and a higher recanalization rate with bipolar diathermy unless the tube is severed. Care must be taken in the presence of thickened tubes or abnormalities; two clips on each tube appear to reduce the risk of failure and should certainly be used where there is any doubt about the application of the first clip.[49]

Staff must be familiar with the equipment, and servicing must be carried out according to the manufacturer's instructions. The Medical Devices Agency recommends that the clip or ring batch number and the applicator number be recorded in the patient notes so that faulty equipment can be identified in cases of failure.[50] The trainee surgeon should read the manufacturer's instructions and study the training videos and CDs. The RCOG suggests that doctors should

perform at least 25 sterilizations under direct supervision by an experienced consultant before independent practice.

Notekeeping and evidence

The Confidential Enquiry into Failed Sterilisation has suggested that there should be a standard national operation record that records important phrases such as 'tubes and fimbriae identified'. It is useful to take a picture after the operation on the tubes and store this information in the patient's notes. Experienced consultants must carry out repeat operations after failed sterilization and the photographic and histological evidence (in the case of tube removal) must be retained for incident reporting and likely legal action.

Reporting failed procedures

Following the RCOG recommendations, there is a voluntary reporting system for failed procedures. Risk managers should report the failure to: Mr V. P. Argent, Secretary, Confidential Enquiry into Failed Sterilisation (CEFS), Eastbourne District General Hospital, King's Drive, Eastbourne, East Sussex, BN21 2UD, UK.

Induced abortion

Induced abortion is the most commonly performed operation by gynaecologists. Adverse outcomes often lead to complaints and litigation, although many patients do not pursue action for confidential reasons. The RCOG evidence-based guideline *The care of women requesting induced abortion*[51] provides a basis for patient information and risk management. Induced abortion in the UK is a relatively safe procedure, but complications depend on gestational age, type of operation, place of operation and skill of the operator. The incidence of complications increases with delay between referral, consultation and operation.[52]

The service

The RCOG guidelines state that there must be prompt access (direct access and self-referral is preferred) to a service providing information, medical assessment, counselling and choice. The best results are obtained in dedicated clinics and by lists run by experienced practitioners, with back-up and follow-up facilities, including a telephone helpline. It is recommended that appointment occurs within 5 days of referral and that the procedure is performed within 7 days of assessment.

Assessment

The gestational age should be determined. Routine ultrasound scanning identifies multiple pregnancy, moles, failed pregnancy and may suggest an ectopic pregnancy, although scanning may be declined if the patient wishes. Photographic records stored in the patient's notes may cause problems at a later date. Routine vaginal examination is not necessary. The possibility of infection should be considered, as part of the strategy to minimize pelvic inflammatory disease, by screening or the use of prophylactic antibiotics.[53]

Information and consent

The RCOG guidelines recommend information on haemorrhage, perforation, cervical trauma, failed abortion, infection, breast cancer, fertility and psychological consequences. The consultation must also deal with the formalities of the Abortion Act including the need for signatures from doctors on the HSA 1 form. Special considerations apply in the case of practitioners who exercise their conscientious objection, mental incapacity, objection from partners or parents, attempted sex selection and in the under-16s, where the Gillick[54] criteria are applied. Many units use special consent forms, specifically mentioning the risk of failed abortion and retained products. Special consent is needed when unlicensed drugs, such as misoprostol, are used.[55]

Complications leading to litigation

The most common reasons for litigation are retained products and trauma; however, litiga-

tion is also likely to occur in the case of failed abortion, missed ectopic, live birth and failure to give anti-D immunoglobulin. Failure to abort is more common after early surgical procedures and follow-up pregnancy tests should be offered. Intra-operative scanning is useful in these circumstances.[56]

Retained products of conception

The occurrence of retained products is a frequent source of complaint. Patients should be informed that post-termination bleeding and pain is common and that some tissue is commonly retained but should pass spontaneously. Cervical preparation, oxytocics, correctly functioning suction equipment and scanning to confirm an empty uterus reduce the problem. Litigation is far more common when recognizable fetal parts are passed at later gestations. Delayed diagnosis and management, and failure to involve senior staff, compound the majority of complaints. Repeat evacuations are seldom necessary, but should be carried out by consultant staff as there is a far higher risk of perforation.

Threats to staff

Risk management also deals with threats to staff and the NHS has a zero tolerance policy on violence. Steps should be taken to protect staff from hostile comments, mailshots or unpleasant protests. Many of the current anti-abortion websites are threatening.[51]

Gynaecological surgery

Gynaecological surgery carries many risks.[57] Particular concerns are unnecessary hysterectomy, removal of the ovaries, damage to the ureter and failed operations for incontinence.

Unnecessary hysterectomy

There is likely to be an increase in the number of claims for alleged unnecessary hysterectomy. Patients suffering with menorrhagia or dysfunctional uterine bleeding, without any major

21

pathology, should be treated medically according to RCOG guidelines, and also offered treatment with the levonorgestrel intrauterine system and second-generation endometrial ablation. A recent study of 37 298 hysterectomies concluded that 75% could have been avoided if endometrial ablation had been offered. The study showed that 1 in 30 patients suffered complications during surgery, with 1 in 130 returning to theatre for treatment of bleeding, with a death rate of 1 in 2500. Half of the operations also involved removal of the ovaries. Some patients will still demand hysterectomy in these circumstances; it is reasonable to grant their wish after a full discussion about alternative treatments and types of hysterectomy.[58]

There is still no consensus on the risks and benefits of subtotal hysterectomy, but there is no doubt that the possible retention of the cervix should be discussed prior to surgery. Unusual cases require particular care. In a case such as a young nulliparous women seeking hysterectomy for pelvic pain, it is vital to seek a second opinion from another senior consultant gynaecologist as well as a psychiatrist and pain specialist; it would be prudent to inform the medical director, risk manager or defence organization.

Removal of the ovaries

Surgical removal of the ovaries may be accidental, incidental or planned. Planned removal may be for existing pathology or for prophylactic reasons. Premature ovarian failure may occur after hysterectomy with conservation of the ovaries. The risk of ovarian cancer after fertility drugs is unclear, but the possibility must be discussed. Fibroid embolization carries a risk of ovarian failure.[59]

There is no doubt that patients should be fully informed about the effects of any treatment on their ovarian function. The removal of ovaries without consent in the presence of endometriosis is unacceptable. Accidental removal is best avoided by careful preoperative discussion with the patient, attention to correct wording on the consent form and the avoidance of abbreviations in patients' notes and on operating list schedules.

Damage to the ureter

Damage to the ureter can happen even in experienced hands during a straightforward hysterectomy. It is, however, difficult to defend these cases. It should be standard practice to warn of the risk of ureteric damage, with a full explanation of the consequences. There is no consensus on the need for routine identification of the ureters at surgery. Extra care must be taken with the counselling of patients with high-risk problems, such as endometriosis and oophorectomy after previous hysterectomy.[60]

Operations for genuine stress incontinence

There are a large number of operative procedures for stress incontinence and, at best, they only achieve about an 80% satisfaction rate in the best hands. Patients must be clearly informed about the likely success rates of procedures and also on the subsequent management in the case of failure. Repeat operations should be carried out by subspecialist urogynaecologists or urologists.

Minimal access surgery

Surgeons must be appropriately trained and experienced, and ideally conform to the RCOG and British Gynaecological Endoscopy Society's three levels of laparoscopy and three levels of hysteroscopy. There are many controversial areas. There are different entry techniques, with gynaecologists preferring blind entry with guarded cannulas, and many abdominal surgeons preferring open entry. The main reason for complaints is the patient's lack of knowledge about what is to be done and what can be done laparoscopically and the unexpected occurrence of laparotomy. The RCOG has stated that patients should be:

- made aware of possible complications prior to surgery
- provided with written information
- warned that a diagnostic procedure may have to be converted to an open procedure
- warned that open surgery may be necessary due to technical difficulties
- made aware that a short hospital stay does not exclude the risk of late complications.[61]

Cervical screening and colposcopy

There have been several high-profile cervical smear scandals[62] and there is an unrealistic public expectation that results should be 100% accurate. More patient education needs to be done about the limitations of screening. The RCOG report on standards in colposcopy and the publications of the British Society for Colposcopy and Cervical Pathology give comprehensive guidance on risk management and quality assurance.[63] These support the principles laid down in the publications of the NHS Cervical Screening Programme. Colposcopists should be accredited and trainees should be taught by preceptors.

Assisted conception

Clinics should provide comprehensive information about their services and treatment based on the information package and code of practice of the Human Fertilisation and Embryology Authority (HFEA). There are many ethical and legal problems and a rapidly increasing number of claims. Wrongful birth and wrongful life claims add to those in negligence.[64] The main problems are:

1. Patients should be informed that a baby conceived by assisted conception is three times more likely to suffer damage or die, principally due to the risk of pre-term labour in multiple pregnancy.
2. There is a possible link between the use of fertility drugs and ovarian cancer. The *British National Formulary* still gives the advice from the Committee on Safety of Medicines: 'The CSM has recommended that clomifene should not normally be used for longer than 6 cycles' although other authorities disagree.[55]
3. The incidence of very high-order multiple pregnancy in controlled ovarian hyperstimulation and intrauterine insemination; this procedure is not regulated by the HFEA.
4. The frequent use of fertility drugs may lead to premature menopause.

5. The cost to the NHS of dealing with patients treated in the private sector.
6. Ensuring adequate checks on practitioners who do not abide by the HFEA code, e.g. the replacement of more than three embryos at in-vitro fertilization (IVF).

Numerous other ethical and legal difficulties surround such issues as contract pregnancy, selective reduction, sex selection, choice of donor characteristics, posthumous conception, identification of gamete donors, upper age limits, treatment of single or gay patients, and cloning.

The focus of this chapter has been on risk management and valid consent. The effective implementation of these, and other aspects of the clinical governance agenda, are essential if high standards are to be safeguarded and improvements made to the quality of care for patients. Successful implementation of clinical governance in obstetrics and gynaecology at the local level will be characterized by:

1. Patient-centred care at the heart of every obstetrics and gynaecology directorate, so that patients are well informed and participate in discussions about their care.
2. The availability of good information about the quality of the obstetrics and gynaecology service, not only to those providing it, but also to the patients and public receiving it.
3. Greatly reduced national variations in outcome and in access to health care.
4. Teams of doctors, midwives, nurses and other health professionals working together to a consistently high standard and identifying ways to provide even better care to their patients.
5. A reduction of risks and hazards to patients to as low a level as currently possible, creating a safety culture throughout the service.

Acknowledgement

Vince Argent acknowledges the support of Professor Aidan Halligan, Director of Clinical Governance for the NHS and Head of the NHS Clinical Governance Support Team.

REFERENCES

1. Department of Health 1998 A first class Service: Quality in the New NHS. Health Service Circular HSC. HMSO, London, p 113
2. Scally G, Donaldson L J 1998 Clinical governance and the drive for quality improvement in the new NHS in England. British Medical Journal 1998: 61-65. Online. Available: http://www.bmj.com/cgi/content/full/317/7150/61 2002
3. The Health Act 1999 Chapter c.8. Stationery Office, London
4. Halligan A 1999 How the National Clinical Governance Support Team plans to support the development of clinical governance in the workplace. Journal of Clinical Governance 14:155–157
5. Halligan A, Donaldson L 2001 Implementing clinical governance turning vision into reality. British Medical Journal 322:1413–1417
6. Clinical Governance Advice No. 2 January 2001 RCOG, London. Online. Available: http://www.rcog.org.uk/mainpages.asp?PageID=317 2002
7. Argent VP 1988 Failed sterilisation and the law. British Journal of Obstetrics and Gynaecology 95:113–115
8. Department of Health 2001 Building a safer NHS for patients: implementing an Organisation with a Memory. HMSO, London. Online. Available: http://www.doh.gov.uk/buildssafenhs 14 April 2002
9. Online. Available: http://www.npsa.org 14 April 2002
10. RCOG 1999 Maintaining good medical practice in obstetrics and gynaecology. RCOG, London
11. Sidaway v. Board of Governors of the Bethlem Royal Hospital and others 1985 1 All ER 643
12. Argent V P, Woodward Z 2001 Consent and the ovary. The Obstetrician and Gynaecologist 3:206–210
13. Kennedy I, Grubb A 2000 Medical law, 3rd edn. Butterworths, London
14. Hawkins C. 1985 Mishap or malpractice. Blackwell Scientific, Oxford
15. Bolam v. Friern. Hospital Management Committee 1957 1 WLR 582
16. Bolitho v. City and Hackney Health Authority 1997 4 All ER 771
17. Canterbury v. Spence D C 1972 464 F 2d 772
18. General Medical Council 1998 Seeking patients' consent: The ethical considerations. General Medical Council, London
19. The Human Rights Act 1998 Capsticks, London
20. Department of Health 1991 Patient's charter. HMSO, London
21. Department of Health 2001 Your guide to the NHS. HMSO, London, p 28
22. Department of Health 2001 12 Key Points on Consent: The Law in England. HMSO, London
23. NHS Executive 2001 Good practice in consent: Achieving the NHS Plan Commitment to Patient-Centred Consent Practice. HSC 2001/023. HMSO, London
24. NHS Executive 2001 Good practice in consent implementation guide: consent to exam or treatment. HMSO, London
25. Full texts of publications on consent (four forms and patients' and clinicians' guides) are online. Available: http://www.doh.gov.uk/consent/index.htm 14 April 2002
26. Lumsden M A, Hickey M 2000 Complete women's health. RCOG, Thorsons, London
27. Stoppard M 2002 Everywoman's lifeguide. Miriam Stoppard Lifetime, London
28. Online: http://www.microsulis.com
29. Fisk N M 2001 Prenatal screening, risk management and litigation in obstetrics and gynaecology. Royal Society of Medicine, London
30. McKay v. Essex 1982 AHA 2 All ER 771
31. RCOG 1997 Ultrasound screening for fetal abnormalities. Report of the RCOG Working Party. RCOG, London
32. RCOG and RCPCh 1997 Fetal abnormalities: guidelines for screening diagnosis and management. Joint Working Party of the Royal College of Obstetricians and Gynaecologists and of the Royal College of Paediatrics and Child Health. RCOG and RCPCh, London
33. Department of Health 1993 Changing childbirth. Report of the Expert Maternity Group. HMSO, London
34. Hannah M E, Hannah W J, Hewson S A et al for the Term Breech Trial Collaborative Group 2000 Planned Caesarean section versus planned vaginal birth for breech presentation at term: a randomised multicentre trial. Lancet 356:1375–1383
35. Gibb D M F 2001 Intrapartum care. Risk management in obstetrics and gynaecology. Royal Society of Medicine, London
36. Cox C, Grady K 1999 Managing obstetric emergencies. Bios, Oxford
37. Lucas D N, Yentis S M, Kinsella S M et al 2000 Urgency of caesarean section: a new classification. Journal of the Royal Society of Medicine 93:346–350
38. James D 2001 Caesarean section for fetal distress. British Medical Journal 322:1316–1317
39. Tufnell D J, Wilkinson K, Beresford N 2001 Interval between decision and delivery by caesarean section – are current standards achievable? British Medical Journal 322:1330–1333
40. Whitehouse v. Jordon and another 1981 1 WLR 246
41. Al-Mufti R, McCarthy A, Fisk N 1996 Obstetricians' personal choice and mode of delivery. Lancet 347:544
42. Keighley M R B, Radley S, Johanson R 2000 Consensus on prevention and management of post-obstetric bowel incontinence and third degree tear. Clinical Risk 6:231–237
43. Adams E J, Fernanado R J 2001 Management of third and fourth degree perineal tears following vaginal delivery. Green Top Guideline No. 29. RCOG, London
44. Dear P R F, Newell S J 2001 Cerebral palsy and intrapartum events in risk management and litigation in obstetrics and gynaecology. RSM Press, London

45. Pharaoh P O, Cooke T, Johnson M A et al 1998 Epidemiology of cerebral palsy in England and Scotland, 1984–89. Archives of Disease in Childhood 79:F21–F25

46. RCOG 1997 Intimate examinations. RCOG, London

47. RCOG 1999 Male and female sterilisation. Evidence based clinical guideline No. 4. RCOG, London

48. Kasliwal A, Farquharson R G 2000 Pregnancy testing prior to sterilisation. British Journal of Obstetrics and Gynaecology 107:1407-1409

49. Filshie clip users manual 1998 Femcare Ltd, Nottingham

50. Medical Devices Agency 1998 MDA SN 9834. MDA, London

51. See online: http://www.nhszerotolerance.nhs.uk 14 April 2002

52. RCOG 2000 The care of women requesting induced abortion. Evidence based clinical guideline No. 7. RCOG Clinical Effectiveness Support Unit, London

53. Penney G C 1996 Prophylactic antibiotic therapy for abortion. The Prevention of Pelvic Infection. RCOG Press, London

54. Gillick v. West Norfolk and Wisbech Health Authority 1985 3 All ER 402

55. BMA and the Royal Pharmaceutical Society of Great Britain 2001 Guidance on prescribing. British National Formulary 42. BMA and RPSGB, London

56. Argent V P 2000 Induced abortion. Risk management. The Obstetrician and Gynaecologist 2:31–36

57. Soutter P 2001 Gynaecological Surgery and Oncology. In: Clements R V (ed.) Risk management and litigation in obstetrics and gynaecology. RCOG/RSM, London

58. Maresh M J A, Metcalfe M A, McPherson K et al 2002 The VALUE national hysterectomy study: description of the patients and their surgery. British Journal of Obstetrics and Gynaecology 109:302–312

59. Stringer N H, Grant T, Park J et al 2000 Ovarian failure after uterine artery embolisation for treatment of myomas. Journal of the American Association of Gynecologic Laparoscopists 7:395–400

60. Clements R V 2000 Urinary tract injury in gynaecology. Clinical Risk 6:89–93

61. RCOG 1994 Training in gynaecological endoscopic surgery. RCOG, London

62. Anonymous 1999 Double jeopardy for women in cervical screening [Editorial]. Lancet 354:1833

63. RCOG 1999 Recommendations for service provision and standards in colposcopy. RCOG, London

64. Human Fertilisation and Embryology Authority 2002 Code of practice. HFEA, London

Surgical wounds and their care

Helena Baxter

CHAPTER

3

Principles of wound healing

All wounds follow a pattern of healing. Immediately after wounding, there is an inflammatory phase when mast cells degranulate, releasing inflammatory mediators, such as prostaglandins and histamine, allowing local blood vessels to dilate. Neutrophils enter to digest bacteria and, later, macrophages flood the wound bed, releasing healing regulators, such as growth factors and prostagandins.[1] At this stage, the wound appears red and swollen, is warm and usually acutely painful.[2] In clean surgical wounds, this inflammatory stage can last from 3 to 7 days, although immunosuppressed patients may not be able to mount an effective inflammatory response, which may cause delays in the healing process.

The second stage of healing is the proliferative phase, where new vessel and tissue growth takes place. Fibroblasts move into the wound and collagen synthesis occurs alongside angiogenesis to fill the defect with granulation tissue.[3] The wound then contracts and epithelial cells migrate across the surface of the wound until full closure is achieved. In wounds closed by primary intention, this process occurs within a matter of days from initial wounding, although the tensile strength of the wound remains poor.

Wound sites regain their strength during the maturation phase. This process starts approximately 20 days after injury and can take up to 18 months (occasionally longer) to complete.[4] In this phase, the scar matures, loses its red pigmentation and lies flatter to the surface of the skin as the collagen fibres reorganize and remodel. Mature scars do not fully regain either the tensile strength or elasticity of undamaged skin. This can leave patients who have suffered pressure sores, or other wounds healing by secondary intention, prone to further breakdown, but is rarely a problem in surgical wounds.

Surgical wound complications

Two main complications arise from surgical wounds—surgical dehiscence and wound infection. Dehiscence can occur in varying degrees, from the splitting open of part of the incision line or the skin layers only, through to full dehiscence of the entire wound down to muscle, fascia and beyond. Worst-case scenarios expose the abdominal or pelvic organs and require prompt, often aggressive management. Occasionally, the muscle and fascia layers break down but the skin layers remain intact and heal perfectly, resulting in an incisional hernia.

Factors affecting surgical dehiscence

Many factors are known or suspected to contribute to surgical dehiscence. Some are patient related, while others are related to surgical technique, site and perioperative complications.

Poole[5] identified male sex, age, malnutrition and long-term steroid use as contributing factors to abdominal dehiscence. Although male sex is not a problem in obstetrics and gynaecology, it is thought that the hormone oestrogen affects collagen deposition and strength, and therefore positively affects wound healing. This may have a detrimental effect on postmenopausal women who are not receiving hormone replacement therapy.

As a person ages, the skin becomes thinner and less elastic, due to a reduction in the quality and quantity of collagen. The older the person, the longer the healing process takes. This is made worse if the patient had been receiving long-term steroid therapy. The skin becomes tissue-paper thin, almost translucent in some cases, and is prone to tearing and breakdown. Other factors, such as diabetes, rheumatoid arthritis and smoking can impair the healing process by adversely affecting the microcirculation.

Malnutrition is another major factor in surgical breakdown and delayed wound healing. Albumin levels are not generally considered to be a useful measure of current nutritional status, as albumin has a long half-life of approximately 19 days. However, albumin levels can indicate chronic protein–energy malnutrition[6] and low albumin levels are frequently found in patients with wound dehiscence. Low protein leads to poor cell growth and the accompanying interstitial oedema impairs the healing process and adds strain to a suture line. Conversely, obesity also presents a problem since the fat layers are largely avascular and significant tension may be put on the suture line. Obese patients are more prone to dehiscence. Research by Derzie et al[7] suggests that continuous fascial closure is associated with fewer deep wound complications than interrupted closure techniques.

Surgical technique and suturing skills can also affect whether or not a wound stays together. Tight suturing can rip the skin and causes damage to the vascularity of the skin edges, resulting in necrosis and breakdown.[8] In patients with friable skin, problems of skin tearing from sutures, staples or clips may be overcome by suturing through Steri-strips® laid parallel to the incision site. This serves to spread the tension over a wider area and was first reported successfully in the management of pre-tibial lacerations.[9]

Underuse of electrocoagulation therapy can result in excessive bleeding and haematoma formation. Blood collections create dead spaces which delay healing, weaken the suture line and are a focus for infection. Conversely, overuse of electrocoagulation can damage the microcirculation and prevent the wound edges knitting together, affecting both the strength and quality of wound healing.

Dehiscence occurs most frequently in abdominal wounds.[8] Abdominal distension and perioperative chest infection have been linked to increased dehiscence and incisional hernia rates,[10] as they increase the tension placed on a new surgical site. Pfannenstiel incisions tend to be preferred in obstetrics and gynaecology, although recent research suggests that there is no advantage in this type of incision in terms of strength or reduction in fascial dehiscence over lower abdominal vertical incisions.[11] However, the cosmetic results from Pfannenstiel incisions tend to be preferred by patients.

Wound infection

Wound infection is a major factor in surgical dehiscence and wound complications. Overall infection rates appear to be rising in surgery, from 4.7% in 1980[12] to 7.3% in 1990.[13] Cruse and Foord[12] further identified differing infection rates for different classifications of surgical wounds. Infection rates of 1.5% were noted in 'clean' operations, such as hysterectomies where no infection is seen, rising to 40% in 'dirty' procedures where a perforated viscus or pus is identified.

However, little standardization was used to determine infection rates between investigators. In 1996, the Nosocomial Infection National Surveillance Service (NINSS) was established to look at standardized infection rates between participating hospitals. By 2001, 152 hospitals were participating, showing infection rates of 2.4% for abdominal hysterectomies, rising to 11% for gastric surgery and 14.8% for limb amputation.[14]

As with dehiscence, several factors have been identified as being associated with increased risks of surgical site infection (Fig. 3.1). Patient-related factors are similar to those affecting surgical dehiscence; however, Mishriki et al[13] also found strong associations between individual surgeons and infection rates. Cruse and Foord[12] found an association with the length of surgery, and suggest that infection rates double for every hour of surgery. This could be due to a higher use of sutures and electrocoagulation, prolonged exposure to potential bacterial contaminants and damage to wound cells that dry out when exposed to air.

Wound drains act as a port for infection, and pre-existing lesions, such as pressure sores or leg ulcers harbour bacteria that can contaminate the surgical wound.[15] Infection risks from pre-existing lesions can be minimized by covering the wound with an occlusive dressing, such as a hydrocolloid, during the immediate perioperative phase.

Identifying wound infection

Wound infection is frequently identified on the basis of a wound swab. Microbiologically

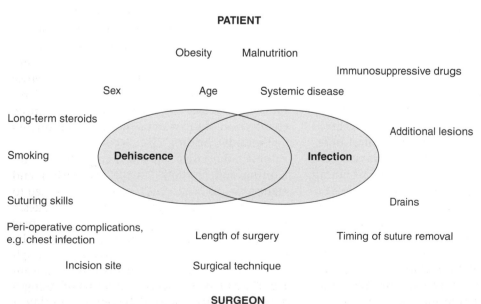

Fig. 3.1 Patient and surgeon factors in wound complications.

speaking, if a wound cultures >10^5 microorganisms, the risk of a surgical site infection being present is markedly increased. However, some more virulent pathogens can cause infection at greatly reduced numbers, and others can be present in large quantities without causing detrimental effect. Equally, some patients are more resistant than others to invading pathogens. Mangram et al[15] described this relationship as:

$$\frac{\text{Dose of bacterial contamination}}{\text{Resistance of the host patient}} \times \text{virulence} = \frac{\text{Risk of surgical site infection}}{}$$

Wound swab results have inherent problems, as they cannot always identify the causative organism. Swabs taken from the surface of the wound pick up colonizing agents and natural flora and may not identify the organism deep in the tissues causing the infection. Anaerobic bacteria are often missed, as the environment at the surface of the wound is too oxygen-rich for their survival. Wound swabs frequently yield false-positive results, particularly in complex surgical wounds where full dehiscence has occurred and the wound is healing by secondary intention.

More accurate results can be obtained by deep tissue sampling through the use of biopsies, as this has the potential to identify causative organisms. However, the process is expensive, requires expertise and is impractical, particularly in the community setting.

Wound swabs have their use, but only when taken in context with clinical signs and symptoms. Many wounds are colonized with bacteria with no detrimental effects on the healing. However, a wound becomes clinically infected when a host response occurs. In surgical wounds closed by primary intention, the signs of clinical infection include spreading erythema, increased pain and tenderness, heat and swelling, with or without a marked pyrexia (Fig. 3.2). These are also the first signs of wound healing in the inflammatory stage, but are normally diminished or absent within 48–72 hours after wounding. Pus or a purulent discharge may be present, and, if not immediately obvious, can often be detected by careful palpation of the suture line. Where known or suspect areas exist, free drainage of the pus can

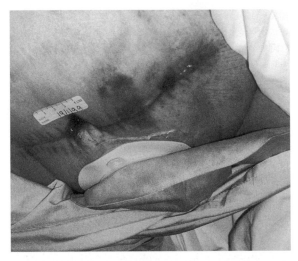

Fig. 3.2 Clinically infected abdominal wound, chacterised by wound breakdown and surrounding erythema.

be encouraged by removing sutures either side of the collection. The wound may begin to break down between the sutures, and it is often advisable to remove the adjacent sutures, allowing the wound to break open completely. Once the infection has cleared, the wound edges can be reapposed with sutures or Steri-strips®, or left to heal by secondary intention.

Removal of intervening sutures in a line of wound breakdown not only makes the wound easier to manage, but prevents secondary complications. Dehiscence often occurs behind the line of the sutures, leaving a track of dead space behind the skin held together with the suture. Additionally, suture material acts as a foreign body and a focus for breeding bacteria, leading to stitch abscesses and the potential for further re-infection of the wound site.

Wounds healing by secondary intention exhibit additional signs of clinical infection. Cutting and Harding[16] identified these further signs as:

- increased exudate or wetness
- change in the appearance of granulation tissue
- odour.

Granulation tissue should be a healthy red or pink colour and slightly bumpy or granular in texture. Healthy granulation tissue should be able to withstand a degree of pressure, but where clinical infection exists, the cells become inflamed and friable. Light pressure, such as removal of a non-adherent dressing or cleansing of the wound bed should not cause bleeding or tissue breakdown. If this occurs, the clinician should be alerted to the possibility of infection. Additionally, the wound edges become inflamed and the wound may become malodorous. Malodour itself does not necessarily equate to infection, since many colonizing organisms, such as *Pseudomonas* sp., give off a distinctive odour and produce a greenish exudate, but may not necessarily be infecting the wound. Streptococcal infections often produce very shiny, smooth, deep-red granulation tissue, which can easily be mistaken for healthy granulation; however, there are often small patches of bleeding or necrosis present within the granulation bed.

In cases of open wounds, swabs should be taken from areas of granulating tissue rather than areas of slough or necrosis if these are present. Necrotic and/or sloughy tissue will grow vast quantities of microbes, but these are not necessarily indicative of the invading pathogen, if there is one. Isolates are best obtained from granulating tissue, as this is the area subject to infection, and a clearer result is likely to be obtained if the wound is cleansed with normal saline prior to the wound swab being taken, as this will clear the wound bed of debris and some of the colonizing organisms.

Antibiotic use in surgical wounds

There is much debate surrounding the use of antibiotics in surgical wounds, and in particular the use of prophylactic antibiotics to prevent surgical site infection. A systematic review of antibiotic prophylaxis for caesarean section suggests that the incidence of endometritis can be reduced by 66–75% if antibiotics are used.[17]

Antibiotic prophylaxis on induction of anaesthesia is a critically timed adjunct to combat the microbial burden of intraoperative contamination and to prevent overwhelming of host defences. However, there is little evidence to suggest that this can overcome postoperative

contamination of the wound site.[15] Overuse of antibiotics can lead to increased antibiotic resistance, and so it is recommended that antibiotics are used only where there are clinical signs of infection, and not on the basis of a positive wound swab alone. Some caution needs to be taken in vulnerable groups, such as diabetics and patients with compromised immunity, as they may not be able to mount an obvious host response to invading pathogens and infection may go undiagnosed.

The Hospital Infection Control Practices Advisory Committee in the USA identified the most common pathogens in surgical wounds associated with different areas of surgery. The most common pathogens in obstetric and gynaecological wounds are Gram-negative bacilli, enterococci, Group B streptococci and anaerobes.[15] *Staphylococcus aureus* is also prevalent, particularly in its methicillin-resistant form (MRSA). This organism frequently colonizes surgical sites but, like other colonizing bacteria, it does not necessarily cause wound infection. Once it does invade and cause infection, however, it is very difficult to treat. Cimochowski et al[18] reported that prophylactic intranasal mupirocin, given 1 day prior to and 5 days following surgery, reduced the incidence of sternal wound infections after open-heart surgery by 66%. There is a suggestion that this inexpensive preventative treatment may reduce MRSA and other staphylococcal surgical wound infections, although this has yet to be determined under trial conditions.

Management of haematoma

Skilled surgical technique can prevent haematoma formation. Some bleeding is expected, but this is generally absorbed and disappears within a few days. In some circumstances, such as emergency caesarean sections where the need to deliver the baby may take precedence over cautious incision techniques, excess bleeding may form a tense haematoma beneath the suture line. The resulting dead space can act as a focus for infection, as well as weakening the suture line and delaying normal healing.

In severe cases, the suture line may have to be reopened and the haematoma evacuated

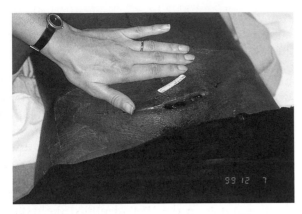

Fig. 3.3 Dehiscence of caesarean section scar with underlying haematoma.

surgically. Often, one or two sutures or clips can be removed to allow the haematoma to drain, but occasionally complete dehiscence of the skin layers occurs (Fig. 3.3).

An open wound with a visible haematoma can be cleaned out quickly and atraumatically with either hydrogen peroxide (3%) solution diluted with normal saline or an enzymatic debriding agent, such as Varidase®, which contains streptokinase and streptodornase. Once clean, the wound edges can be reapposed or, more commonly, left to heal by secondary intention.

The management of open wounds

The first rule of wound management is holistic assessment of the patient. Simply, if the patient conditions are right, the wound will generally heal. Therefore, any existing co-morbid states, such as diabetes, malnutrition, systemic or local infection, should be addressed and managed before the wound can heal properly.

Prior to Winter's[19] work on cutaneous wounds, most open wounds were managed using dry dressings or by being left exposed to the air to form a protective scab. However, Winter discovered that epithelialization of acute wounds was almost twice as fast if the wound surface was kept moist. Further work by Dyson et al[20] showed that moist wounds moved through the inflammatory phase of healing more quickly than dry wounds, producing more macrophages and fewer neutrophils. Additionally, more endothelial cells were present, indicating increased capillary growth. Epithelialization is slower in dry wounds with scab formation as the new skin epithelial cells have to effectively burrow underneath the scab to cover the wound. In moist wounds, however, they are unimpeded and can 'skate' across the surface of the moist wound bed.

Since this early work, the wound-care market has become flooded with moist wound healing, or 'modern' dressings. Advancing technology and understanding of wound healing has led to a new era of wound management products, which aim to manipulate the environment at the wound bed, to improve healing, particularly in chronic, recalcitrant wounds. Modern wound dressings aim to provide the ideal environment for wound healing. This includes:

- patient comfort and atraumatic removal
- maintaining a moist environment but absorbing excess exudate
- providing an environment at the correct pH and temperature to facilitate healing
- protecting from the outside environment (infection and trauma)
- leaving no particulate matter in the wound bed
- cost-effectiveness.

Categorization by tissue types

There are more than 125 different dressings available on the UK market. Absolute categorization of these different dressings is difficult, and so dressing choice is largely dependent upon the type of tissue present in the wound. There are four basic categories of wound tissue, excluding infected tissue:

1. *Necrotic tissue*: this is black, brown and dry or leathery in appearance. It has a distinctive odour when wet and is the result of tissue death secondary to ischaemia. Wounds in this state are prone to infection as bacteria invade the dead tissue, and healing is delayed as the wound becomes stuck in the inflammatory phase.

2. *Slough*: this is yellow/white runny or fibrous material made up of dead cells. This is common

in the inflammatory stage when cellular debris collects at the wound surface. Wounds can continue to heal in the presence of small amounts of slough; however, large amounts can delay healing and need to be removed.

3. *Granulation*: comprises a macrophage- and fibroblast-rich tissue, with an extracellular matrix composed of hyaluronic acid, collagen and fibronectin. It is healthy red or pink, granular tissue.

4. *Epithelial tissue*: the new layer of epidermis that covers the defect and achieves wound closure. The cells are pinky/white and are most often seen at the edges of the wound. The cells also migrate across the surface of the wound and cluster around hair follicles, resulting in small epithelial islands on the surface of the wound.

Different wound tissue types require different dressing properties. Fig. 3.4 gives a simplistic breakdown of the different main properties of dressing groups. This list is not exhaustive and some dressings may fall into more than one group.

Dressings for sloughy and necrotic wounds

The main aim of treatment is to rid the wound bed of necrotic material or slough. The cheapest and fastest way to do this is by sharp debridement. However, unless the patient is taken to theatre for proper surgical débridement, it is unlikely that all this unwanted material will be eradicated in one go. The body will try to facilitate this removal by a process of autolytic debridement, but this can be enhanced by the use of moisture-giving dressings. This group of dressings donates water to the necrotic/sloughy tissue, making it wet and easy to separate from healthy granulation tissue.

Moisture-donating dressings include the hydrogels and hydrocolloid wafers. Hydrogels ideally need a wound depth of greater than 0.5 cm to maximize their full potential and prevent maceration of the surrounding healthy skin. Conversely, hydrocolloids only work to a depth of 0.5 cm, but need to be kept in place for 3–5 days to allow the hydrocolloid to gel and debride. Hydrocolloids are occlusive and are contraindicated in infected wounds. Other debriding agents include the enzymatic debriding agents, such as Varidase®, but these are largely ineffective on dry or hard eschars and need to be changed twice daily. Cadexomer iodine pastes are designed to donate moisture and iodine in a controlled release to the wound bed, which may be required in a heavily colonized wound bed or a high-risk patient.

Some necrotic or sloughy wounds are particularly wet. A thorough assessment of the wound needs to be carried out to eliminate this increased wetness as being a sign of wound infection. In these wet wounds, autolytic débridement is already under way, and rarely do they require extra moisture donated through a wound dressing. In these cases, the moisture-absorbing dressings usually used in granulating wounds are required, although these wounds should be re-assessed regularly, as they are likely to lose this excess exudate and require some additional moisture.

Maggots (larvae therapy or biosurgery) can also be used to debride necrotic or sloughy wounds. *Lucilia sericata* (greenbottle fly) larvae are used because they produce powerful enzymes that break down only dead tissue, and do not burrow into healthy tissue.[21] They cannot be used in the presence of fistulae or wounds close to major blood vessels, and the larvae themselves do require some care and attention in order to survive.

Fig. 3.4 Three basic categories of wound dressings

- Moisture-giving (necrotic/sloughy wounds):
  — hydrogels
  — hydrocolloids
  — saline soaks.
- Moisture-absorbing (granulating wounds):
  — alginates
  — hydrofibres (hydrocolloid fibres)
  — hydropolymers
  — foams.
- Wound contact layers (epithelializing wounds):
  — foams
  — non-adherent wound contact layers
  — paraffin gauze
  — semi-permeable films.

Dressings for granulating wounds

The main aim of treatment is to maintain a moist, not wet or dry, environment and to minimize interruptions to the healing process through unnecessary dressing changes. To facilitate this, a moisture-absorbing dressing is needed which will absorb enough exudate to not require frequent dressing changes. Commonly used dressings include the alginates, the new hydrocolloid fibre dressings (hydrofibres) and hydropolymer dressings. Hydrocolloid wafers can also be used on superficial granulating wounds, but have limited absorbency.

Occasionally, granulating wounds can become very dry, particularly if the patient is dehydrated. In these cases, moisture-giving dressings, such as the hydrogels, can be used to create an improved environment for tissue repair.

Where possible, if the wound is healing and healthy, the dressing should be kept as simple as possible and any potentially irritant substances, such as iodine or silver, should be avoided.

Dressings for epithelializing wounds

Once granulation tissue reaches the surface and epithelialization begins, the exudate level normally reduces and the wound bed must be kept free from trauma. Dressings for this phase of wound healing are usually the wound contact layers, which are non-adherent, maintain a moist environment and offer some protection to the delicate epithelial cells. These dressings include the foams, thin hydrocolloids, non-adherent contact layers, paraffin gauze and hydropolymers. Paraffin-gauze dressings need to be applied in several layers as there is a tendency for them to dry out and stick to the wound bed.

Dressings for infected wounds

There is an argument that if a wound is clinically infected, then a dressing applied topically will have no effect on the infective organisms deeper in the tissues. This is true in part, and any treatment should be used in conjunction with appropriate antibiotic therapy. However, dressings may have a crucial role to play in reducing bacterial counts at the surface of the wound, or preventing a heavily colonized wound from becoming infected.

Traditionally, dressings for infected wounds have centred around iodine, and the use of povidone-iodine-soaked gauze is still common practice in many areas. The problem with povidone-iodine soaks is that the iodine is rapidly deactivated in the presence of pus or excess exudate, and may therefore be limited in its effectiveness against bacteria.[22] However, there is no known documented evidence to suggest resistance to iodine, and so it continues to be used as an antimicrobial. Iodine-based dressings bound to cadexamer molecules are readily available, and these have a slower release of iodine into the wound, thereby extending their antiseptic properties, as well as having the ability to absorb exudate. Povidone-iodine soaks, however, may have some benefit in very large, dirty wounds, but it should be remembered that these need to be changed a minimum of three times per day.

Antibiotic creams or gels may have some place in the short-term treatment of colonized wounds, but the evidence of their superiority in infected wounds over other treatments is scanty.[23] However, they do have some use in controlling wound odour, discussed later in the chapter.

Recently, attention has been focused on silver-based dressings and honey. Silver has been used for a long time to eradicate surface bacteria. Silver ions inhibit the reproduction of bacteria, and so, rather than killing them by toxicity, they naturally reduce in numbers and eventually disappear. Silver sulphadiazine cream has been used for many years in the treament of burns and to eradicate Gram-negative bacilli, such as *Pseudomonas* sp. More recently, a surge of dressings containing silver has hit the market, although their efficacy in managing colonized or infected wounds is as yet largely untested in robust clinical trials. Some are unlikely to have a significant effect as the silver is contained in the backing of the dressing, and so is unlikely to reach the wound bed in ionic form until the dressing is soaked in exudate. This usually heralds the need for a dressing change!

Honey is the newest antimicrobial on the market, despite being used for centuries, prior to the advent of antibiotics, to manage infected wounds. Honey works because it is a saturated sugar solution and therefore generates a very high osmotic potential, dehydrating all bacteria in its path, including MRSA. Honey impregnated dressings are currently under production. In European countries, granulated sugar poured straight into wounds has been used with much success, both as an antimicrobial and as an 'absorbing' material for excess exudate. In the UK, granulated sugar is rarely used from the packet, but a similar product is available through pharmacies as sugar paste.

Odour

Malodour occurs for a reason and can be distressing for the patient as well as unpleasant for staff and visitors. Necrotic tissue, by its nature, can be extremely unpleasant when it is undergoing autolytic débridement. Similarly, infected wounds, or those heavily colonized with *Pseudomonas* sp., for example, can be rather less than fragrant. It is worth remembering that, as health care professionals, we can walk away from a smelly wound, but the patient experiences a continuous unpleasant odour which can exacerbate nausea and cause loss of appetite.

The cause of the odour needs to be addressed. If necrotic tissue is a factor, it may be worth removing as much as possible by sharp débridement. If the wound is infected, antibiotic treatment needs to be instigated. Heavy colonization may not warrant antibiotic use and all necrotic tissue may not be removable, and so attention should be paid to the dressing. Charcoal-impregnated dressings are often used to control malodour; however, their effectiveness is limited. Charcoal is only active against odour while it is dry. Once wet by exudate, the wound will begin to smell again. For this reason, it is often advisable to dress the wound accordingly and then apply a charcoal dressing over the top of the dressing.

Alternatively, or additionally, the wound bed can be treated with a topical antibacterial. Silver sulphadiazine cream (e.g. Flamazine®) is extremely effective at removing *Pseudomonas* sp. as well as other bacteria. Metronidazole gel is particularly effective against the anaerobes found in liquefying necrotic tissue, although, as with silver sulphadiazine, its use should not be prolonged once the odour has been controlled or eradicated.

Pain

Large, deep wounds do not necessarily equate to similar pain levels. Very often, superficial wounds are exceptionally painful as the nerve endings are exposed, whereas in large, deep wounds the nerve endings are obliterated, rendering them relatively pain free. Wound pain is often managed successfully with simple analgesia, but occasionally wounds remain painful even with seemingly adequate analgesia. Superficial wounds may benefit from hydrocolloid dressings, as these keep the nerve endings moist and occluded to air. For extremely painful wounds, local anaesthetic dressings, such as bupivacaine-soaked gauze, can be beneficial, and some success has been reported with diamorphine mixed with hydrogels. However, it is not certain how much systemic uptake of diamorphine there is through an open wound.

Pain can be controlled when changing dressings by use of short-acting, powerful analgesics, such as dextromoramide or inhaled nitrous oxide.

Overgranulation

Overgranulation or 'proud flesh' arises when the granulating bed continues unchecked and exceeds the level of the surrounding skin. It is thought to occur as a result of chronic wound infection, although it can occur in some cases in the absence of any known infection. The aim of management is to flatten the overgranulation and to encourage the wound to epithelialize. In the past, silver nitrate has been used to cauterize the tissue, but this can be extremely painful and traumatic to healing tissue. Foam dressings have been advocated to flatten overgranulation, but take some time to achieve the desired result. A more successful method is to use a steroid and antibiotic ointment (Terra-Cortril®) for a short period of 5–7 days, applied directly to the wound bed. This will flatten overgranulation and encourage the wound to epithelialize.

Maceration

Macerated tissue of the area around the wound usually occurs because of excess exudate from the wound, or as a result of the wound dressing being used. The problem of maceration needs to be addressed, as it can lead to further tissue breakdown or secondary infection. If the problem is the dressing, either donating too much moisture or not absorbing enough, it may be appropriate to reassess the dressing regimen and change to an alternative product. If the wound bed still requires a particular type of dressing product, then the skin surrounding the wound needs to be protected. This can be achieved either by using a barrier cream (often used for nappy rash in babies) or by using a protective film barrier spray, such as Cavilon®.

Large, complex and difficult to manage wounds

This section will cover deep cavity wounds, wounds that have become chronic or recalcitrant and wounds that occur in the vulval/perianal area.

Large cavity wounds can pose problems in terms of healing and exudate management. In wounds with large amounts of necrotic or sloughy tissue present, it may be more cost-effective to use saline soaks rather than several applications of hydrogels or other débriding agents per dressing change. Saline soaks will débride necrosis and slough by donating moisture to the wound bed. In addition, some mechanical débridement takes place as the soak becomes drier and devitalized tissue adheres to the dressing material. Saline soaks should not be allowed to dry out completely and must be changed three times per day to be effective and to prevent trauma on removal.

One of the most successful treatments for large wounds is vacuum-assisted closure (VAC®). VAC therapy works by applying a subatmospheric, or negative, pressure to the wound bed through an open-cell polyurethane foam. The open-cell polyurethane foam dressings allow equal distribution of the negative pressure over the whole wound bed. In addition, it allows exudate to flow through the dressing freely for removal and collection in the cannister, and it provides effective packing for undermining areas and open cavity wounds. The pore sizes of the VAC foam dressing differ from other foam dressings, and are larger to maximize tissue growth.[24]

Applying subatmospheric (negative) pressure to a wound bed via the VAC pump achieves three main objectives:

- it controls exudate
- it reduces the bacterial count
- it promotes granulation.

In animal studies, blood flow levels to the wound bed increased fourfold when 125 mmHg subatmospheric pressure was applied.[24] Granulation tissue formation was increased by approximately 64% on 125 mmHg continuous pressure, and 103% on 125 mmHg intermittent pressure. This therapy is particularly successful in surgical dehiscence and can be used on infected wounds with antibiotic cover. VAC therapy can be used for any depth of wound, but is contraindicated in wounds with fistulae, known or suspected malignancy and needs particular caution in patients with bleeding disorders. VAC should be used on clean granulating wounds, or wounds with minimal amounts of slough. It cannot débride large quantities of slough or necrotic tissue. The highly vascularized wound bed is expected to bleed when the VAC dressing is removed. It is not a sign of clinical infection.

Some wounds become chronic in nature and delayed wound healing can be a problem. VAC can be used on recalcitrant wounds, as can other substances, such as hyaluronic acid and growth factors. Hyaluronic acid is a naturally occurring extracellular matrix molecule and major component of human skin. It is non-immunogenic and so is unlikely to provoke adverse responses in even the most sensitive patients. The hyaluronic acid dressing (Hyalofill®) is an esterified form of pure hyaluronic acid and has a similar appearance to an alginate. Essentially, it dissolves in the wound bed on contact with exudate and create a hydrophilic gel, which overlays the wound and creates a hyaluronic acid rich tissue interface.[25] It has been shown to enhance angiogenesis[26] and to improve the phagocytic response of macrophages.[27,28]

Growth factors are under much debate in the management of chronic or recalcitrant wounds.

They are generally expensive and are still undergoing modifications and clinical trials. While research continues in this area, many of the growth factors in current use have inconsistent results in clinical practice. One of the problems is that growth factors are often degraded if there are high levels of matrix metalloproteinases (MMPs) in the wound bed, rendering the growth factors inactive. A new dressing under review on the market is an MMP inhibitor (Promogran®) and is thought to boost stagnant wounds by blocking inhibitory substances, rather than adding growth factors to the wound bed. Research into growth factors and MMP inhibitors for complex wounds continues.

Some wounds become difficult to manage due to their anatomical positioning. Wounds in the vulval or perianal areas are particularly difficult, as it is virtually impossible to dress this area. Many wounds heal without any intervention; however, occasionally problems arise. The greatest problem is that these areas are classed as dirty areas and wounds are more prone to infection or contamination. Personal hygiene is paramount to preventing infection, and conventional dressings are relatively useless. In some cases, silver sulphadiazine cream can be applied to wounded areas and Surgipads®, held in place by underwear, can be used as a secondary dressing. Some success has also been noted using natural yogurt to prevent or treat infections due to *Candida* sp., and this treatment has the added advantage of being cooling and soothing to the area. Other treatments for wounds in the vulval area have included mouth ulcer preparations, such as Orabase®, which can be applied as a short course to provide a protective film.

Wound cleansing

Traditionally, wounds have always been cleaned with saline at every dressing change. This practice is no longer advocated as it causes unnecessary cooling and potential trauma to the wound bed. Wound cleansing is only advised when there is cellular debris in the wound bed, e.g. sloughy, necrotic tissue, or debris from the dressing material. Wounds should be gently irrigated with warmed normal saline, rather than wiped over with moistened gauze swabs. It may be necessary to clean wounds more thoroughly with wet swabs if the wound bed needs to be inspected closely to determine depth, or to examine for undermining or for sinus/fistula formation.

Much has been written about the use of antiseptics to clean wounds. Many in vitro and in vivo studies[22,29] have condemned the use of antiseptics in wound cleansing, as chlorhexidine (0.05%), savlodil, povidone-iodine (10%) and hydrogen peroxide (3%) were all found to be toxic to fibroblasts at concentrations used for wound cleaning. Routine cleansing with antiseptics is therefore not advisable, particularly when the antiseptic solution, particularly povidone-iodine, cetrimide and savlodil, is in contact with the wound for such a short period of time that it has no discernible effect on the presence of bacteria.[30,31]

Hydrogen peroxide solution works by releasing oxygen when it comes into contact with a wound bed. Some caution is needed as there have been anecdotal reports of air emboli entering the bloodstream when used in cavity wounds with sinuses or fistulae present. Although not recommended for routine cleansing of wounds, due to its fibroblast toxicity, it is an effective method for removing slough, debris and haematomata from the wound bed. It is also very effective against Gram-negative bacilli, such as *Pseudomonas* sp. Since necrotic or sloughy wounds, or those with infected tissue, tend to be stuck in the inflammatory phase, it is unlikely that short-term cleansing with hydrogen peroxide will have any detrimental effects on wound healing. However, it should be stopped once the desired effect has been achieved.

Salt baths

There is no evidence to suggest that salt baths improve healing in surgical wounds. Surgical wounds healing by primary intention are usually kept covered and dry for the first 24 hours; after that, the wound can be uncovered and the patient able to shower. Showering is preferable to bathing as the water gently cleanses the wound without immersing it totally in water for too long. Wounds healing by secondary intention

37

can also be cleaned in the shower prior to dressing changes. This also allows the patient to maintain some degree of normality in personal hygiene and has not been reported to have adverse effects on wound healing or an increase in wound infection rates.

Unintentional, secondary wounding

Patients undergoing surgery expect to have a surgical wound following their procedure. Unfortunately, all too often secondary wounding can occur in the form of pressure sores.

Pressure sores used to be thought of as a nursing issue, but the responsibility is multidisciplinary. Patients are most at risk on the operating table, but damage is unlikely to become apparent until 2–3 days following surgery. Another major risk factor for pressure sore development is epidural analgesia. Roche and Walker[32] conducted a retrospective analysis of postoperative epidural analgesia and pressure sore development and found that gynaecology accounted for only 7% of the total epidurals used in surgery (compared to 34% general and 56% orthopaedics), but had 25% of the total number of pressure sores reported, three times the expected rate. Conversely, obstetrics had no pressure damage reported, but this may be due to the relatively short duration of the epidural. The areas most at risk of pressure damage under epidural analgesia are the sacrum and heels.

Preventative management is paramount in these cases. A wide range of pressure-relieving mattresses is available and these should be utilized before the patient goes to theatre. Too often patients are placed on pressure-relieving equipment once the damage has already occurred. Multidisciplinary communication and team working could identify patients most at risk, or those expected to have epidural analgesia, and plans for appropriate equipment could be made.

Conclusion

The majority of surgical wounds heal without incident. However, some wounds can be more challenging, resulting in dehiscence and/or infection, with associated morbidity and, occasionally, mortality. Skilled surgical technique can eradicate some of these problem wounds, but the real skill of the clinician lies in the ability to identify the patients at risk and to act promptly and appropriately at the first sign of complication.

Wound healing is a dynamic field, with advancing technology and increased understanding of wound complications. However, it is not rocket science, and a sound understanding of the basic principles of healing and the application of good wound care practices will heal most wounds and prevent secondary complications.

REFERENCES

1. Nathan C F 1987 Secretory products of macrophages. Journal of Clinical Investigation 79:319–326
2. Tortora G J, Grabowski S R 1996 Principles of anatomy and physiology, 8th edn. HarperCollins, New York
3. Eckersley J R, Dudley H A 1988 Wounds and wound healing. British Medical Bulletin 44(2):423–436
4. Clark R A F 1988 Overview and general considerations of wound repair. In: Clark R A F, Henson P M (eds) The molecular and cellular biology of wound repair. Plenum, New York
5. Poole G V 1985 Mechanical factors in abdominal closure. Surgery 97:631–640
6. Dealey C 1996 The care of wounds. Blackwell Science, Oxford
7. Derzie A J, Silvestri F, Liriano E, Benotti P 2000 Wound closure technique and acute wound complications in gastric surgery for morbid obesity: a prospective randomised trial. Journal of the American College of Surgeons 191(3):238–243
8. Westaby S 1985 Wound closure and drainage. In: Westaby S (ed.) Wound care. William Heinemann, London
9. Silk J 2001 A new approach to the management of pretibial lacerations. Injury, International Journal of Care of the Injured 32:373–376
10. Bucknall T E, Cox P J, Ellis H 1982 Burst abdomen and incisional hernia: a prospective study of 1129 laparotomies. British Medical Journal 284:931–933
11. Hendrix S L, Schimp V, Martin J et al 2000 The legendary superior strength of the Pfannenstiel incision: a myth? American Journal of Obstetrics and Gynecology 182:1446–1451
12. Cruse P J, Foord R 1980 The epidemiology of wound infection, a ten year prospective study of 62,939 wounds. Surgical Clinics of North America 60(1):27–40
13. Mishriki S F, Law D J, Jeffrey P T 1990 Factors affecting the incidence of post-operative wound infection. Journal of Hospital Infection 16:223–234

14. NINSS 2002 Surveillance of surgical site infection in English hospitals 1997–2001. PHLS, London

15. Mangram A J, Horan T C, Pearson M L et al 1999 Guideline for prevention of surgical site infection, 1999. Infection Control and Hospital Epidemiology 20(4):247–278

16. Cutting K, Harding K 1994 Criteria for identifying wound infection. Journal of Wound Care 3(4):198–201

17. Smaill F, Hofmeyr G J 2000 Antibiotic prophylaxis for cesarean section. In: The Cochrane Library Issue 1. Update Software, Oxford

18. Cimochowsky G E, Harostock M D, Brown R et al 2001 Intranasal Mupirocin reduces sternal wound infection after open heart surgery in diabetics and nondiabetics. Annals of Thoracic Surgery 71:1572–1579

19. Winter G D 1962 Formation of the scab and the rate of epithelialisation of superficial wounds in the skin of the young domestic pig. Nature 193:293–294

20. Dyson M, Young S, Pendle C et al 1988 Comparison of the effects of moist and dry conditions on dermal repair. Journal of Investigative Dermatology 91(5):434–449

21. Jones M, Andrews A 1999 Larval therapy. In: Miller M, Glover D (eds) Wound management: theory and practice. NT Books, London

22. Leaper D, Cameron S, Lancaster J 1987 Antiseptic solutions. Community Outlook April:30–34

23. Drugs and Therapeutics Bulletin 1991 Local applications to wounds: 1. Cleansers, antibacterials, debriders. Drugs and Therapeutics Bulletin 29(24):93–95

24. Morykwas M J, Argenta L C, Shelton-Brown E I et al 1997 Vacuum-assisted closure: A new method for wound control and treatment: Animal studies and basic foundation. Annals of Plastic Surgery 38(6):553–562

25. Ballard K, Baxter H 2000 Developments in wound care for difficult to manage wounds. British Journal of Nursing 9(7):405–412

26. West D C, Hampson L N, Arnold F et al 1985 Angiogenesis induced by degradation products of hyaluronic acid. Science 228:1324

27. Bernake D N, Marwald R R 1979 Effects of hyaluronic acid on cardiac cushion in collagen matrix cultures. Texas Respiratory Biological Medicine 39:271–285

28. Ahlgren T, Jarstrand C 1984 Hyaluronic acid enhanced phagocytosis of human monocytes in vitro. Journal of Clinical Immunology 4(3):246–249

29. Cameron S, Leaper D 1988 Antiseptic toxicity in open wounds. Nursing Times 84(25):77–78

30. Mertz P M, Alvarez O M, Smerbeck R V, Eaglestein W H 1984 A new *in vivo* model for the evaluation of topical antiseptics in superficial wounds. The effect of 70% alcohol and povidone-iodine solutions. Archives of Dermatology 120(1):58–62

31. Gorden M, Aikman L, Little K, Luke D 1989 Prevention of wound infection in the accident and emergency department: does povidone iodine spray reduce infection rates? British Journal of Accident and Emergency Medicine 4:11–13

32. Roche S, Walker S 2000 Retrospective analysis of postoperative epidural analgesia and pressure sores. Acute Pain 3(2):77–83

Perioperative care

Kate Harding

Introduction

The safety of a woman undergoing surgery depends on good preparation and anticipation of potential complications. Communication between the surgeon and the anaesthetist is essential, particularly if the case is likely to be complicated in any way. The woman must be fully informed as to what is going to be done to her, the reasons for the procedures and the possible complications. With good planning most procedures will be successful for both the patient and the medical team.

Most women who undergo either obstetric or gynaecological surgery are young and healthy. In this chapter we will discuss the management of various surgical and medical complications, both those that are pre-existing and those that arise secondary to the procedure.

Preoperative considerations

It is important that the woman knows what procedure is going to be done, why, and the possible complications. Informed consent can only be obtained by someone who understands these issues, and it is therefore not a suitable job for an SHO in his or her first week. Information leaflets written in conjunction with patient groups and in languages other than English can be of great help in ensuring that women are well informed about both the procedure and common complications.

The woman needs to be in good health for her operation and, unless the operation cannot wait, she should not have an anaesthetic while suffering from a chest infection. All black women need to have a sickle test done preoperatively, and all women should have a full blood count done in the month prior to their operation. Further investigations will depend on the procedure and the woman's health (see below).

There is some controversy about how long a woman needs to be starved prior to an operation. The traditional teaching is for 6 hours' starvation, but this is probably not sufficient for those in pain, with intra-abdominal sepsis or pregnant, and is too long for the normal healthy woman having an elective procedure. Pain, opiate analgesics and intra-abdominal sepsis significantly decrease gastric motility and one has to assume that the stomach is not empty despite starvation and the use of metoclopramide. A healthy woman having an elective procedure should stop eating 6 hours before the operation, but she may continue to drink clear fluids up until 3 hours preoperatively (water is absorbed from the stomach within 30 minutes of ingestion if the stomach is empty).

In pregnancy, aspiration pneumonitis is a concern due to decreased lower oesophageal tone, increased abdominal pressure and decreased gastric pH. Therefore starvation is important, as is the use of metoclopramide and H_2-blockers (e.g. ranitidine) preoperatively. The usual regime for women undergoing an elective caesarean section is 6 hours' fasting, ranitidine 150 mg preoperatively (at 22.00 and 07.00 hours) and metoclopramide 10 mg at 07.00 hours. The use of sodium citrate to neutralize the stomach contents is common, although it may be unnecessary prior to a regional block.

Care of the elderly patient

Care of the healthy woman over the age of 65 is not significantly different from that of the younger woman. Based on physiological parameters and operative outcome, 80 is a more appropriate age at which to consider taking extra precautions, as the risk of both morbidity and mortality are increased. Around 10% of all elderly patients show cognitive dysfunction 2 years following abdominal surgery.

Careful assessment of coexisting medical problems is vital and should be done in conjunction with the anaesthetist and the elderly care team. Preoperative medication must be continued throughout the hospital stay (inadvertent discontinuation of drugs is a common problem). Surgery may need to be delayed until health is optimized (although realistic goals are important). The overall risks and benefits of surgery need to be carefully considered with the patient (and her relatives). Apart from an electrocardiogram (ECG) in women over the age of 50 (to detect silent cardiac disease), investigations should be directed by the woman's medical condition. A chest X-ray is unnecessary unless she has respiratory symptoms (or underlying chest disease). Blood tests (other than full blood count) should only be performed where indicated, for example U&Es for women on diuretics, liver function tests for alcoholics or those with malignant disease.

Intra-operative risks include fluid overload and dehydration, heat loss and pressure sores. Recent National Confidential Enquiry into Peri-operative Death (NCEPOD) reports have highlighted the risk of fluid overload in the elderly, precipitating cardiac failure and pulmonary oedema. The elderly patient may be unable to counteract heat loss, and shivering may increase oxygen demand. Conservation of heat with the use of active warm-air heaters and warmed intravenous fluids helps to maintain body temperature and aids recovery. Pressure sores develop within the first 24 hours of surgery and care must be taken in theatre with positioning the patient and preventing skin damage or excess pressure, especially in areas where the circulation is poor (e.g. bony points or areas of oedema). Hypotension may exacerbate the tendency to develop pressure sores.

Acute confusional states are common postoperatively for a variety of reasons, including pain, hypoxia and cessation of smoking or alcohol. Pain control in the elderly may be difficult, as they are more sensitive to opiates (they require less with increased risk of respiratory depression). Regional anaesthetic techniques and the use of patient-controlled analgesia (PCA) may help. Non-steroidals should be used with care as they may precipitate renal failure or gastrointestinal haemorrhage.

Mobilization and rehabilitation postoperatively are vital, with discharge being carefully planned with the family or home care team.

Diabetes

Diabetic women need to be assessed preoperatively for co-morbidity, such as nephropathy and coronary heart disease. Investigations should include renal function tests and, if over 35 years of age, an ECG. Diabetics need to have their disease as well controlled as possible preoperatively. They need to be first on the operation list if possible. Non-insulin-dependent diabetics may need little specific care, as they are unlikely to run into problems while kept starved. They should omit their morning oral hypoglycaemic medication, and 2-hourly sugars and urine testing should be done postoperatively to ensure that they become neither ketotic nor hypoglycaemic. For insulin-dependent diabetics, an intravenous infusion of insulin and glucose is titrated against the woman's serum sugar level (using a glucometer). This regime should be continued until the woman is eating and drinking normally. The insulin requirements of a pregnant woman are likely to diminish greatly after delivery of the placenta, and the insulin infusion can usually be reduced by 50%.

Sickle-cell disease

Sickle-cell trait affects 8–20% of women of African origin. Sickling can occur in women with haemoglobin SS, haemoglobin SC and in severe hypoxia (or cold) with sickle trait. Most adults with Hb SS will be aware of this, but those with Hb SC may be unaware as they are often asymptomatic in pregnancy but can suffer the same problems as women with Hb SS.

To prevent perioperative complications, attention needs to be paid intra-operatively and postoperatively to maintaining adequate hydration, oxygenation and analgesia. This can be done by maintaining facial oxygen until 24 hours, even after minor procedures, giving intravenous (i.v.) fluid at a rate of 3 litres daily and using space blankets and hot-air blowers to prevent hypothermia. Exchange transfusion preoperatively is not usually required; these women are used to a low haemoglobin and are not usually transfused unless their haemoglobin drops below 5 g/dL. It is useful to liaise with the haematologist prior to performing any elective or emergency procedure.

Cardiac disease

Women with structural cardiac abnormalities (either congenital or acquired) are at risk of bacterial endocarditis following obstetric and gynaecological procedures. The risks are greatest for those with prosthetic heart valves (especially mitral) and least for those with atrio-septal defects. The current recommendation is for these women to be given amoxycillin 1 g and gentamicin 120 mg i.v. at induction of anaesthesia, followed by amoxycillin 500 mg orally or i.v. 6 hours later (if allergic to penicillin give vancomycin 1 g over 1 h and gentamicin 120 mg at induction). Women with mechanical heart valves will be fully anticoagulated, and their management should be undertaken in consultation with haematologist, cardiologist and anaesthetist.

Jehovah's Witnesses

Members of this Christian sect believe that it is wrong to be given blood or blood products. Many of these women will decline transfusion even in the face of death. It is important to have discussed all possible situations with the patient prior to surgery, so that the clinicians can be sure to follow her wishes, as to give a transfusion in these circumstances could be construed as assault. To prevent misunderstanding, the most senior member of the team should discuss the operation with the woman (without her family present so they cannot use undue influence). Overall, a Jehovah's Witness has a 44 times increased risk of maternal death. Each woman can make an individual choice as to whether or not to accept blood or any blood products. Some Witnesses will accept autologous transfusion, and some will accept blood that has not become disconnected with the body. In the latter circumstances it may be worth taking a unit of blood from the patient at the beginning of the procedure and transfusing it at the end of the procedure (while keeping the line in continuous contact with the woman). Another technique is to use a cell-saver to 'suction' and 'wash' the woman's own blood perioperatively (this technique is commonly used for aneurysm surgery).

Many other techniques can be used to minimize blood loss at both gynaecological procedures and in the face of postpartum haemorrhage (see 'Shock' below and Chapter 14).

Medication

Oral oestrogens, in particular the oral contraceptive pill, increase a woman's risk of venous thrombo-embolism. If elective surgery is planned, a woman could be asked to stop her oestrogens, although it must be remembered that she may still require adequate contraception, and that pregnancy is associated with a higher risk of thrombosis.

Oral steroid therapy can cause adrenal suppression and inhibit the normal physiological stress response, resulting in an Addisonian crisis. It is recommended that women on more than 5 mg of prednisolone daily for more than 1 month are given hydrocortisone, 150 mg i.v. 8-hourly for 24 hours. This will cover the physiological stress of the procedure. If the procedure is relatively minor (e.g. diagnostic laparoscopy) steroid cover is not required.

Operative considerations

Shock

Blood loss is an inherent risk in any operative procedure, although the amount will depend on the operation, previous surgery, pathology and operative technique. How well the woman copes with the blood loss depends on her physiological state and management of the loss (i.e. fluid replacement). The effect on the woman can be minimized with good preparation and careful intra-operative and postoperative fluid management. Even in the case of a Jehovah's Witness, there are many techniques that can be used

both to minimize blood loss and to reduce the consequences.

Blood pressure is maintained by a combination of stoke volume, heart rate and arteriolar resistance. If the blood volume reduces (for example due to blood loss) there is an initial decrease in arterial pressure. This decreases the stimulation of the baroreceptors, which causes excitation of the sympathetic and inhibition of the parasympathetic nervous systems, resulting in an increased heart rate, an increased strength of contraction (stroke volume), constriction of non-vital arterioles (not cardiac or cerebral) and venous constriction. Together these factors raise the cardiac output, increase resistance and increase venous return, and therefore return the blood pressure towards normal. The physiological response depends on the amount of fluid loss and the measures taken to replace it. The effect of blood loss shock becomes noticeable with a loss of more than 15% of circulating volume, and becomes pronounced only when the loss is greater than 30% (Fig. 4.1). Initial resuscitation is usually with crystalloid (0.9% saline or Hartman's solution) followed by a colloid such as Haemaccel® or Gelofusine®. This will restore the circulating volume but will not optimize either oxygen delivery (for which haemoglobin is required) or replace clotting factors, which are quickly consumed (or lost). If the blood loss is greater than 1500 mL, consideration should be given to blood replacement, keeping the patient warm and central haemodynamic monitoring. When giving blood, it is best done through a blood warmer (stored blood is cold and some of the damage from hypovolaemia is due to reduction in the microcirculation due to cold). Fresh frozen plasma should be given in a ratio of one unit to every four of blood up to 8 units of blood, then a ratio of 1:2 up to 12 units, then in a ratio of 1:1. The use of platelets and other blood products should be informed by a haematologist, but may be needed earlier than anticipated in obstetric cases.

The requirement for homologous blood may be reduced with the use of a cell-saver. This is particularly useful in cases where massive haemorrhage can be anticipated (such as huge fibroids or Grade IV placenta praevia and a previous

Blood loss	Class 1	Class 2	Class 3	Class 4
Percentage	<15	15–30	30–40	>40
Volume (mL)	750	800–1500	1500–2000	>2000
Blood pressure				
Systolic	Unchanged	Normal	Reduced	Very low
Diastolic	Unchanged	Raised	Reduced	Unrecordable
Pulse	Slightly raised	100–120	120 (thready)	Very thready
Respiratory rate	Normal	Normal	Tachypnoeic	Tachypnoeic
Urinary flow (mL/h)	>30	20–30	10–20	0–10
Complexion	Normal	Pale	Pale	Ashen

Fig. 4.1 Classification of hypovolaemic shock according to blood loss (Baskett 1990)

caesarean section). This equipment needs to be prepared before the case starts and effectively returns washed blood to the patient from the suction bottle.

Pharmacological methods to reduce blood loss include the use of agents such as tranexamic acid and aprotinin. The former is a synthetic agent and the latter is a naturally occurring protease inhibitor. They both bind to plasminogen and plasmin, blocking the ability of fibrinolytic enzymes to bind at lysine residues of fibrinogen. Their main action is to prevent re-bleeding by inhibiting the breakdown of already formed clot.

Hypothermia

Perioperative hypothermia is a common consequence of a long operative procedure. It occurs due to decreased thermoregulation in the anaesthetized patient (both general and regional), cool ambient theatre temperature, heat loss secondary to fluid evaporation from the wound site, infusion of cold fluids and respiratory heat loss. Perioperative hypothermia can have adverse outcomes, especially in the elderly patient. There is an increase in cardiac morbidity (6% versus 1%) in high-risk patients. Hypothermia reduces enzymatic reactions. This is of importance when considering coagulation, and can increase the severity of a coagulopathy. Hypothermia also has an adverse impact on wound healing, the immune response, recovery from anaesthesia, increased oxygen requirement due to shivering and can augment the potency of volatile anaesthetic agents.

Hypothermia can be reduced by various means. Reducing the amount of skin exposed to air will reduce cooling, as would increasing the air temperature. Theatre heating should not be excessive as the staff will be unable to work effectively, thus heating the air surrounding the patient (using forced-air warming devices) is more suitable. Space blankets in recovery can reduce heat loss by 30%. Fluid warming should be used if more than 2 litres of fluid are to be given, especially if the fluid is blood as this is usually cold. Heat loss from the airway can be reduced with a heat moisture exchange filter (HME).

Prevention of infection

Infection is a common complication of both obstetric and gynaecological procedures. The risks can be minimized by scrupulous surgical technique and adherence to basic aseptic principles.

Preparation by the surgeon

Hand washing is an important part of the prevention of wound infection, as it removes 'resident' skin bacteria. Nails only need to be scrubbed before the first case of the day. All jewellery should be removed, as bacteria have been shown to reside beneath all rings, this is particularly important for rings with irregular surfaces, as scrubbing them will not remove all bacteria. The wearing of face masks is of limited value, especially in 'dirty' operations, but will protect the wearer from blood splashes.

45

Preparation of the surgical site

It is preferable to shave the abdominal skin immediately preoperatively as this prevents the skin bacteria from having the time to multiply in the skin abrasions. Depilatory creams could be used, but these can cause skin reactions. The skin should be cleaned with an antiseptic solution such as chlorhexidine gluconate 0.5% or iodine 1%. These should be aqueous solutions as (if allowed to pool) alcohol solutions can be ignited by sources such as diathermy or operative light sources. Urinary catheterization should be performed with care to prevent ascending infection.

Pharmacological antimicrobials

Postoperative infections, both superficial and deep, can be reduced with the use of prophylactic antibiotics. The causative organisms include both aerobes and anaerobes (staphylococcal, streptococcal, coliform and *Bacteroides* species in particular). If antibiotics are to be used, they should be given to achieve a peak of activity intraoperatively or at the time of highest bacteraemia (e.g. removal of infected material). The antibiotics should be given either 1 hour preoperatively or at induction of anaesthesia, except at caesarean section when they should be given after umbilical cord clamping to prevent unnecessarily treating the neonate. The value of antibiotic prophylaxis has been established for both obstetric and gynaecological operations. In a review of 66 trials, the use of prophylactic antibiotics was shown to reduce the risk after caesarean section of endometritis (relative risk (RR) 0.37), urinary tract infection (RR 0.55) and serious infection (RR 0.44). Overall the relative improvement in outcome was the same for intrapartum and elective caesarean section. The reduction after gynaecological surgery, especially vaginal surgery, is also well established.

Common regimes are either metronidazole 1 g and cefuroxime 750 mg or co-amoxiclav (Augmentin®) 1.2 g, given at induction of anaesthesia. One dose at the time of surgery is sufficient in most cases. If this has been overlooked, there is no advantage to giving prophylaxis

several hours later, it is safer to await sepsis and treat it if it occurs. For penicillin-sensitive individuals either erythromycin or clindamycin can be used. When using prophylaxis, it must be remembered that the risk–benefit balance favours non-intervention when extra risks, such as penicillin sensitivity, in an individual are included.

Wound closure

Wound healing is affected by a number of factors, including obesity, diabetes, infection, malignancy and length of operation. Surgical expertise and technique are obviously important as haematoma formation can interrupt the healing process.

Wound healing is a four-stage process of inflammation, epithelialization, fibroplasia and maturation. The inflammatory process includes blood clot formation with a phagocytic response (migration of phagocytes and macrophages into the surrounding area). Within 72 hours (unless infection or continued blood loss occurs) the wound surface will be sealed and epithelialization will be complete. Fibroblasts form a collagen matrix over 3–5 days that becomes the scar; this takes approximately 9 weeks to mature. By week three the scar will have attained 20% of its pre-wound strength, and this reaches 60% by 9 weeks.

The sutures for the skin need only achieve approximation of the wound edges and can be removed after 5 days (when epithelialization should be complete). Choice of suture material (Fig. 4.2) depends on the surgeon's preference. In general, monofilament (e.g. Prolene®) causes the least tissue reaction, although subcuticular Dexon® (polyglycolic acid) is popular as no material needs to be removed. The fat layer does not need closure, although haemostasis is vital.

Fig. 4.2 Absorbable suture materials

- Catgut, no longer manufactured
- Polyglycolic acid, Dexon®
- Polyglactin, Vicryl®
- Polydioxanone-S, PDS®

The sheath should be closed with a delayed absorption suture material (e.g. polyglycolic acid or polyglactin 910). If there is concern about wound breakdown (e.g. in cases of recurrent surgery, previous herniation, malignancy or infection) a material such as polydioxanone-S (PDS®) can be used as it is not absorbed for approximately 6 weeks. The risk of hernia after midline incision is similar (10–20%) with interrupted polyglactin and continuous polyglactin, polydioxanone-S or nylon. The patients who have closure with nylon have a higher risk of later wound pain and suture sinus formation.

Postoperative considerations

Venous thrombo-embolism

Venous thrombo-embolism remains the most common cause of maternal mortality in the UK, although it is gratifying to read, in the 1996–1999 confidential enquiry into maternal mortality, that the incidence would appear to have decreased since the introduction of guidelines

Fig. 4.3 Risk factors for thrombo-embolism
• Age >35 years
• Body mass index (BMI) >30
• Weight >80 kg
• Malignancy
• Sepsis
• Pregnancy
• Pelvic surgery
• Thrombophilia (e.g. antiphospholipid syndrome)
• Family history of thrombosis
• Previous thrombosis
• Pre-eclampsia
• Dehydration (e.g. hyperemesis)

from the Royal College of Obstetrics and Gynaecology. Thrombo-embolism occurs when there is an increase in venous stasis, damage to vessel walls or an increase in coagulability (Virchow's triad). These events can be precipitated by various conditions, such as pregnancy, pelvic surgery, malignancy and ongoing sepsis (Fig. 4.3).

Such risk factors have led to various risk tables being devised to plan the minimal types of antithrombotic precautions to be taken (Fig. 4.4).

Fig. 4.4 A risk table devised to plan the minimal types of antithrombotic action to be taken postpartum

Points	Age (years)	Weight (kg)	Risk factor Delivery	Other
0	<36	<81	Vaginal	
1	36–40	81–100 (BMI >25)	Elective caesarean section	>para3, gross varicose veins, current infection, pre-eclampsia, immobility prior to surgery >4 days, major current illness (e.g. heart disease)
2	>40	>100 (BMI >30)	Emergency caesarean section	Sickle-cell disease
3		>120		Extended major abdominal or pelvic surgery (e.g. hysterectomy), personal or family history of thrombosis or thrombophilia, antiphospholipid syndrome

Total points	Action
0	No action
1	Flowtron™ boots, early mobilization and hydration
2	TED® stockings and consider heparin
3	Heparin prophylaxis

the abdominal wound. This will reduce superficial wound pain and can be a useful adjunct in women not having an epidural. The local anaesthetic should be injected into the lateral aspect of the wound in a fan distribution, to block the nerves that supply the skin.

Pre-eclampsia

The postoperative pre-eclamptic patient requires careful and close monitoring. She is at risk of several specific complications, including venous thrombosis, fluid overload and pulmonary oedema, eclampsia, hepatic and renal failure, and postpartum haemorrhage. Attempting to prevent one of these complications can increase the risk of another (e.g. pulmonary oedema versus renal failure). These women should therefore be managed in a high-dependency area. With careful management of fluids, seizure control and thromboprophylaxis, most women will improve and suffer no long-term complications. Non-steroidal anti-inflammatory drugs should not be used for at least 24 hours as they can precipitate renal failure.

Seizure control

Eclampsia is an uncommon complication of pre-eclampsia, occurring in about 1–2% of women with pre-eclamptic toxaemia (PET). The role of magnesium sulphate in the treatment and prevention of further fits is now well established, following the Eclampsia Trial in 1996. The regime is 4 g of magnesium sulphate over 20 minutes, followed by an infusion of 1 g/h until 24 hours after delivery or 24 hours after the last fit, whichever is the longer. The Magpie study has shown that prophylactic use of magnesium sulphate will decrease the risk of eclampsia and may reduce the risk of maternal mortality. In the UK, three fits can be prevented for every 1000 women with severe PET.

Fluid balance

Pulmonary oedema, and subsequent adult respiratory distress syndrome, is the most common cause of death from pre-eclampsia in the UK. Most cases are due to iatrogenic fluid overload in the presence of renal impairment and oliguria. Women with a low albumin (<20 g/L) and significant peripheral oedema are particularly at risk. Care must be taken to restrict fluids (especially i.v. fluid) and avoid worrying unduly about oliguria. The use of non-steroidal anti-inflammatory drugs for postoperative pain relief can exacerbate the problem by enhancing renal impairment. A useful fluid regime is total fluid of 85 mL/h, or urine output plus 20 mL/h (whichever is the lesser). If the urine output falls below 80 mL over 4 hours, renal function should be checked (urea and creatinine) before any fluid challenge is given. This has the useful benefit of 'buying' time for the normal physiological postoperative oliguria to correct itself. If the renal function tests are normal, then it is safer to reduce i.v. fluids and await diuresis, rather than to give extra fluids and cause pulmonary overload. If the urea or creatinine levels are rising, or if there has been significant blood loss and fluid replacement is required, a central line should be inserted and used to monitor fluid replacement. The central line can be via the jugular vein or a long line from the brachial vein, depending on local expertise and the woman's risk of coagulopathy (see Fig. 4.7).

Hypertension

Hypertension must also be controlled in pre-eclampsia. This should be done with a mixture of colloid and a vasodilating drug such as hydralazine (5 mg boluses or an infusion at 10 mg/h up to 40 mg/h). If the hydralazine is ineffective, or if its use is limited by tachycardia, labetalol is a useful alternative drug (infusion of 40 mg/h up to 160 mg/h).

Thromboprophylaxis

Thromboprophylaxis is important in the pre-eclamptic postoperative patient as she is at increased risk of thrombosis. This is complicated by the fact that she may have low platelets or incipient (or full) disseminated intravascular coagulation (DIC). If her clotting profile is normal and her platelet count greater than 50×10^9

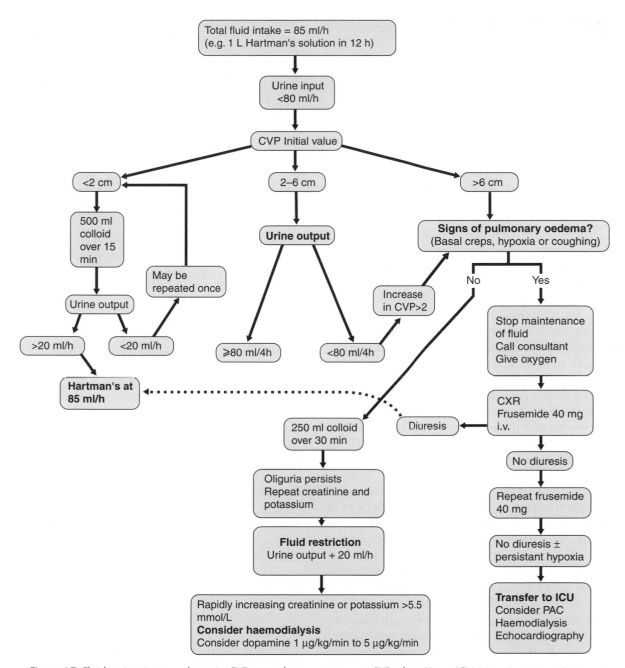

Figure 4.7 Fluid regime in pre-eclampsia. CVP, central venous pressure; CXR, chest X-ray; ICU, intensive care unit; PAC, pulmonary artery catheter; i.v., intravenous

she should be given heparin (e.g. dalteparin 5000 IU). If her APTT ratio or INR is greater than 1.5, this should be corrected with fresh frozen plasma and anticoagulants should be withheld.

Nausea and vomiting

Postoperative nausea and vomiting (PONV) are common and distressing symptoms, which typically last for up to 24 hours after surgery 51

Fig. 4.8 Incidence of nausea and vomiting

- Hysteroscopy, dilatation and curettage (D and C), 13%
- Vaginal surgery, 60%
- Abdominal hysterectomy, 67%
- Laparoscopy, 52%

(Fig. 4.8). Postoperative nausea and vomiting can lead to discomfort, embarrassment, exhaustion, dissatisfaction, electrolyte imbalance and fear of further surgery. It is a common cause for admission after day surgery. Gynaecological patients are particularly prone to this, with up to 42% of women suffering PONV. This increased incidence may be due to the nature of the surgery (laparoscopy is associated with a high incidence) or the otherwise reported greater incidence in women.

Postoperative nausea and vomiting can be decreased by the following measures. Limiting preoperative fasting to the required 6 hours—prolonged fasting can increase the volume of liquid in the stomach. Gastric distension can occur as a result of inadvertent oesophageal intubation, it can also occur if the anaesthetic is prolonged, due to absorption of nitrous oxide which causes distension of the gut. Adequate analgesia (especially non-opiate analgesia) will help minimize PONV. Anti-emetics also play a role in decreasing nausea, although they are better given prophylactically rather than once nausea has developed. Metoclopramide may be useful as it not only controls nausea but also enhances gastric motility, which may be impaired postoperatively due to handling, sepsis or intra-abdominal blood. Ondasetron appears to be an excellent anti-emetic although expensive. Acupuncture and acupressure bands have not been shown to reduce postoperative nausea.

In women undergoing caesarean section with a regional block the nausea may be due to hypotension and is best managed with adequate fluid replacement and vasoconstrictors such as ephedrine.

Postoperative neuropathies

Damage to nerves is uncommon during surgery but can occur due to poor patient positioning or pressure on various nerves during surgery.

Femoral neuropathy

The femoral nerve can be compressed by a self-retaining abdominal retractor. The patient may complain of weakness in her knee, pain anterior to her hip or decreased sensation over the antero-medial aspect of her thigh. She may be unable to climb stairs. Different suggestions have been made as to how to prevent this complication, including the use of smaller (narrower) blades on the retractor and placing a pack under the lateral blades; intermittent release of the retractor to decrease pressure on the nerve; or palpation of the femoral artery, as if it is palpable the pressure on the nerve is unlikely to be excessive. In the event of the development of classic signs, prompt physiotherapy is likely to lead to full recovery.

Sciatic and peroneal neuropathy

Injury to the sciatic or peroneal nerves occur in approximately 1–3 per 500 cases of pelvic surgery. Symptoms include lateral foot drop and leg numbness. It is due to stretching of the nerve during improper patient positioning. Tension on the nerve is least when the hips and knees are flexed and the hip mildly externally rotated. Excessive rotation or abduction when placing the woman in lithotomy or Lloyd-Davis position can cause damage, as can sudden movement (such as dropping a limb). It is best if both legs are lifted together and placed in the correct position. Should damage occur, symptoms tend to arise early and abate within 6 months with physiotherapy.

Brachial plexus damage

The brachial plexus can be damaged if the arm is poorly positioned. It may be overabducted by the anaesthetist to enhance venous access and displace it from the operating field (or out of the surgeon's way). Symptoms include arm or shoulder pain, or upper limb weakness. Most injuries resolve spontaneously.

Pressure sores

Pressure sores are due to poor circulation, obesity or lack of subcutaneous fat, poor skin condition or inadequate nutrition, exacerbated by continuous pressure. They are therefore more common in the elderly or those suffering from chronic disease, but can occur in anyone. They can be prevented by scrupulous attention to patient position, cushioning pressure points (especially if they are already in poor condition or the procedure is lengthy), both on the operating table and in recovery. Once sores develop, a specialist tissue viability opinion should be sought.

Obstetric high-dependency unit

The surgical and obstetric high-dependency units (HDU) can both improve patient's outcome and decrease the requirement for intensive care unit (ICU) admission. The advantages of an obstetric HDU include midwifery care for the mother and neonate, midwifery care for the antenatal sick mother and a close working relationship between highly skilled midwifery staff and the medical team. The unit is defined by the staff working in it, rather than the physical space, as it is availability of skilled staff that makes the difference to outcome. By keeping sick women within the labour ward (rather than being moved to an intensive care unit) the mother and baby can be kept together, the psychological pressure on the partner is reduced, and the woman is cared for by a team that understands the physiology of both pregnancy and the index illness.

Guidelines

Guidelines for the management of various common (and more importantly uncommon) conditions should be agreed by the obstetric, anaesthetic, medical and midwifery teams. These should be (as far as possible) reference based. There are guidelines available for the management of conditions such as massive haemorrhage, pre-eclampsia, diabetic keto-acidosis, asthma and pneumonia (see Fig. 4.7 for the guideline for fluid management in pre-eclampsia).

Staffing

High-dependency units commonly work on a staffing level of one nurse (or midwife) for every two beds. These staff need to be familiar with the unit, the protocols and the medical staff. If the unit is staffed as part of the general ward, then although one can maintain the staff to patient ratio, the other advantages of HDU care (such as understanding how equipment works, knowledge of protocols and clear lines of communication with the medical staff) are lost. The midwifery team needs a leader to keep the protocols up to date and to ensure that staff are suitably trained. New staff may need to spend some time undergoing training in HDU techniques (e.g. care of central lines). This training can be done in critical care areas around the hospital (e.g. ICU and recovery).

Admission criteria

Women who benefit from being admitted to HDU include:

1. Severe PET (BP > 140/90, proteinuria > 0.3 g/24 h, biochemical or haematological abnormality and the decision has been made to deliver).
2. Blood transfusion >3 units or blood products.
3. Shocked, oliguric, hypotensive.
4. Deranged liver function associated with diagnosis of haemolytic anaemia elevated liver enzymes and low platelets (HELLP) or acute fatty liver.
5. Cardiac disease.
6. Pulmonary embolus and hypoxic in air ($sP_{O_2} < 94\%$).
7. Pulmonary oedema.
8. Peripartum hysterectomy.
9. Ventilatory requirements e.g., continuous positive airway pressure (CPAP), non-invasive positive pressure ventilation (NIPPV) or intermittent positive pressure ventilation (IPPV).
10. Sickle-cell crisis.
11. Severe thrombocytopenia (platelets $< 20 \times 10^9$/L).

Using the above criteria, approximately 2–3 in 100 will require admission to the obstetric HDU. Indications for HDU admission in the first year of the obstetric HDU being opened at

St Thomas' hospital in London (1997–1998) were as follows (delivery rate 3750):

- pre-eclampsia, 23%
- postpartum haemorrhage, 21%
- post general anaesthetic, 11%
- diabetic stabilization, 6%
- sickle-cell crisis, 5%
- other, 34%.

HDU admission was predictable from pre-delivery morbidity (e.g. hypertension) in 33% of cases.

FURTHER READING

Anderson I 2001 Care of the critically ill surgical patient. Royal College of Surgeons, London

Anonymous 1999 Practice guidelines for preoperative fasting and the use of pharmacological agents for the prevention of pulmonary aspiration: application to healthy patients undergoing elective procedures. Anaesthesiology 90:896–905

Eclampsia Trial Collaborative Group 1995 Which anticonvulsant for women with eclampsia? Evidence from the Collaborative Eclampsia Trial. Lancet 345:1455–1463

Frank et al 1997 Perioperative maintenance of normothermia reduces the incidence of morbid cardiac events. Journal of the American Medical Association 277:1127–1134

Moller et al 1998 Prolonged post-operative cognitive dysfunction in the elderly. Lancet 351:857–861

National Confidential Enquiry into Perioperative Deaths. November 1999. HMSO, London

Report on Confidential Enquiry into Maternal Deaths in the UK 1996–1999. HMSO, London

Smaill F, Hofmeyr G J 2000 Antibiotic prophylaxis for caesarean section. Cochrane database of systemic reviews, CD000933

Obstetric techniques

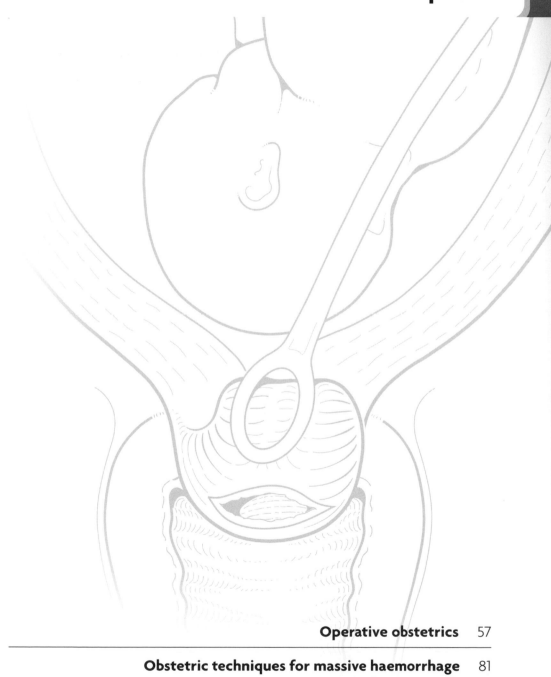

2

Operative obstetrics

Donald Gibb

CHAPTER

5

General principles of obstetric surgery

Surgery is a further challenge to the pregnant woman, already in a condition of physical and psychological stress. Good pain relief, asepsis, minimal tissue handling and the use of appropriate materials with good technique are the cornerstones of good surgery. Limitation of the period of tissue handling is important, but speed is only valuable in association with meticulous technique. Planning, good lighting in the correct environment, appropriate instruments, skilled assistance and support are all essential.

During training, each surgeon should develop their preference for instruments and suture material. The support staff should then be ready with the appropriate tray of instruments and materials on each occasion they are required. Instruments are a personal choice, but are selected to minimize tissue handling and allow precision of technique. Retractors of the correct size are useful, but when applied with strength, sometimes unrecognized, can cause significant bruising. Any trainee would benefit by referring to the essential principles of gynaecological surgery as stated by Bonney.[1]

The appropriate choice of the suture material promotes healing. Catgut is no longer available in the UK. Synthetic materials are superior, in causing less tissue reaction, less infection and having more consistent tensile strength. They are of monofilament or multifilament structure. The most commonly used monofilament materials are polypropylene (Prolene®), polydioxanone (PDS®), polyglyconate (Maxon®) and poliglecaprone 25 (Monocryl®). The popular multifilament sutures are polyglactin 910 (Vicryl®) and polyglycolic acid (Dexon®). Monofilament material is smoother and a knot on such material has a greater tendency to run than on a multifilament suture. Knot security is important; however, multiple knots should be avoided. As it is the material that provokes a tissue reaction, its volume should be limited. Knot-holding capacity is optimal with three throws on any knot.[2] It is also known that the gauge of the material rather than the number of throws on the knot adds more foreign body and tissue reaction.[3] The gauge should therefore be small but appropriate for the tissue being closed and the tensile strength required. A secure knot is tied by reversing the direction of tying for the second throw, creating a reef knot rather than a sliding knot. A further throw creates a square knot which is probably most secure with a third turn on the third throw.[4] The inclination to add further throws and further volume should be resisted. Single sutures with ends cut short should be used for discrete bleeding points. Diathermy is also valuable for this purpose. Sutures for tissue approximation should not be tied too tight because pain and strangulation of the tissues may occur. There is always some postoperative tissue swelling and oedema, which leads to discomfort. A few good large bites of tissue approximating tissues are better than multiple small stitches. Nature is a good healer. The purpose of suturing is to achieve haemostasis and bring tissue together for natural healing to occur. Local physical pressure should be applied to bleeding tissue for several minutes. If the bleeding is not from a discrete vessel, then this may suffice without suturing. On the anterior abdominal wall, a subcuticular closure can be finalized with Steri-strips® and a light, dry dressing suffices.

The protection of health professionals has become important in recent years on account of the threat of blood-borne infections such as hepatitis B and human immunodeficiency virus (HIV). For more major surgery, disposable waterproof gowns and drapes are useful. The drapes may include pockets for fluid collection. Goggles and double gloves should be used in situations of greater exposure. Every effort should be made to avoid needlestick injury. Rigorous discipline in instrument and needle handling is preferable to the use of blunt needles, which can lead to tissue tearing and a suboptimal surgical result.

Repair of episiotomy and tears

The extent to which women may suffer after childbirth has previously not been acknowledged.[5] It is estimated that over 85% of women sustain some perineal damage during vaginal birth[6] and of these 60–70% will require suturing.[7,8] In a diminishing number of cases in this country, this will be an episiotomy, most often in the medio-lateral position. A midline episiotomy will heal better but presents the added risk of extension to the anal margin. There are wide variations in the rates of episiotomy. After a peak in the 1970s in the UK, use of an episiotomy has declined. This was due to more critical analysis of the result, and studies such as the West Berkshire perineal management trial.[7] A Cochrane Review[9] has concluded that a policy of episiotomy restricted to clear fetal or maternal indications is recommended. This is associated with a reduced risk of posterior perineal trauma, an increased risk of anterior perineal trauma, no difference in the risk of severe vaginal or perineal trauma and no difference in the risks of pain, dyspareunia or urinary incontinence. In Eastern European countries and other parts of the world episiotomy rates remain very high. In the prevention of perineal trauma, consideration should be given to a programme of perineal massage in late pregnancy. In a randomized controlled trial, one group were instructed to massage the perineum daily for 10 minutes, using almond oil, from 34–35 weeks' gestation. This group had a significantly lower rate of perineal damage when it was a first delivery, but not when there had been a previous vaginal birth.[10] A more upright, mobile position of the mother in labour facilitates an easier birth. During the expulsive phase a low squat, such as a partner to partner squat, is effective in aiding descent of the head. The partner in this instance is a midwife or doctor, not the woman's partner, who is better placed providing physical support from behind the woman. Once the head is on the perineum, the use of a birthing stool may lead to excessive perineal oedema, tearing and postpartum haemorrhage. As the head crowns, the woman should be lifted from a low squat to a more upright position: this protects the perineum from excessive tearing. An all fours position is probably the position most effective in promoting an intact perineum. A conservative approach to the perineum allows for the possibility that there will be an intact perineum with all its advantages. However, the pursuit of an intact perineum should not result in irregular large tears that are difficult to repair. A large baby in an occipitoposterior position and a prolonged second stage are more obvious examples when an episiotomy might be beneficial. A conservative approach to the perineum may result in anterior perineal trauma, particularly with a prolonged period of expulsive effort in a squatting position.

Recommended technique

After delivery of the placenta and membranes the perineum and vagina should be inspected for damage. This should not interfere with the initial physical contact and bonding of the parents with the baby, unless there is obvious significant bleeding. Full inspection requires good light and exposure. Adequate exposure of small tears is often obtained without placing the woman in a lithotomy position; however, it should be used as necessary. Gauze swabs should be used for examination rather than cotton wool, which becomes saturated and is easily lost. Swabs are counted by the operator at the beginning and the end. Any swab inserted into the vagina to aid inspection should be attached to a string. A systematic inspection from front to back is important: traumatic division of the labia minora can be missed. After inspection a decision is made about the need for suturing, the position necessary to perform it effectively and the need for analgesia. Extension of damage to the anal

area requires inspection in lithotomy. If anal sphincter damage is recognized, then special arrangements should be considered for repair. There should be no reluctance to perform anal examination, informing the woman of the need and seeking verbal consent. Analgesia should then be obtained by topping up an existing epidural or by generous use of 1% lidocaine (lignocaine) infiltration. The use of Entonox® should be avoided at this time as it is neither adequate nor pleasant in these circumstances. Patience and available time is important for the operator, both in obtaining analgesia and the process of repair.

There are two immediate objectives in suturing the perineum:

- haemostasis
- approximating disrupted tissue to aid natural healing.

This should be done with the minimum of foreign suture material, whether by gauge or volume. The best stitch is 'no stitch'. Several studies of material used in perineal suturing have been reviewed in The Cochrane Library.[11] Synthetic suture material such as polyglycolic acid or polyglactin is the optimal material. Vicryl rapide® 2/0 or 3/0 is an appropriate and commonly used material for the perineum. An obvious arterial or venous bleeding point should be secured individually. Small lacerations with capillary ooze, especially anteriorly, will benefit from a few minutes of pressure with a gauze swab and may not then require suturing. The area near the urethra and clitoris is a particularly sensitive area for healing. Nature heals remarkably well and it is probably better to leave small, non-bleeding tears unsutured, as long as good tissue approximation is likely. Small studies in the midwifery literature[12-14] and personal experience, with careful follow-up, suggests that this is good practice.

Having identified and secured the apex of the tear, a continuous stitch is applied to the vaginal tissues. Although some suggest a continuous locking stitch,[15] a continuous non-locking technique is more commonly used. A locked throw being applied if there is a bleeding point or if there is asymmetry of the tissues, requiring adjustment by shortening. Lateral asymmetrical damage should be assessed for the landmarks of the remnants of the hymenal ring and the change of pigmentation at the perineal area. If exposure is difficult, a Weislander retractor is useful to hold back the vaginal edges. Tissue bites should be of significant volume but not too tight. When the fourchette is reached, the needle should be inserted though the skin tissue on one side but brought out in the deeper subcutaneous tissue on the other side. The first muscle stitch finishes the vaginal repair. The knot is therefore buried under the skin, obviating a painful knot in this sensitive area. If the muscle layer is damaged more deeply, then single interrupted sutures should be placed to approximate the tissues. Specific bleeding points should be secured with individual sutures. Looser sutures will approximate tissue that is not bleeding to close space. Superficial muscle should be closed with a continuous stitch, starting near the fourchette with the end kept long for finishing after subcuticular closure. The continuous muscle suture emerges at the distal apex of the skin and then, in a reversed direction, closes the subcuticular tissue just under the skin edge. The loose end at completion is then tied to the starting stitch end and buried (Fig. 5.1). Women find exposed knots painful, and they should be minimized. Haemostasis should be verified, the anus should be checked and, with consent, a diclofenac pessary administered rectally for pain relief. At the conclusion of any suturing, swabs, needles and instruments should be checked. Less experienced staff may use interrupted sutures on the skin. This provides a less satisfactory result than a subcuticular technique.[11] Training should be encouraged in the subcuticular technique.

An alternative approach to skin closure was suggested in the Ipswich Childbirth Study.[16] These authors compared a traditional three-stage repair (vagina, deep tissues and skin) with a two-stage repair, leaving the skin unsutured if there was a less than 0.5 cm gap between the skin edges with the woman in the lithotomy position. This may be satisfactory as long as there is not too much material left in the subcutaneous tissues; however, in this study there was an incidence of gaping perineum in the group who

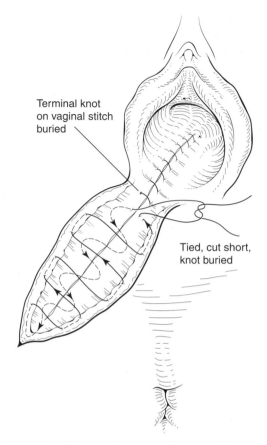

Terminal knot on vaginal stitch buried

Tied, cut short, knot buried

Fig. 5.1 Perineal closure. Interrupted line, muscle layer; continuous line, subcuticular layer.

did not have skin sutures. This approach should be used with great care.

The use of a tissue adhesive appears attractive in obviating painful stitches. Preliminary work[17] appears encouraging.

The after care of perineal repair includes basic hygiene, local application of herbal treatments and pain relief. The midwife will check the stitches before and after discharge. If there has been any difficulty, then the operator should arrange follow-up. Some women find that the stitches are more uncomfortable than expected. A review of the perineum after 3–8 days may reveal loose stitches or long knots that should be removed or trimmed. Although uncomfortable when being done this can lead to enormous benefit. The taking of a swab and prescription of antibiotics are of limited value when a perineum is infected. Removal of suture material and good hygiene is the key. Salt baths are of no value, but herbal baths may be useful.

A first-degree tear involves only the skin, whereas a second-degree tear involves the perineal muscles. More problematical are third-degree tears, involving partial or complete disruption of the anal sphincter, and fourth-degree tears, involving complete disruption of the external and internal anal sphincter and mucosa.[18] Severe perineal tears may occur in up to 9% of deliveries where a medio-lateral episiotomy has been performed.[19] However, since the introduction of endoanal ultrasound, occult damage to the anal sphincter has been identified in up to 36% of women after vaginal delivery in prospective studies.[20-22] The clinical relevance of asymptomatic defects is unclear. All women having a vaginal delivery should have a systematic examination of the perineum, vagina and rectum to assess the severity of damage prior to suturing. All women having instrumental delivery, or who have extensive perineal injury, should be examined by an experienced obstetrician, trained in the recognition and management of perineal tears.[23] The repair of third- or fourth-degree tears should be carried out in an environment, possibly the operating theatre, where there are appropriate instruments, adequate light and assistance. Pain relief is important, with epidural or general anaesthesia, to encourage the anal sphincter to relax, allowing retrieval of the retracted torn ends. This allows the ends of the anal sphincter to be brought together without any tension.[24] There is no reliable evidence to show that the overlap method[23] is superior to the end-to-end (approximation) method of repair. A randomized controlled trial found no differences in continence symptoms, anorectal manometry or ultrasound appearances of the anal sphincter at 3 months' follow-up.[25] Monofilament suture material such as polydioxanone (PDS®) or Dexon® should be used to repair the sphincter itself because of a longer half-life and lower likelihood of infection than if a braided material such as Vicryl® is used. The use of antibiotics intra-operatively and postoperatively is recommended because of the serious consequences of infection and wound break-

down. Broad-spectrum antibiotics with the addition of metronidazole are appropriate. Laxatives are recommended in the recovery period to soften the stool: lactulose 15 mg twice a day and a bulking agent such as Fybogel® are used.

Careful follow-up is important, with the use of endoanal ultrasound and electromyography if indicated. Early referral should be made to a specialist, usually a colorectal surgeon. An unsatisfactory result will require further surgery, often involving the adjunctive use of a defunctioning colostomy. Careful notekeeping and audit are obviously important throughout the process of treatment, bearing in mind the potential for complaint and litigation. Prevention is better than cure, with judicious use of episiotomy in high-risk situations and meticulous attention to repair.

Secondary repair

Secondary repair of the perineum should not be undertaken too early. The mother should be encouraged to undertake pelvic floor exercises for several months. If she then persistently complains of the vagina being too loose or complains of vaginal flatus, then a secondary repair should be undertaken electively. A transverse incision on the perineum with excision of redundant vaginal and perineal skin, followed by reclosure of the vagina with Vicryl®, achieves restoration of the perineum. Care is essential to ensure that it is not too tight. The skin should be closed with unabsorbable interrupted sutures, such as silk, which are removed on the fourth day.

The management at her next birth of the woman with previous significant perineal damage should be individualized. If she has had a third-degree tear with significant morbidity then a caesarean section may be justified. If she has had a complicated repair, but not of a third degree, then careful assessment of her perineum should be made at 37 weeks' gestation in her next pregnancy. If her baby is not big and she is well motivated, then vaginal delivery is reasonable under careful supervision. Ideally the perineum will not tear, but if a tear of a fibrous, scarred perineum appears imminent, then an episiotomy should be performed. This requires expert repair. 61

Great attention to detail must be exercised in record keeping because of the risk of complaint and litigation. A diagram of the damage and the repair is indispensable. A note of follow-up arrangements should be made.

Excellent care of the perineum is essential to enhance the quality of modern maternity care. Some women choose caesarean in part because of fear of perineal damage. Programmes of education and training of doctors and midwives should be implemented to allow women to make a choice of delivery secure in the knowledge that their vagina and perineum will be looked after in a skilled and expert way.

Cervical cerclage

Cervical incompetence, more sensitively referred to as cervical weakness,[26] has been a controversial subject for many years. It is relatively unusual, with an incidence 0.5–2.0% of all pregnancies.[27] Historically it has been overdiagnosed and consequently overtreated with cerclage. A problem lies in the definition and diagnosis. Traditionally it has been postulated as a cause when there has been a mid-trimester pregnancy loss, presenting with rapid painless dilatation of the cervix. There are many causes of mid-trimester pregnancy loss, of which cervical weakness is but one. Multiple pregnancy, persistent bleeding, uterine anomaly, multiple fibroids and genital tract infection should all be excluded before a diagnosis of cervical weakness is entertained.[26] Cervical weakness is usually acquired and very rarely congenital. It may be congenital in association with connective tissue diseases. The presence of previous trauma to the cervix at childbirth, miscarriage or abortion, or surgery on account of cervical neoplasia may be significant. There may have been a miscarriage proceeding with a cervical suture remaining in place. Damage may also occur in association with a complicated second stage of labour. Forceps delivery, breech extraction and mechanical dilatation have all been linked to cervical weakness. Conization of the cervix is not commonly associated with cervical weakness: it is more commonly associated with subsequent progress to a normal gestational age or, indeed, to failure of cervical dilatation in labour due to cervical stenosis.[28] A minority of cases will suffer pregnancy loss due to cervical weakness. This may relate to the type of conization and subsequent healing.[29–34] Caution should be exercised in counselling patients who have had repeat surgical procedures on the cervix. It may be prudent to recommend cerclage, particularly with advancing age.

Diagnostic tests of cervical strength, such as the passage of a Hegar dilator in the non-pregnant state,[35] a traction test with Foley catheter,[36] X-ray hysterography[37] and the use of a cervical resistance measuring device[38] have generally not proved useful, and it remains an empirical diagnosis.

The cervix may be repaired or strengthened in the non-pregnant state by interval procedures, or by cerclage in pregnancy. Lash introduced the term 'incompetent cervix' in 1950,[35] describing a surgical procedure of trachelorrhapy in the non-pregnant state. Palmer attempted to define the role of the cervical isthmus in habitual abortion.[39]

McDonald and Shirodkar were the first to report the insertion of a cervical suture to prevent miscarriage and preterm birth. McDonald, visiting from Australia, was an obstetric registrar at the North Middlesex hospital. He observed a woman in the emergency department with a dilating cervical os. The first cerclage he performed was an emergency procedure.[40] Shirodkar, working in Bombay, without knowledge of McDonald's work, was pursuing the same management. His technique was different, requiring more dissection to reach the internal os.[41] The popularization of cerclage as a prophylactic manoeuvre led to its overuse. Three randomized controlled trials failed to show much benefit from the technique.[42–44] The Medical Research Council/Royal College of Obstetricians and Gynaecologists (MRC/RCOG) study was flawed by liberal inclusion criteria obscuring the true high-risk cases. The subgroup of subjects in this study with three mid-trimester pregnancy losses did benefit from cerclage. The study was further weakened by lack of specificity about the procedure, which was usually a McDonald approach.

Management must be individualized, bearing in mind age, fertility, appearance of the cervix and other factors. There is now a small group of women who have had cervical amputation as a conservative procedure for early cervical cancer. Some surgeons place a nylon stitch at the time of cervical amputation.[45] If this should become extruded, consideration is made of transabdominal cervical cerclage. The role and type of cervical cerclage is currently defined by clinical indications.

The type of cerclage

It is accepted that weakness of the cervix is critical at the level of the internal os rather than lower on the cervix. It is also accepted that the upper vagina contains microorganisms that are a potentially pathogenic threat to the intrauterine contents. Placing a suture high on the cervix and distal from vaginal organisms is therefore logical. Both approaches require a reasonable bulk of cervix on which to operate. When the cervix can be effectively grasped, a vaginal approach is appropriate. Theoretically a Shirodkar suture achieves better placement but requires more expertise, a longer operating time and there is a greater potential for bleeding. Patients who have lost a previous pregnancy with a McDonald suture in place generally prefer to have a Shirodkar, and may ask for a transabdominal approach (Fig. 5.2). Although failure of a vaginally placed suture has been cited as an indication for a transabdominal approach, this is only logical if the previous vaginally placed suture was a Shirodkar. This can lead to difficulties in counselling. There are cases where there has been failure of pregnancy with a McDonald approach when there has been no good indication for any cervical strengthening. It is difficult to convince these patients that they do not require cerclage: they can be offered serial cervical length ultrasound scans. It is disappointing when they present with a damaged cervix on account of a suture remaining in place during a miscarriage when they have originally had no good reason to have a cerclage. The suture has led to a problem rather than solved one.

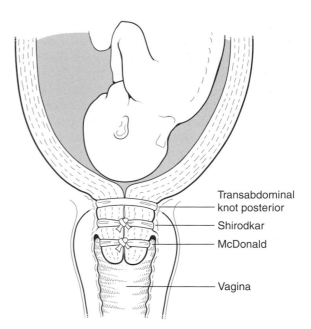

Fig. 5.2 Sites of cervical cerclage.

Labels: Transabdominal knot posterior; Shirodkar; McDonald; Vagina

Vaginal cerclage

The couple are fully counselled about the operation. They should realize that there is no guarantee that it will result in a successful outcome. In most instances the procedure can be done conveniently as a day case. Shortly before the operation ultrasound scan should confirm fetal viability. The technique should have been discussed and selected some days or weeks before the operation. The operator should have examined the cervix in order to confirm feasibility for a vaginal approach. With the patient under anaesthesia in the operating theatre it is the wrong time to decide that a vaginal approach is not possible. Most operators select a McDonald approach as the method of first choice. If the woman has already had such a procedure in a previous unsuccessful pregnancy, then she will not wish to have the same procedure a second time. Most specialists would consider a formal Shirodkar procedure in this situation. There has been no randomized controlled trial of McDonald versus Shirodkar technique. The procedure may be performed under general or regional anaesthesia. Although the objections to general anaesthesia are not as compelling in early pregnancy as in late pregnancy, regional anaesthesia is probably preferable. It can be a matter of choice for the women, with those of a more nervous disposition choosing to be asleep. A lithotomy position with the possibility of a head down tilt is chosen. Prior to washing and draping, a labial shave should be performed, as profuse hair interferes with access and may introduce infection. It is optimal if the operator positions the patient and shaves the vulval area. Time and patience are important to achieve a good result.

McDonald suture

The vulva and perineum are washed with antiseptic. The vagina and cervix are washed under direct vision, removing discharge and often some mucus. The bladder should not be emptied. An Auvard speculum with the correct angle is the best means of visualizing the cervix, which is grasped with a two-sponge holding forceps, one on the anterior lip and one on the posterior lip. A vulsellum forceps should not be used as this tends to traumatize the cervix. Most specialists then use Mersilene tape RS22 (Ethicon, Edinburgh) to insert the stitch. RS22 has a smaller needle than RS21, which should not be used. All recently manufactured Mersilene is now a 40 cm length, rather than the original 30 cm length: this facilitates handling. The cervix is then pierced in the four quadrants sequentially to take a bite of each part. This is a pursestring suture which is tied anteriorly in the midline. The knot is tied with three throws, fairly tightly but not so tightly as to cause ischaemia. Surgeons' knots are rarely too tight but may be too loose. The ends are then cut reasonably short, with approximately 0.5 cm tails. An excessive length of material in the upper vagina may exacerbate infection and cause a discharge. The woman is warned that there may be a small amount of bleeding later that day and the next day. Patients are happy if a Doptone examination demonstrates a fetal heart before discharge from hospital. She can be discharged home with advice to restrict her activities for a couple of days and report to the hospital if she has pain, bleeding or vaginal loss. Couples are counselled to avoid penetrative sex in the early

weeks after cerclage and usually do not have a problem with this.

A McDonald suture is removed at 37–38 weeks. This can be done in the labour ward using a lithotomy position without specific anaesthesia. There is no particular indication to induce labour at the same time and the patient can be sent home shortly thereafter, reassured by a normal fetal heart tracing. In some cases there may be a surprising interval before labour occurs. This does not mean the suture was not necessary: it may mean that the suture has caused some fibrosis. It is not unknown for a caesarean section to become necessary for failure to progress in labour.

Shirodkar suture

The following is a modification of Shirodkar's original description, in that Mersilene tape is used rather than fascia lata.

The same preparations of shaving and antisepsis are made as for a McDonald cerclage. The cervix is visualized and cleaned with antiseptic. The cervix is grasped with sponge holding forceps anteriorly and posteriorly, rather than with vulsella. Adrenaline (epinephrine) is diluted in 20 mL of saline to achieve a dilution of 1:200 000. Lidocaine (lignocaine) with adrenaline (epinephrine) can also be used. This is infiltrated with a green needle in the anterior and posterior vaginal fornices. The purpose of this infiltration is to open tissue planes and to promote haemostasis. A 2-cm transverse incision is made in the anterior vaginal fornix, at the point where the vagina meets the cervix. (Fig. 5.3a). This is best made with cutting diathermy, although it can also be made with a pointed blade. The stroke should be bold, so that the incision is several millimetres deep, to allow reflection of the forniceal skin. It should be at least 2 cm long, extending to the lateral border of the cervix and the paracervical tissues. A pledget (peanut swab) is mounted on a vulsellum and the incision is further opened by reflection of the vaginal skin with the mounted pledget. An ellipse is opened that is at least 1 cm in its shorter length, which is vertical to the horizontal incision already made (Fig. 5.3b). Attention is now

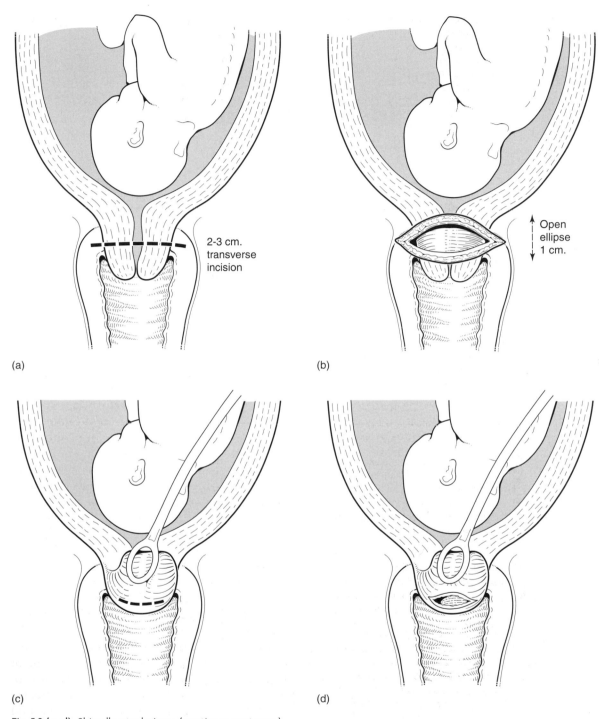

(a)

2-3 cm. transverse incision

(b)

Open ellipse 1 cm.

(c)

(d)

Fig. 5.3 (a–d) Shirodkar technique. (*continues next page*)

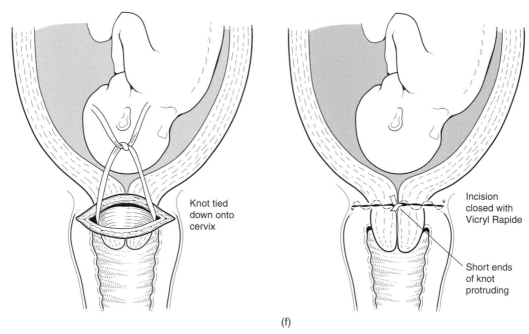

(e)

(f)

Knot tied
down onto
cervix

Incision
closed with
Vicryl Rapide

Short ends
of knot
protruding

Fig. 5.3(e–f) Shirodkar technique.

turned to the posterior fornix with the cervix being lifted forwards. Although Shirodkar originally described a vertical incision in the posterior fornix, a horizontal incision of 1–2 cm is more appropriate (Fig. 5.3c). This is then opened with the mounted pledget as an ellipse to a vertical diameter of about 1 cm (Fig. 5.3d). The finger and thumb are then inserted to pinch the paracervical tissue antero-posteriorly at the paracervical area just right lateral to the cervix. This determines the direction of approach for the needle with the Mersilene tape. The Mersilene tape has a needle on both ends, which are not necessary but both of which should be kept until the suture is safely in place. The needle is then passed antero-posteriorly through the paracervical broad ligament. As the needle tip appears posteriorly, the needle tip is picked up with a Spencer Wells forceps and guided safely through, while the needle holder is removed from its original position on the needle and then replaced on the needle replacing the Spencer Wells forceps. The procedure in the reverse direction is then used on the left lateral paracervical area and the same needle is passed postero-anteriorly. Greater than expected resistance is met when the needle actually goes through the cervix itself, or if there

is scarring from previous surgery. The needle may become detached in these circumstances and the other needle may then be useful. The two ends of the tape are then crossed in front of the cervix and tied in the midline (Fig. 5.3e). During the tightening and tying of the knot, the patient should be placed in a maximal head-down position and the cervix massaged to encourage any funnelling of the membranes to retreat. The stitch should then be flush with the cervix anteriorly and posteriorly. The ends should be cut to a length of less than 1 cm. The cut ends of the stitch are then held in a Spencer Wells forceps in the midline. Continuous 2/0 Vicryl® is then used to close the anterior incision with the end of the Mersilene protruding in the midline (Fig. 5.3f). Ideally, the cervix should then be drawn forwards and the posterior incision closed in the same way. If there is no bleeding and/or the operation is already prolonged, then this step can be omitted. The patient should be warned to expect some dark discharge until 6 weeks after the operation and this may include pieces of Vicryl® being discharged. It is almost impossible for the Mersilene to be extruded. The patient should be reassured of this and shown a piece of Mersilene for her own information.

66

A decision is made regarding mode of delivery at the end of the pregnancy. If an attempt at vaginal delivery is considered appropriate, then the suture should be removed at 37–38 weeks' gestation. This should be done as a day case in the labour ward. It will require preferably spinal or general anaesthesia and should be done by a doctor who is familiar with the placement of these sutures. The ends of the Mersilene are located and grasped with a Spencer Wells forceps. The ends are drawn down to expose part of the loop of the stitch which is then cut, released and removed. The patient may return home a short time later, reassured by a normal fetal heart recording.

If labour does not ensue in a few days, it is not because the stitch was unnecessary. The stitch itself can cause some fibrosis. In some cases, to the surprise of the patient, the onset and the progress of labour is delayed, with a caesarean delivery becoming necessary. Women often feel very uncomfortable in the later weeks while the stitch remains in place. There is sometimes a great release of discomfort when it is removed.

If there is an independent indication for caesarean section, then the suture can be left in place for a subsequent pregnancy. Supervision should be continued between pregnancies because of the risk of infection. Intermenstrual bleeding and postcoital bleeding may occur. There have been several successful pregnancies after leaving the suture in place. In other cases, symptoms have necessitated suture removal with possible re-insertion in a later pregnancy.

Modified Shirodkar technique

The use of this has been prompted by the need to place the knot posteriorly and to bury it. The idea arose because of experience with the trans-abdominal suture (see below), where the knot is tied posteriorly in the pouch of Douglas. This can be considered if there have been prominent bladder symptoms attributed to an anterior knot: this is very uncommon. It can also be considered if infection has been prominent with a previous vaginal cerclage. The technique is similar to the Shirodkar technique but the pouch of Douglas is opened and the knot placed posteriorly in the

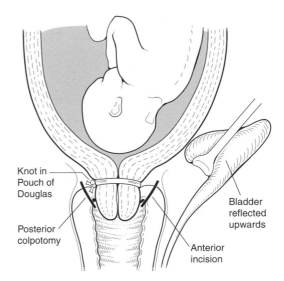

Knot in Pouch of Douglas

Posterior colpotomy

Bladder reflected upwards

Anterior incision

Fig. 5.4 Modified Shirodkar technique.

pouch (Fig. 5.4). The pouch of Douglas is then closed. This suture is very difficult to remove and these cases are considered for caesarean section for delivery. These patients also carry explanatory warning notes with them in case they require emergency treatment.

Choice of vaginal technique

As so often is the case in medicine, treatment is decided based on the previous experience of the doctor. In the UK, McDonald cerclage is performed more commonly than Shirodkar cerclage. This may not matter because both may have similar high success rates in 'usual' cases. The MRC/RCOG study suggested that many procedures were unnecessary, and successful, probably reflecting a previous lack of critical analysis of so-called cervical incompetence. The data in this study suggested very heterogeneous entry criteria, manifesting as uncertainty of the specialist. There has never been a randomized study comparing the two techniques. Harger[46] retrospectively reviewed 251 cervical cerclage procedures and found similar success rates with the two techniques. There was an eightfold improvement in pregnancy outcome when these procedures were performed in women with two or more second trimester losses. The MRC/RCOG data suggested a similar effect.

McDonald cerclage therefore is usually effective. However, it may be that a McDonald cerclage fails in a subgroup where there is clearer evidence of cervical weakness. There is a rationale for performing a McDonald cerclage as a first procedure as a routine and then undertaking a Shirodkar cerclage in the next pregnancy, if that pregnancy fails. The disadvantage of this approach is obvious in older patients who may have difficulty in conceiving. There is also the problem that during miscarriage with a McDonald suture in place the cervix may become badly torn, compromising a future pregnancy. Cases should therefore be selected for Shirodkar cerclage as the first procedure, particularly in 'unusual cases'.

Emergency cervical cerclage

Some patients present with a history of lower abdominal discomfort and pink vaginal discharge. On speculum examination the membranes are found to be bulging through the cervix. It may be difficult to know how dilated the cervix is, and in some cases there is a herniation with only a slight degree of cervical dilatation. This may be an acute problem or one of more long standing. If it is acute and associated with pain, then there may be an underlying precipitating factor. Closing the cervix may not be useful in promoting continuation of the pregnancy. It is worth waiting for 24 hours, with the patient resting, to see if an acute problem declares itself further. In some cases contractions, vaginal bleeding and inevitable miscarriage supervene. If this does not occur, then emergency cerclage is considered.

A McDonald technique is generally used in cases of emergency cervical cerclage, in order to shorten the operating time. Some recommend decompression by ultrasound-guided amnio-drainage, with the patient in a steep Trendelenberg position to facilitate suture placement.[47] This can also serve the purpose of providing a sample for microbiological analysis. If the result is positive and further symptoms develop, then the suture can be removed expeditiously. When a cervix is more than 3 cm dilated and fully effaced, then emergency cervical cerclage is unlikely to con-

tribute to an improved outcome. Care should be exercised in not converting a miscarriage into a very premature delivery with a child that may become handicapped. Orr[48] reported a technique of using a Foley catheter balloon with the tip cut off as a counter pressure to the bulging bag of membranes. This is pushed into the lower uterus and a McDonald stitch placed round the cervix (Fig. 5.5a, b). The stitch is tied as the catheter is removed. Fetal survival rates of 89% have been reported when antibiotics and tocolytics were used with emergency cervical cerclage.[49] The prognosis is influenced by cervical dilation and gestational age.[50]

Transabdominal cervical cerclage

In some cases a transvaginal technique may not be possible, because of an anatomically deficient cervix, and a transabdominal approach is necessary. The original description of this technique was by Benson and Durfee in 1965.[51] Subsequent modifications have been made in patient selection criteria, surgical technique, timing of the operation and subsequent management.[52–58] The deficient cervix may be due to previous conization or other gynaecological surgery. There are now several women who have had conservative treatment, such as trachelectomy, for cervical cancer. It has been argued that previous failed vaginal cerclage is an indication for transabdominal cerclage. This may be true if the previous suture was a well-placed Shirodkar suture. If it was a McDonald, then it will be worth considering a Shirodkar suture before resorting to the more invasive transabdominal approach.

Most reports in the literature are of transabdominal cerclage performed in the pregnant state. The hazards of operating at this time include provoking a miscarriage and encountering serious bleeding from the tissues affected by pregnancy. However, the enlarging uterus and the effect of pregnancy homones on the tissues clarifies the anatomy for placement of the suture at the cervico-isthmic junction (Fig. 5.6a). The tissues are more pliable and the paracervical window is more easily opened for placement of the suture (Fig. 5.6b). The high success rates of the procedure have been satisfying; however,

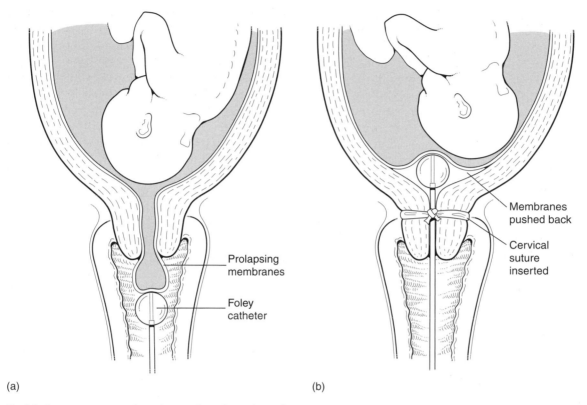

(a)   (b)

Fig. 5.5 Emergency cervical cerclage with prolapsed membranes.

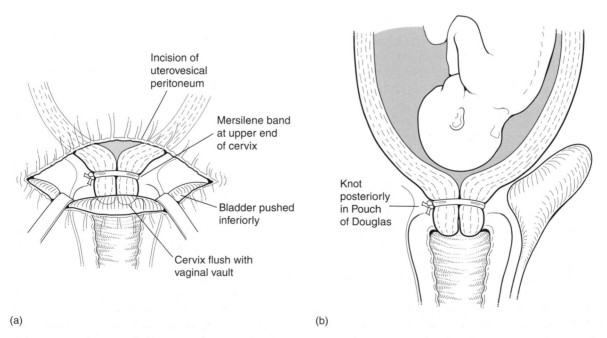

(a)   (b)

Fig. 5.6 Transabdominal cerclage: (a) antero-posterior view; (b) lateral view.

more experience is now being gained in the procedure performed outside of pregnancy as an interval procedure.

An insertion during pregnancy is performed between 11 and 13 weeks. This avoids the time of early miscarriage and also permits an early scan for major fetal abnormality, including Down syndrome assessment, to be done before the operation. Surgery at later than 12 weeks is more problematic because access to the lower part of the uterus is more difficult. General anaesthesia is necessary because the significant intra-abdominal manipulation renders regional block inadequate. A Foley catheter is placed in the urinary bladder at the start of the operation. As well as draining the bladder, this is useful as a marker. A transverse suprapubic incision is usually adequate, although access can be difficult in the scarred or overweight patient. This may necessitate a vertical incision. The peritoneal cavity is opened and the intestine packed superiorly, with the patient in a Trendelenburg position. The pelvic organs are inspected and palpated. The uterovesical fold of peritoneum is exposed and divided. The bladder and paravesical tissue is reflected to expose the supravaginal cervix. The uterine vessels are displaced laterally, opening the paracervical connective tissue window. The lower portion of the isthmus at the level of the internal os is palpated between thumb and index finger, with the uterus in the palm of the hand. Three anatomical features are identified to locate the site of suture insertion: the widening of the cervix into the soft isthmus, the uterine vessel passing longitudinally and the point of insertion of the uterosacral ligaments into the uterus. The needle is passed anteroposteriorly through the paracervical tissues immediately adjacent to the cervix, superior to the insertion of the uterosacral ligaments, taking care to avoid the uterine vessels. This is done on both sides. An alternative approach is to make fenestrations in the paracervical area with an instrument. The tape is then passed through the fenestration on an instrument obviating the risk of using a needle and having to locate it, often with a finger, as it passes through. The band of suture material is adjusted to ensure that it lies flush on the anterior aspect of the cervico-isthmic region before being tied with a knot posteriorly. The suture therefore lies in an extraperitoneal position anteriorly and intraperitoneally posteriorly. The free ends of the suture are cut to 2 cm, secured with some non-absorbable suture and placed in the pouch of Douglas, to aid access by posterior colpotomy if this becomes necessary. Closure is routine and the vulva is checked for blood loss at the end of the procedure. Postoperative pain relief is standard but there is no specific use of tocolytic or antibiotic therapy. Patients remain in hospital for 5 days and have a scan for fetal viability before discharge.

Care is continued in a high-risk clinic. Transvaginal scans are unnecessary in the absence of symptoms. If there is a high level of anxiety at the gestation of previous pregnancy losses, then admission to hospital may be beneficial. Steroid therapy may be considered if the pregnancy is unstable. Most cases are able to reach 37/38 weeks' gestation before elective caesarean section. At caesarean section the suture is visualized and left in place until the patient has considered her reproductive future. The suture can be used for consecutive pregnancies. Alternatively, if she has completed her family the suture is removed at caesarean section.

Removal of transbdominal suture and vaginal delivery has not been reported. It might be technically difficult, and the patients are at such high risk that they request caesarean section. They have been counselled about the necessity some time previously.

Complications of transabdominal cerclage

Surgical haemorrhage is a matter of concern. Careful selection and assessment are important. Obese women should be seen pre-pregnancy and encouraged to lose weight. Those with previous abdominal surgery should be assessed, if necessary with pre-pregnancy laparoscopy, to evaluate adhesions and feasibility. The main area of difficulty can be the paracervical tissue: there can be venous bleeding. This is most often resolved by oversewing. Only rarely is blood transfusion necessary. None the less patients are consented for hysterectomy to be used as a life-saving procedure. This has never been necessary.

The uterus may become unstable if the operation is prolonged, as it might be with a fibroid, difficult uterus. In this case extensive manipulation may be necessary. When the vulva is inspected at the end of the operation, there may be significant bleeding, and miscarriage occurs through the stitch. The fetus may extrude and the placenta can be aspirated through a Karmann cannula. The suture may be kept in place for a future pregnancy.

Membrane rupture soon after the operation can be dealt with as above. Membrane rupture a few days after the operation may mean that the fetus is too big to extrude through the suture. This is also the case if there is an intrauterine death for other reasons in mid-pregnancy. In these cases, it is necessary to remove the stitch and deliver vaginally or to perform a hysterotomy. There is a difficult choice in this matter. If the patient is keen to retain the suture for a future pregnancy, then a hysterotomy can be performed with the resultant hazard of a scar on the uterus. Alternatively, a decision can be made to perform a posterior colpotomy under general anaesthesia, with removal of the suture and subsequent vaginal miscarriage. The possibility would remain of re-insertion in a future pregnancy. This has been done on two occasions.

As mentioned above, a transabdominal suture is left after caesarean delivery and potentially used for subsequent pregnancies. An early miscarriage does not present a problem in a subsequent pregnancy. A pre-11-week pregnancy can miscarry, and an evacuation of retained products can be performed, through a stitch.

Transabdominal sutures remaining in place during a non-pregnant interval do not generally cause symptoms.

Adjuncts to management

There is no role for tocolysis in early gestation cervical cerclage. In later gestations, beyond 18 weeks, particularly if performed as an emergency procedure, then a tocolytic in a carefully controlled dose may be useful. The uterus seems to be resilient to handling as long as there has not been previous instability, manifest as vaginal bleeding. The differential diagnosis of mid-trimester preg-

nancy loss includes genital tract infection: as a consequence, adjunctive antibiotics are used, particularly when a vaginal approach for cerclage is used. Erythromycin is the antibiotic of choice, with the possible addition of metronidazole. There are no data available on the role of local vaginal antibiotics such as clindamycin. In high-risk cases, a course of erythromycin and Canesten® can be given perioperatively and again at 20 weeks' gestation. A single course of metronidazole can be given at 24 weeks' gestation.

Reduction of physical activity may be of value in an acute situation or when a patient's lifestyle may involve particular physical or psychological stresses. This should not extend to prolonged bed rest, which is of no value and can be associated with physical and psychological complications. Once a suture is in place, the patient often comments that the 'baby feels higher up' and they feel more secure. They are often surprised at the normalization of their activities compared to a previous pregnancy. Penetrative sexual intercourse is generally discouraged, particularly at the time of greatest risk to the pregnancy. While there is no strong evidence for this, it seems sensible, both to the couple and their obstetrician. The theoretical risk would be disturbance of the cervix and lower uterus with prostaglandin release both from mechanical effects and from semen. There might also be the disturbance of the vaginal flora and possibility of infection.

The support of, and access to, a nurse/ midwife/counsellor is important during the ongoing pregnancy.

Interval cerclage

Several operations have now been undertaken in non-pregnant women. This may be their choice or for convenience. It may also be because they have had a mixture of early and late miscarriage and are particularly anxious about the risk of perioperative miscarriage. There are a small group of women who have had radical trachelectomy with insertion of a nylon suture at the time, which has later extruded. A transabdominal suture is then required to strengthen the cervix. During this laparotomy the pelvic-abdominal lymph nodes can be assessed.

Mersilene tape RS22 has been used in these cases. The patient is placed in a semi-lithotomy (Lloyd-Davies) position. The anatomy is more difficult to define, as there is effectively no cervix present and distortion of the tissues with fibrosis: this is particularly true in the previous trachelectomy cases. A Spackman cannula or a dilator is placed in the cervix. An assistant manipulates the lower uterus from below. In the few cases where this has been done, there appears to be some delay in conception. It is not clear whether this due to the original condition or an effect of the stitch. Laparoscopy, performed 18 months later on one case, showed a free pelvis and the suture in the correct position. Peritonealization of the knot of the stitch was clearly seen. Pregnancy is now proceeding at 32 weeks gestation.

Laparoscopic cerclage

Developments in minimal-access surgery have opened the way for laparoscopic insertion of a cervical suture. Reports of this have been confined to the non-pregnant state.[59,60] This is obviously less invasive and requires less time in hospital. Other advantages remain to be proven. Although theoretically possible, the insertion of a cervical suture laparoscopically in pregnancy would be difficult. Access would be difficult, and the possibility of manipulation using an instrument in the cervix would be denied. Any effect of a transbdominal suture on fertility, whether done laparoscopically or by an open method, remains to be quantified.

Transabdominal suture removal

A final question is, when should a transabdominal suture be removed? The late development of a recto-uterine fistula along the track of a long-standing suture is a real possibility. Foreign material should not remain in the human body in the long term without a specific purpose. Such sutures should therefore be removed when the woman has concluded her reproduction, and certainly when she approaches her menopause. This can be done by one of two routes, both of which require day-case general anaesthesia.

The suture can be removed laparoscopically[61] or by posterior colpotomy.[58]

Caesarean section

Caesarean section was performed in ancient times but no woman survived caesarean section until the 19th century. Fascinating accounts of the history are available.[62,63] The origin of the term lies in Latin and ancient Rome; however, it was not the mode of delivery of Julius Caesar, whose mother was alive at the time the Romans invaded Britain. During the past century there has been a rapid rise in caesarean section rates, which continues and amounts to an epidemic in most countries. In industrialized countries, about one in four births is by caesarean section. This rise can be attributed partly to its ease and relative safety. None the less complications do occur, and medical staff must take steps to minimize the risk.

Preoperative measures

The main risks, which must be discussed in the consent process, are surgical (organ damage and bleeding), anaesthetic, thrombotic and infective. Preventive steps are outlined and written consent should be obtained. The risk of blood transfusion is low in an uncomplicated caesarean section. Blood group and save serum is an adequate precaution, unless specific bleeding risks such as placenta praevia are identified when an ultrasound should be performed shortly before the operation, so that the operator knows the intrauterine anatomy with as much precision as possible. There is a clear association between previous caesarean section and placenta praevia.[64] In a case of anterior placenta praevia and previous caesarean section, the significant risk of placenta accreta must be recognized.[65] Possible caesarean hysterectomy should be mentioned in the consent process. Beware of the Internet! Many patients will have accessed the Internet and done their own research. The risk of fetal damage should not be forgotten, although not mentioned in the consent process. Don't cut the baby!

Organ damage and haemorrhage can be minimized by the good surgical technique of experienced operators. Recognition of the specific risks of anatomical distortion due to previous surgery, the natural dextrorotation of the uterus, and the rotation of the uterus due to tilt of the table. There is no good evidence that tilt of the table is useful.[66,67] Measured pace rather than excessive speed is appropriate. Regional anaesthesia is safest. It is also most appropriate, as mothers, in general, like to be awake when their baby is born and it encourages early mobilization in the interest of minimizing the risk of venous thrombosis. The specific precautions of using intermittently inflating pneumatic boots perioperatively and elastic stockings postoperatively are now standard. In higher-risk cases, subcutaneous heparin should be used, according to the guidelines issued by the Royal College of Obstetricians and Gynaecologists.[68] The risk of infection has been reduced by the use of prophylactic antibiotics during caesarean delivery.[69] This is probably more important during emergency surgery than elective. During a prolonged labour, especially with prolonged membrane rupture, care should be taken to perform pelvic examination with sterile precautions. The standard dose of antibiotics is one dose of Augmentin® (co-amoxiclav) 1.2 g, or a cephalosporin, just after placental delivery. This can conveniently be given with the prophylactic Syntocinon® 10 units to reduce the risk of haemorrhage. Although most units have a standard protocol for this treatment, the surgeon should always verify with the anaesthetist that it has been given. The use of such antibiotics reduces the risk of postpartum endometritis and wound infection. If there has been prolonged membrane rupture or fever during labour, then a full course of 5 days of antibiotics is appropriate.

It is now considered appropriate to use double-glove technique at caesarean section. It is seen as a high-risk operation for needlestick injury and double gloving affords a degree of protection. Gloves half a size apart should be used, with the larger pair put on first. Sharp needles are most effective but carry the greatest risk of needlestick injury. However, blunt needles can traumatize the tissues, of the uterus in particular, leading to more difficult haemostasis. Needleholders, dissecting forceps, thimbles and instruments functioning as needle guides may be used. Safety should not be sacrificed for speed. Absorbable braided material is used for all layers at caesarean section.

An indwelling urinary Foley catheter is placed, in the operating theatre after the anaesthesia has taken effect. This is important postoperatively to keep the bladder empty while the epidural continues to function. It is also sometimes useful to locate the bladder with the balloon in situ during the operation. Skin preparation should be non-toxic, fast acting, easy to apply and have broad-spectrum antibacterial activity. Povidone iodine or chlorhexidine gluconate is usually used.

Recommended operative technique

Historically, caesarean section was performed through a longitudinal (vertical) skin incision. This was because originally the uterine incision was in this direction. Rarely, a longitudinal incision is used when upper abdominal exploration is required, in cases of massive haemorrhage and at perimortem caesarean section. In cases requiring speed, most operators are as comfortable with a transverse incision. The transverse incision can be that of Pfannenstiel or Joel Cohen (Fig. 5.7). The Pfannenstiel incision was introduced in 1900, providing a low incidence of wound infection, breakdown and hernia formation. It also provides a better cosmetic result than the longitudinal incision. Joel Cohen introduced a transverse incision, for gynaecological surgery, with the deeper layers opened by stretching with the fingers in 1954.[70]

There are various modifications of the incisions. A low vertical incision in the uterus (De Lee) can be done through a transverse skin incision. This may be useful in a premature breech caesarean section.

Repeat caesarean sections, which are increasingly frequent, require more of a sharp dissection technique, possibly including excision of a previous scar. The rectus sheath will usually require dissection off the rectus muscle in these cases. If a previous caesarean section has been

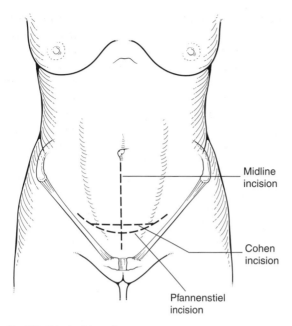

Midline
incision

Cohen
incision

Pfannenstiel
incision

Fig. 5.7 Skin incisions for caesarean section.

done through a longitudinal skin incision, as is still done in some countries, then a discussion should take place about whether to re-open the previous scar or make a new transverse scar. If the old scar has keloid formation which might be improved, then re-entry through it is reasonable. In other circumstances a new transverse incision should be made. There is sometimes confusion during antenatal assessment about the scar in the skin and the scar in the uterus. A longitudinal incision in the skin does not mean there is a vertical incision in the uterus. In many African countries and in Japan transverse lower segment caesarean section is still done though a longitudinal, subumbilical skin incision. This may be because some caesarean sections are done by those with less experience and training and even by general surgeons! If a true classical caesarean section has been done in a term pregnancy, then there will have been a high longitudinal incision in the skin. It may have been paramedian to access above the umbilicus.

The incision for caesarean section today, usually transverse, should be big enough to allow the exit of the baby's head: about 15 cm.

The incision, by Joel Cohen method, should not be too high or too low. It should be about 1 cm below the pubic hair line. If it is too low, then there may be tissue distortion with healing near the symphysis pubis. It should not be curved more than slightly. Care is taken to position the incision, bearing in mind the tilt of the table, making it symmetrical to the linea nigra. The abdominal wall skin should be pushed down from above to see the natural skin folds. This is where the incision is placed. The exception to this is the obese patient, where the disappearance of the scar into a damp skin fold will not aid healing. In this case the incision may be placed at a point in the skin where it will be more exposed for healing. There are few significant vessels just below the skin, but they should be secured carefully with diathermy. It is important not to use diathermy just at the skin edge. This may result in a small skin burn which takes time to heal and is unsightly. The incision is continued in the middle of the incision to the deep tissues, where the rectus sheath is incised for about 3 cm. The subcutaneous tissue and rectus sheath are opened by stretching with the fingers. The muscles are not separated from the sheath. The peritoneum is picked up superiorly with an instrument and pinched with the thumb and finger to ensure that there is no bowel adherent. It is then incised and the fingers inserted to open by traction in a transverse direction. The operator and assistant must make a very firm pull at this point.

The operator must then make an assessment of the position of the uterus, which will probably be dextrorotated. Some correction of this can be made. A Doyen retractor, of which more than one size should be available, is then inserted to allow full exposure of the lower part of the uterus. The uterovesical peritoneum is then incised and opened transversely. This is best done with a blade of the scissors, but not using the scissors to cut. The lower edge of the peritoneal incision and the attached bladder is then pushed inferiorly with a swab on a holder. The uterus itself is exposed at this point. The couple are then informed that the baby is about to be born. The incision should not be made too low. This is a risk after a long labour with a very stretched lower segment. The cervix has been drawn up and the incision may be in the anterior vaginal fornix. This leads to surgical difficulties during the closure. There can be confusion by the in-experienced between the edge of the incision and the curtain-like edge of the dilated cervix, with suturing of the wrong tissues. An incision is then made curving with the ends superiorly in the lower segment. This incises only super-ficially into the thickness of the uterus. It is then deepened carefully in the midline over 1–2 cm. Using the belly of the knife rather than the point, and a swab in the other hand, the incision is con-tinued until the decidua appears and the mem-branes bulge (Fig. 5.8a). These are carefully perforated and the fingers are then used to bluntly extend the incision laterally (Fig. 5.8b). Intra-operative haemorrhage is reduced by this blunt expansion of the uterine incision.[71] This is the technique that avoids the cardinal sin of cutting the baby. Particular care is required when the membranes have already ruptured or there is oligohydramnios for other reasons. It can also be difficult when there is a thick, fleshy lower segment which bleeds profusely during the inci-sion. Patience is important. The head should appear in the incision with fundal pressure and the use of a hand to cup the posterior aspect of the head. It is not necessary to pull vigorously on the head especially after the shoulders have traversed

the incision. Fundal pressure suffices for the baby to emerge gradually as the anaesthetist gives intra-venous Syntocinon®. The baby may benefit from the pressure on the chest and it also seems more like a natural delivery. Some women appreciate the concept of natural birth by caesarean!

The direction of incision in the uterus should not be decided until the abdomen is open and the uterus has been visualized (Fig. 5.9). If there is a premature breech baby and there is a narrow lower segment, then a low vertical (De Lee) incision in the uterus may be appropriate. Multiple fibroids or adhesions from previous surgery may dictate a less usual incision in the uterus. Fibroids may lead to rotation of the uterus,[72] which once resulted in an inadvertent posterior lower segment caesarean section. The patient in question proceeded to a myomectomy and vaginal birth in a subsequent pregnancy!

There may be difficulties in delivering the baby. When there is an abnormal lie the foot should be identified and the baby delivered as a breech extraction. The same principles are applied as at vaginal breech delivery, although the use of the Mauriceau–Smellie–Veit manoeuvre is most appropriate for the delivery of the head, rather than forceps. With a cephalic presentation, the head may be so low or so high that delivery is difficult.

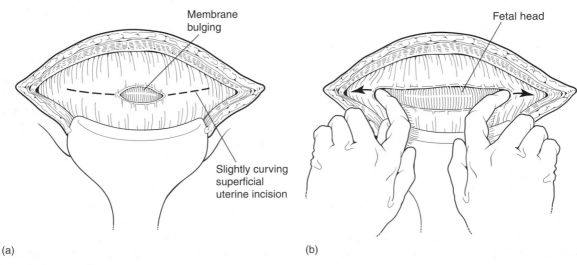

Membrane bulging

Slightly curving superficial uterine incision

Fetal head

(a)

(b)

Fig. 5.8 Opening the uterus.

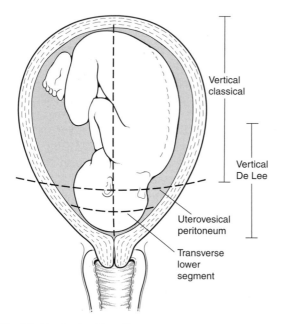

Vertical
classical

Vertical
De Lee

Uterovesical
peritoneum

Transverse
lower
segment

Fig. 5.9 Uterine incisions for caesarean section.

The head may sometimes be difficult to deliver at caesarean section. It may be too low or too high. After a long, augmented labour and possibly an attempted instrumental delivery, the head may be low in the pelvis. This should be recognized at the beginning of the operation. The head should be pushed up from below at the beginning and an assistant should apply pressure from below during the operation if there is difficulty reaching the head. The abdominal hand should be passed in front of the head and used like a shoe horn. On occasion the hands of the operator and assistant may meet. During such a manoeuvre the lower segment may be torn vertically and a careful inspection should be made for damage. If the head is high and does not descend with fundal pressure then forceps or a small vacuum device such as a Kiwi cup can be applied. If the head is difficult to reach, then a leg can be grasped and an internal version and breech extraction performed. The incision should be extended as necessary.

The placenta and membranes may be expelled spontaneously after the anaesthetist has given the Syntocinon®. This can be aided by fundal compression and controlled cord traction but it will rarely be necessary to place a hand in

the uterus to deliver the placenta. It has been suggested that this leads to greater blood loss and increases the risk of infection.[73] It is, however, wise to check the cavity before closure, to ensure there is no extra part of the placenta remaining.

The uterus should not be exteriorized unless surgical difficulties are encountered. Exteriorization is likely to be painful. It will be necessary if there is lateral extension of the uterine incision. One hand can then be placed behind the uterus to facilitate visualization of the bleeding area. A Doyen retractor is usually not necessary to facilitate closure of the uterus: it may cause bruising if not carefully handled. The uterus is normally closed in two layers, although there has recently been a tendency to consider one layer closure. This is to be part of the subject of a study by the National Perinatal Epidemiology Unit, in Oxford, called the CAESARean trial.

Individualization of care seems to be important. If there is a thick, fleshy lower segment, then two-layer closure seems appropriate. The first layer is done with a locking continuous stitch for haemostasis. The ends of the suture material are held with a Spencer Wells forceps until the second layer is placed and the angles are inspected for haemostasis. The second layer does not require to be closed with a locking stitch. The secured angles are used for traction to verify haemostasis. Additional haemostatic sutures are applied as necessary. Diathermy should be used with caution near suture material. A large pack can be applied with pressure for haemostasis before inspection of the ovaries and tubes and final closure.

A classical incision needs to be closed in three layers (Fig. 5.10). Traditionally several 'all-layer' interrupted sutures are placed but not tied. The deep and middle layers are then closed with a locking, continuous suture. The superficial layer is closed with a continuous suture. The 'all-layer' interrupted sutures are then closed.

If sterilization is performed at caesarean section, it should be by the Pomeroy method, with excision of segments of each tube, which are then sent for histology. Absorbable suture material such as Vicryl rapide® should be used.

It is unnecessary to close the peritoneum. This is also being considered by the CAEARean trial. Care is taken to identify and locate the lateral

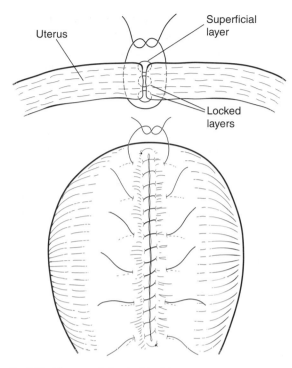

Fig. 5.10 Closure of classical incision.

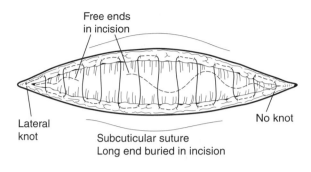

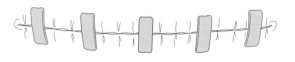

Supporting 0.5" steri-strips

Fig. 5.11 Closure of skin at caesarean section.

ends of the opened rectus sheath by the application of a tissue forceps. The rectus sheath is closed with size 1 Vicryl® absorbable suture material. A drain to the rectus sheath is generally unnecessary, although this is also being considered by the CAESARean trial. Individualization of care is important, but it should be stressed that effective haemostasis is better than drainage. Closure of the fat layer will not contribute to the tensile strength of the incision, but will approximate the skin for closure under less tension. The skin should be closed with a subcuticular closure such as 2/0 Monocryl®. A knot can be tied and buried at one end, with the other end being brought back through half of the incision and not tied (Fig. 5.11). A few Steri-strips® vertically, or one horizontally, suffice to finalize closure. A hand should support the incision while removing the drapes and washing is done. It is prudent to swab the vagina to release any clot and to check that some lochia is draining. Rarely, there may be no lochia draining because of incorrect apposition of the uterine incision to the cervix or back wall of the

uterus. Timely recognition of this is important. Further surgery is necessary.

Caesarean section for placenta praevia presents a special challenge. The operator should have seen a preoperative ultrasound scan to map the intrauterine anatomy. The baby should be approached around the edge of the placenta, with the operator's hand drawing the main body of the placenta to one side to locate the membranes adjacent to it and the most direct approach to the baby. It should not be necessary to incise the placenta. An anterior placenta praevia may be accreta when associated with previous caesarean section. It may be difficult to remove all of this placenta without provoking serious bleeding. Haemostasis is secured by undersewing vessels or by techniques discussed in the next chapter. Consent should have been taken for possible hysterectomy.

Caesarean section with a fibroid uterus may involve an unorthodox incision to access the uterine cavity and deliver the baby. Myomectomy should not be undertaken unless the traumatized base of a fibroid is bleeding, or unless there is a clearly pedunculated fibroid that has been causing symptoms and can be removed with ease.

Caesarean section for twins requires care with the asymmetry of the very distended abdomen. The technique is routine. The first twin, lower in the uterus, is delivered first. After clamping and cutting the cord, the membranes of the second sac are normally visualized and ruptured. The next baby is then delivered according to the presenting part, with a likelihood of breech extraction by identifying and exerting traction on a foot. A hand should be rapidly returned to the uterus! Triplets and higher-order babies are delivered in succession.

Caesarean section for premature babies and breech presentation requires an appropriate incision for access and atraumatic delivery.

Caesarean section on the obese woman requires particular care to be taken in thromboprophylaxis. It also requires extra assistance to hold the abdominal wall, and sometimes a larger operating table! Access may be difficult and the availability of the most experienced surgeon is important.

There is a clear place for a Syntocinon® infusion to maintain contraction of the uterus after delivery in certain situations. This would be when the uterus has been overstretched with a large baby, multiple pregnancy or polyhydramnios. It is also necessary when the uterus has been contracting poorly in labour. This occurs in prolonged labour with induction or augmentation of labour. At least 50 units of Syntocinon® in 1 litre of fluid are used over 4 h.

The normal postoperative course

The woman will be relatively immobile, requiring pain relief for 24 h. The epidural can be used to administer this or, alternatively, strong opiate analgesia is necessary. During this time the urinary catheter and intravenous infusion remain in place. Under normal circumstances oral fluids can be taken after 4 h and light diet after 10 h. Movement of the legs should be encouraged with mobilization after 24 h. The wound can be washed in a shower or a bath, with the Steri-strips® left in place for 7 days. They can then be soaked and removed in the bath. Haemoglobin can be checked on the third day if blood loss has been considered to be significant. Dietary supplements usually suffice to correct this, but blood transfusion should be considered if the haemoglobin in under 8.5 g/dL.

Follow-up should be arranged 6 weeks later for debriefing, discussion and general advice about reproductive health and future childbearing.

Conclusion

The pregnant woman requires special attention when challenged by surgery. Haemorrhage and infection are the main threats to her continuing wellbeing. Careful, meticulous technique observing basic principles should achieve the results that our patients deserve.

REFERENCES

1. Bonney V 1974 General operative considerations. In: Howkins J, Stallworthy J (eds) Bonney's gynaecological surgery, 8th edn. Balliere Tindall, London, pp 1–5
2. Brown R P 1992 Knotting techniques and suture materials. British Journal of Surgery 79:399–400
3. van Rijssel E J C, Brand R, Admiraal C et al 1989 Tissue reaction and surgical knots: the effect of suture size, knot configuration and knot volume. Obstetrics and Gynaecology 74:64–68
4. van Rijssell E J C, Trimbos B, Booster M H 1990 Mechanical performance of square knots and sliding knots in surgery. A comparative study. American Journal of Obstetrics and Gynecology 162:93–97
5. Glazener C M A, Abdalla A, Stroud P et al 1995 Postnatal maternal morbidity: extent, causes, prevention and treatment. British Journal of Obstetrics and Gynaecology 102:286–287
6. Department of Health 1998 National Maternity Statistics, England 89–90 to 94–95. HMSO, London
7. Sleep J, Grant A, Garcia J et al 1984 West Berkshire Perineal Management Trial. British Medical Journal 289:587–690
8. McCandlish R, Bowler U, Van Asten H et al 1998 A randomised controlled trial of care of the perineum during second stage of normal labour. British Journal of Obstetrics and Gynaecology 105:1262–1272
9. Carroli G, Belizan J 2003 Episiotomy for vaginal birth (Cochrane Review). In: The Cochrane Library Issue 1. Update Software, Oxford
10. Labreque M, Eason E, Marcoux S et al 1999 Randomised controlled trial of the prevention of perineal trauma by perineal massage during pregnancy. American Journal of Obstetrics and Gynecology 180(3):593–600
11. Kettle C, Johanson R B 2003 Absorbable synthetic versus catgut suture material for perineal repair (Cochrane Review). In The Cochrane Library Issue 1. Update Software, Oxford

12. Lundquist M, Olsson A, Nissen E, Normal M 2000 Is it necessary to suture all lacerations after a vaginal delivery? Birth 27(2):79–85

13. Head M 1993 Dropping stitches. Do unsutured tears to the perineum heal better than sutured ones? Nursing Times 89(33):64–65

14. Clement S, Read B 1999 To stitch or not to stitch? Practising Midwife 2(4):20–28

15. Ethicon Training Pamphlet 1996 Perineal repair. Ethicon Limited, PO Box 408, Bankhead Avenue, Edinburgh EH11 4HE

16. Gordon B, Mackrodt C, Fern E et al 1998 The Ipswich Childbirth Study: 1. A randomized evaluation of two stage postpartum perineal repair leaving the skin unsutured. British Journal of Obstetrics and Gynaecology 105:435–440

17. Rogerson L, Mason G C, Roberts A C 2000 Preliminary experience with twenty perineal repairs using Indermil tissue adhesive. European Journal of Obstetrics and Gynaecology and Reproductive Biology 88.2:139–142

18. Sultan A H, Kamm M A, Bartram C I et al 1994 Perineal damage at delivery. Contemporary Reviews in Obstetrics and Gynaecology 6:18–24

19. Thacker S B, Banta H D 1983 Benefits and risks of episiotomy: an interpretative review of the English language literature, 1860–1980. Obstetrical and Gynecological Survey 38:322–338

20. Sultan A H, Kamm M A, Hudson C N et al 1993 Anal sphincter disruption during vaginal delivery. New England Journal of Medicine 329:1905–1911

21. Faltin D L, Boulvain M, Irion O et al 2000 Diagnosis of anal sphincter tears by post partum endosonography to predict fecal incontinence. Obstetrics and Gynecology 95:643–647

22. Donnelly V, Fynes M, Campbell D et al 1998 Obstetric events leading to anal sphincter damage. Obstetrics and Gynecology 92:955–961

23. Adams E J, Fernando R J 2001 Management of third and fourth degree perineal tears following vaginal delivery. Royal College of Obstetricians and Gynaecologists Guideline No.29. Guidelines and Audit Committee of RCOG, London

24. Sultan A H, Monga A K, Kumar D et al 1999 Primary repair of obstetric anal sphincter rupture using the overlap technique. British Journal of Obstetrics and Gynaecology 106:318–323

25. Fitzpatrick M, Behan M, O'Connell P R et al 2000 A randomised clinical trial comparing primary overlap with approximation repair of third degree tears. American Journal of Obstetrics and Gynecology 183:1220–1224

26. Palaniappan V, Gibb D 1999 Cervical cerclage. Fetal and Maternal Medicine Review 11:55–68

27. Baden W F, Baden E E 1960 Cervical incompetence: current therapy. American Journal of Obstetrics and Gynecology 79:545–551

28. Jones J M, Sweetnam P, Hibbard B M 1979 The outcome of pregnancy after cone biopsy of the cervix: a case control study. British Journal of Obstetrics and Gynaecology 86:913–916

29. Leiman G, Neville A H, Rubin A 1980 Pregnancy following conization of the cervix: complications related to the size of the cone. American Journal of Obstetrics and Gynecology 136:14–18

30. Luesley D M, Wade-Evans T, Nicolson H O et al 1985 Complications of cone biopsy related to the dimensions of the cone and the influence of prior colposcopic assessment. British Journal of Obstetrics and Gynaecology 92:158–164

31. Bigrigg A, Codling B W, Pearson P et al 1991 Pregnancy after surgical loop diathermy (Letter). Lancet 337:119

32. Haffenden D K, Bigrigg A, Codling B W 1991 Pregnancy following large loop excision of the transformation zone. British Journal of Obstetrics and Gynaecology 100:1059–1060

33. Ferenzy A, Choukroun D, Falcone T et al 1995 The effect of surgical loop electrosurgical excision on subsequent pregnancy outcome: North American experience. American Journal of Obstetrics and Gynecology 172:1246–1250

34. Hagen B, Skeildestad F E 1991 The outcome of pregnancy after laser conization of the cervix. British Journal of Obstetrics and Gynaecology 100:717–720

35. Lash A F, Lash S R 1950 Habitual abortion: the incompetent internal os of the cervix. American Journal of Obstetrics and Gynecology 59:68–76

36. Bergman P, Svenerrund A 1957 Traction test for demonstrating incompetency of the internal os of the cervix. International Journal of Fertility 2:163–170

37. Jeffcoate T N, Wilson J K 1956 Uterine causes of abortion and premature labour. New York State Journal of Medicine 56:680–690

38. Anthony G S, Calder A A, MacNaughton M 1982 Cervical resistance studies in patients with previous spontaneous mid trimester abortion. British Journal of Obstetrics and Gynaecology 89:1046–1049

39. Palmer R 1950 Physiology of the uterine isthmus and its parts in sterility and habitual abortion. Revue Française de Gynecologie et d'Obstetrique 45:218–220

40. McDonald I A 1957 Suture of the cervix for inevitable miscarriage. Journal of Obstetrics and Gynaecology of the British Empire 64:346–350

41. Shirodkar J N 1955 A new method of operation for habitual abortions in the second trimester of pregnancy. Antiseptic 52:290–300

42. Rush R W, Issacs S, McPherson K et al 1984 A randomised controlled trial of cervical cerclage in women at high risk of preterm delivery. British Journal of Obstetrics and Gynaecology 91:724–730

43. Lazar P, Guerguen S, Dreyfus J et al 1984 Multicentred controlled trial of cervical cerclage in women at moderate risk of preterm delivery. British Journal of Obstetrics and Gynaecology 91:731–735

44. MRC/RCOG Working Party on Cervical Cerclage 1993 Final Report of the Medical Research Council/ Royal College of Obstetricians and Gynaecolgists multicentre randomised controlled trial of cervical cerclage. British Journal of Obstetrics and Gynaecology 100:516–523

45. Shepherd J H, Mould T, Oram D H 2001 Radical trachelectomy in early stage carcinoma of the cervix: outcome as judged by recurrence and fertility rates. British Journal of Obstetrics and Gynaecology 108:882–885

46. Harger J H 1983 Comparison of success and morbidity in cervical cerclage procedures. Clinics in Perinatology 10:321–341

47. Goodlin R C 1979 Cervical incompetence, hourglass membranes and amniocentesis. Obstetrics and Gynecology 54:748–750

48. Orr C 1973 An aid to cervical cerclage. Australian and New Zealand Journal of Obstetrics and Gynecology 13:114–116

49. Novy M J, Haymond J, Nichols M 1990 Shirodkar cerclage in a multifactorial approach to the patient with advanced cervical changes. American Journal of Obstetrics and Gynecology 162:1412–1420

50. Aarts J M, Brons J T, Bruinse H W 1995 Emergency cerclage: a review. Obstetrical and Gynecological Survey 50:459–469

51. Benson R C, Durfee R B 1965 Transabdominal cervicouterine cerclage during pregnancy for the treatment of cervical incompetency. Obstetrics and Gynecology 25:145–155

52. Mahran M 1978 Transabdominal cerclage during pregnancy: a modified technique. Obstetrics and Gynecology 52:502–506

53. Novy M J 1982 Transabdominal cervico isthmic cerclage for the management of repetitive abortion and premature delivery. American Journal of Obstetrics and Gynecology 143:44–54

54. Olsen S, Tobiassen T 1982 Transabdominal isthmic cerclage for the treatment of the incompetent cervix. Acta Obstetrica et Gynecologic Scandinavica 61:473–475

55. Van Dongen P W J, Nijhius J G 1991 Transabdominal cerclage. European Journal of Obstetrics, Gynecology, and Reproductive Biology 41:97–104

56. Novy M J 1991 Transabdominal cervic isthmic cerclage: a reappraisal 25 years after its introduction. American Journal of Obstetrics and Gynecology 164:1635–1642

57. Heron M A, Parer J T 1988 Transabdominal cerclage for fetal wastage due to cervical incompetence. Obstetrics and Gynecology 71:865–868

58. Gibb D M F, Salaria D A 1995 Transabdominal cervicoisthmic cerclage in the management of recurrent second trimester miscarriage and preterm delivery. British Journal of Obstetrics and Gynecology 102:802–806

59. Scibetta J J, Sanko S R, Phipps W R 1998 Laparoscopic transabdominal cervicoisthmic cerclage. Fertility and Sterility 69:161–163

60. Lesser K B, Childers J M, Surwit E A 1998 Transabdominal cerclage: a laparoscopic approach. Obstetrics and Gynecology 91:855–856

61. Scarantino S E, Reilly J G, Moretti M L, Pillari V T 2000 Laparoscopic removal of a transabdominal cervical cerclage. Americal Journal of Obstetrics and Gynecology 182:1086–1088

62. Young J H 1944 Caesarean section: The history and development of the operation from earliest times. HK Lewis, London

63. Trolle D 1982 The history of caearean section. CA Reitzel, Copenhagen

64. Ananth C V, Smulian K C, Vintzileos A M 1997 The association of placenta praevia with history of caesarean delivery and abortion: a meta analysis. American Journal of Obstetrics and Gynecology 177:1071–1078

65. Clark S L, Koonings P P, Phelan J P 1985 Placenta previa/accreta and prior caesarean section. Obstetrics and Gynecology 66:89–92

66. Wilkinson C, Enkin M W 2002 Lateral tilt for caesarean section (Cochrane Review). In: The Cochrane Library, Issue 1. Update Software, Oxford

67. Matorras R, Tacuri C, Nieto A et al 1998 Lack of benefits of left tilt in Cesarean sections: a randomised study of cardiotocography, cord acid–base status, and other parameters of the mother and the fetus. Journal of Perinatal Medicine 26:284–292

68. RCOG 1995 Report of a Working Party against Thromboembolism in Gynaecology and Obstetrics. RCOG, London

69. Smaill F, Hofmeyr G J 2002 Antibiotic prophylaxis for cesarean section (Cochrane Review). In: The Cochrane Library, Issue 1. Update Software, Oxford

70. Stark M, Finkel A 1994 Comparison, between the Joel Cohen and Pfannenstiel incisions in Caesarean section. European Journal of Obstetrics, Gynecology, and Reproductive Biology 53:121–122

71. Magann E F, Chauhan S P, Bufkin L et al 2002 Intra-operative haemorrhage by blunt dissection versus sharp expansion of the uterine incision at caesarean delivery: a randomised clinical trial. British Journal of Obstetrics and Gynaecology 109:448–452

72. Rich D A, Stokes I M 2002 Uterine torsion due to a fibroid, emergency myomectomy and transverse upper segment caesarean section. British Journal of Obstetrics and Gynaecology 109:105–106

73. Wilkinson C, Enkin M W 2002 Manual removal of the placenta at caesarean section (Cochrane Review). In: The Cochrane Library, Issue 1. Update Software, Oxford

Obstetric techniques for massive haemorrhage

Philip Steer

Definition and incidence

What is massive obstetric haemorrhage? Primary postpartum haemorrhage is usually defined as a blood loss of more than 500 mL in the first 24 hours after birth,[1] but it is known that estimation of blood loss at delivery is inaccurate.[2,3] There is a tendency to overestimate blood loss when it is less than 150 mL and underestimate it when it is over 300 mL.[3] The American College of Obstetricians and Gynecologists has therefore suggested that a more appropriate definition would depend on the number of units of blood it is thought necessary to transfuse in each individual case. Figure 6.1 shows the mean and 95%

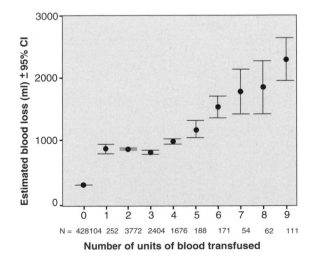

Fig. 6.1 The mean and 95% confidence interval of the estimated blood loss (mL) in 436 794 pregnancies recorded on the North West Thames database from 1988 to 1998 inclusive.

confidence interval of the estimated blood loss in 436 794 pregnancies recorded on the North West Thames database from 1988 to 1998 inclusive. It can be seen that the estimated blood loss did not change according to whether 1, 2 or 3 units of blood were thought necessary.

Figure 6.2 shows that the most common number of units transfused was two, rather than one. The reason for the custom that if any blood transfusion is thought necessary, one generally gives two rather than one unit, is unclear and it has no basis in either logic or evidence. The percentage of women requiring blood transfusion is shown in Fig. 6.2; overall it amounts to 2.4%. In parts of the world where blood transfusion is not readily available, major obstetric haemorrhage still results in about 125 000 deaths per year.[4] Fortunately, the number in the UK is only about 2–3 per year.

It is well known that parity affects the risk of postpartum haemorrhage, but it is not always appreciated that the risk falls after the first birth and then does not exceed the risk in the first birth again until the sixth birth! (Fig. 6.3; numbers for parity >7 are too small to be meaningful and have therefore been omitted).

Further analysis reveals that any method of operative delivery increases the need for trans-

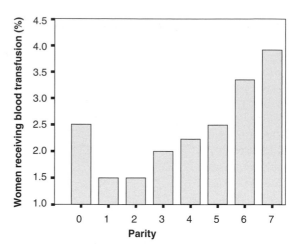

Fig. 6.3 Percentage of women requiring a blood transfusion according to parity in 436 794 pregnancies recorded on the North West Thames database from 1988 to 1998 inclusive.

Fig. 6.4 Effect of method of delivery on the need for transfusion	
Method of delivery	**Percentage transfused**
Spontaneous	0.9
Assisted breech	1.7
Ventouse	3.1
Elective caesarean	3.9
Breech extraction	4.6
Lift out forceps	4.9
Rotational forceps	6.2
Emergency caesarean	6.3

fusion (Fig. 6.4). Both mode of delivery and the need for transfusion are linked to the duration of labour (Figs 6.5 and 6.6).

Techniques for controlling haemorrhage

Medical

Unless the mother refuses, the third stage should be actively managed (administration of a prophylactic oxytocic before delivery of the placenta, and controlled cord traction of the umbilical cord), because this results in a 62% reduction

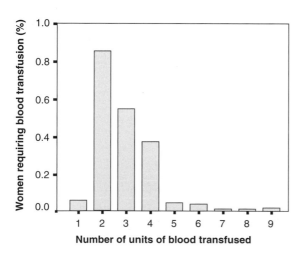

Fig. 6.2 Percentage of women requiring blood transfusion for obstetric haemorrhage in 436 794 pregnancies recorded on the North West Thames database from 1988 to 1998 inclusive.

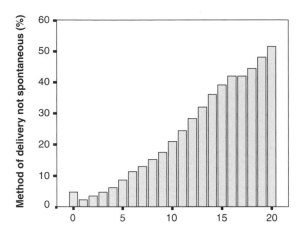

Fig. 6.5 Relationship between duration of labour (in hours) and proportion (%) of non-spontaneous deliveries (i.e. instrumental or caesarean delivery). Data from 436 794 pregnancies recorded on the North West Thames database from 1988 to 1998 inclusive.

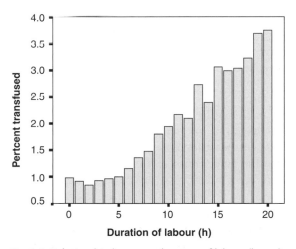

Fig. 6.6 Relationship between duration of labour (hours) and percentage of patients receiving a blood transfusion. Data from 436 794 pregnancies recorded on the North West Thames database from 1988 to 1998 inclusive.

in the incidence of postpartum haemorrhage >500 mL.[5] The usual oxytocic used in the UK is Syntometrine® (5 IU of Syntocinon® plus 0.5 mg of ergometrine), given either intramuscularly or intravenously. Some studies have suggested that Syntocinon® alone is as effective as Syntometrine®,[6,7] whereas others have suggested that Syntometrine® is more effective,[8] albeit with more side-effects (nausea and vomiting, hypertension).

If bleeding per vaginam following delivery persists despite active management, then a careful examination should be undertaken to check that there is not a traumatic cause for the bleeding, such as a vaginal or cervical tear. Such an examination needs to be carried out with the mother in the lithotomy position and with a good light, and this often means moving the mother to the operating theatre. Once local trauma has been ruled out, the possibility of uterine atony and/or retained placental parts should be considered. It is useful to give a further intravenous dose of ergometrine 0.5 mg (provided the mother is not hypertensive) and set up an infusion of Syntocinon® 10 units in 500 mL of saline, infused at 80 mL/h. Bimanual compression of the uterus, with one hand in the vagina and the other hand applying pressure per abdomen, will usually staunch the flow, at least temporarily (Fig. 6.7). The anaesthetist should be summoned and blood crossmatched. Once adequate anaesthesia has been established or restored, the uterine cavity should be explored digitally to ensure that any removal tissue is evacuated. Care should be taken not to perforate the uterus. No attempts should be made to evacuate a placenta that is obviously accreta. In this case, it is usually best to leave the adherent placenta in place and concentrate on making the uterus contract.

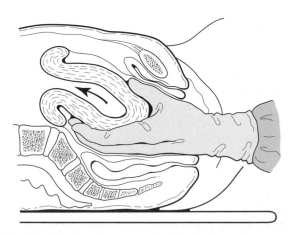

Fig. 6.7 Manual replacement of an inverted uterus.

If the uterus still remains atonic, the use of prostaglandins should be considered, although the place of these agents is not fully established at the present time. Injection of 15-methyl prostaglandin $F_{2\alpha}$ (Hemabate®) via the abdominal wall into the uterine muscle was introduced over 10 years ago[9] and has been claimed by some to be effective, although the author's personal experience of its use has been disappointing. It can be used intramuscularly into the mother's thigh, but given by this route is no better than ergometrine and produces profuse diarrhoea.[10] More recently, use of agents such as misoprostol orally,[11,12] rectally[13] or intrauterine[14] have all been suggested, with varying claims for success. The proper place of such agents can only be established by further prospective studies.

Surgical

Re-insertion of an inverted uterus

Inversion of the uterus is an uncommon event, but can occur when the lower segment of the uterus fails to contract well, the fundus of the uterus is broad (as with a bicornuate uterus) and the placenta is situated in the fundus. It is often said that it can result from excessive cord traction, but the author's experience is that it is just as likely to occur spontaneously when the above circumstances apply. The best immediate management is, if maternal analgesia permits, immediate reinsertion of the uterus by pressure on the everted fundus, using a fist (Fig. 6.8). The alternative is to use O'Sullivan's hydrostatic method, which involves instilling warmed normal saline into the vagina until the hydrostatic pressure replaces the uterus.[15] Leakage of the saline from the vagina is prevented by keeping the fist in the vagina, through which is passed the tubing carrying the saline. An even better seal can be produced by passing the saline through a silc® cup ventouse extractor, which is passed into the middle part of the vagina and held in place by hand.[16]

Packing

Packing the uterus is a traditional procedure, which largely fell out of favour in the 1970s.

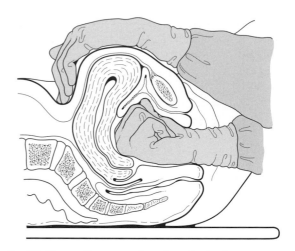

Fig. 6.8 Bimanual compression of an atonic uterus.

However, several series of cases have been published suggesting that it can be effective if performed correctly.[17,18] The author's experience is that it is most valuable when the upper segment of the uterus is well contracted, but the lower segment is not; or when the cervix itself is bleeding, as may occur following the removal of a low-lying placenta. In this situation, there is a firm upper part of the uterus against which the pack can be pressed, and the volume to be packed is not very large. It is also necessary for there to be sufficient tension in the cervix to keep the pack in place; if it remains fully dilated, there is a tendency for the pack to keep slipping down into the vagina. In one case that the author dealt with, a pack was clearly being effective at staunching the bleeding so long as it was being pressed from below, but the cervix was fully dilated, so that the pack would not stay in place when the applied pressure was discontinued. The solution was to place a nylon suture circumferentially around the cervix, in the manner of a cervical cerclage. When this was pulled tight, the cervix decreased to only 4 cm in diameter, thus providing a platform upon which the pack could sit and continue to exert pressure inside the uterus. The cervical opening remained sufficient to remove the pack the following day.

There are several important aspects to the technique. First, one must obtain a firm hold on the cervix, usually requiring the use of a vulsellum forceps. Second, one should use roll gauze that is fed into the uterus over the operator's fingers, which are inserted along the posterior wall of the vagina. Usually, several rolls of gauze are needed, which can be joined together by knotting. Specially designed gauze tampons are available for the purpose,[19] but the author has no experience of their use (Fig. 6.9).

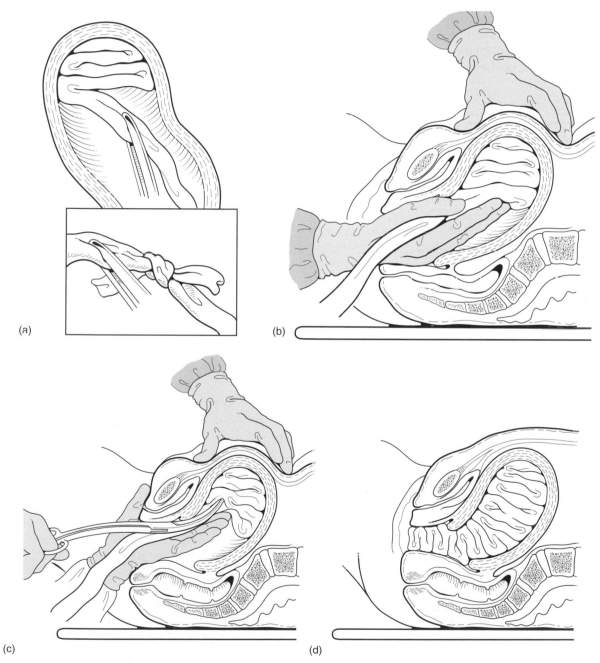

(a)

(b)

(c)

(d)

Fig. 6.9 Packing the uterus. (a) making sure the pack goes in as far as posible; join packs as necessary (b) ensure firm packing (c) apply fundal counter pressure when feeding in the pack (d) cavity completely packed with no spaces remaining.

Tamponade of the uterus using balloons

When adequate pressure in the uterus cannot be achieved using a gauze pack, it may be possible to staunch the bleeding by inflating an appropriately designed balloon inside the uterus.[20,21] If a specially designed balloon is not available, the author has successfully used the gastric balloon of a Sengstaken–Blakemore tube (designed to arrest bleeding from oesophageal varices), as have others.[22]

Uterine compression sutures (Brace sutures, B-Lynch sutures)

In 1997, B-Lynch et al[23] described the use of uterine compression sutures to treat uterine atony (Figs 6.10 and 6.11) in five cases of massive obstetric haemorrhage.

The objective of this technique is to compress the uterus without occluding either the uterine arteries or the uterine cavity. Several subsequent publications reporting six more cases have attested to its efficacy.[24,25] Key points in the technique are:

- The abdomen is opened via a Pfannenstiel incision (although a modified Cohen's procedure would be just as appropriate).
- Bimanual compression is applied to check that this arrests bleeding, before the suturing is performed.

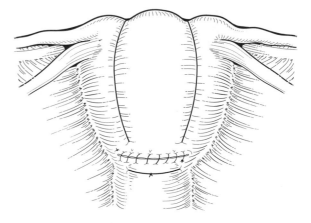

Fig. 6.11 Suture tied.

- A lower-segment incision in the uterus is made or re-opened to allow the suturing to be performed.
- The uterine cavity is not crossed.
- Vicryl® or Dexon® sutures are used.
- The sutures must be pulled tight to achieve appropriate compression.

I have now performed six cases of uterine compression suturing, and can suggest the following modifications to the technique:

- It does not appear to be necessary to open the uterus or avoid crossing the uterine cavity.
- Vicryl® or Dexon® are strong and unlikely to cause external adhesions to the uterus.

In this simplified approach, adopted independently by Richard Hayman and Professor Subaratnam Arulkumaran in Derby, a number 2 Vicryl® or Dexon® suture on a straight, blunt needle is used to transfix the uterus from front to back, just above the reflection of the bladder (Fig. 6.12), and is then tied at the fundus of the uterus. This can be done as one suture on each side of the uterus, or more than one suture if the uterus is particularly broad, and more than one suture appears to be necessary to obtain adequate compression (Fig. 6.13).

If only two sutures are needed, there is sometimes a tendency for the sutures to slide off the side of the uterus, like the braces off a round-

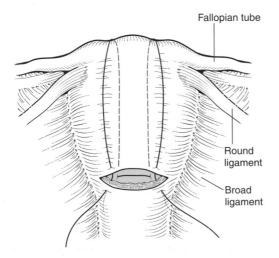

Fallopian tube

Round ligament

Broad ligament

Fig. 6.10 Insertion of suture.

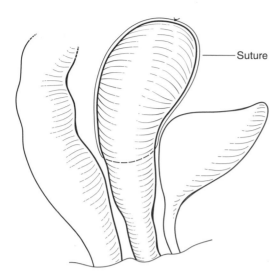

Fig. 6.12 Lateral view of uterus, showing where the compression suture is placed.

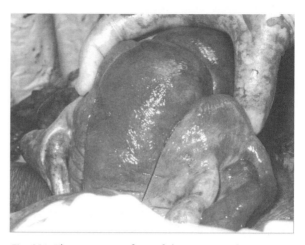

Fig. 6.14 The anterior surface of the uterus with compression sutures applied postpartum—illustrating the sutures tied together at the fundus of the uterus to prevent them slipping down the side of the uterus.

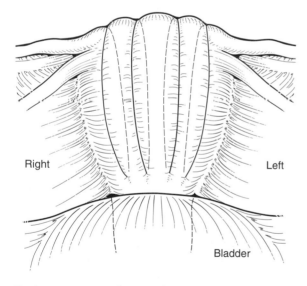

Fig. 6.13 Front view of uterus, showing where the compression sutures are placed.

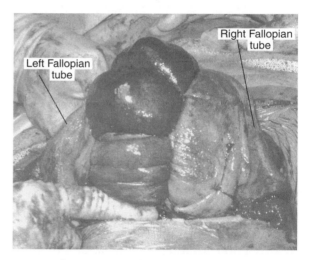

Fig. 6.15 The posterior surface of the uterus, showing additional ties to increase compression.

shouldered man. To prevent this, the simplest technique is to tie the knots at the top of the uterus and then tie the loose ends together, as shown in Fig. 6.14.

If the uterus in between the two lateral sutures still appears to be in need of further compression, then side-to-side ties can be inserted in between the lateral sutures (Fig. 6.15).

The indications for which I have performed these sutures include an atonic uterus following uterine inversion, an atonic uterus following prolonged labour, an elective caesarean section in a woman with heart disease in whom the use of oxytocics was contraindicated, and a woman with an anterior placenta praevia implanted on to a previous caesarean section scar. Despite the fact that the suture is passed through the uterine cavity, all the women have passed normal lochia and there has been no delay in the resumption of normal menstruation following the cessation of breast-feeding. One woman required laparoscopy just over a year following the birth, for intermittent lower abdominal pain. Some adhesions were noted from the uterus to the anterior abdominal wall, but these were easily divided, and the woman subsequently had no further symptoms.

Other conservative techniques

The confidential inquiry into maternal death generally lists as one of the avoidable factors in deaths from postpartum haemorrhage, unnecessary delay in performing a caesarean hysterectomy in the presence of massive obstetric haemorrhage.[26] However, there are circumstances in which it is probably appropriate to attempt conservative procedures. For example, the mother may be very young and be in her first pregnancy, so that preservation of the uterus for future childbearing is a major concern. Alternatively, if the risk of haemorrhage has been foreseen, conservative measures can be planned in advance. For example, a diagnosis of adherent placenta may have been made on ultrasound scanning or magnetic resonance imaging, or there may be a history of previous massive postpartum haemorrhage (greater than sixfold increased risk of a further such haemorrhage, to 8%).

Vascular catheters and embolization

The technique of arterial embolization to arrest major postpartum haemorrhage was reported as long ago as 1979[27] and sporadic reports appeared during the 1980s.[28-30] However, more systematic use has only been reported in the past few years. Most reports suggest it is useful in expert hands.[31-38] Embolization requires the placement of intravascular catheters under radiological control, usually into the internal iliac arteries. This is preferably done before surgery if a problem with haemorrhage is anticipated (for example, caesarean section for placenta accreta shown on ultrasound or magnetic resonance imaging). Flow can be interrupted temporarily (for example, by inflating balloons at the end of the catheters) to arrest haemorrhage, and then allowed to resume once haemostasis has been achieved surgically.[39] However, experience with this technique is small, and some workers have not found it very valuable.[40] In most reported series, the placement of catheters was used to inject granules, such as gelfoam pledgets, promoting thrombosis in the terminal arteries and arterioles.[36] Occlusion can be made permanent by the injection of 3 mm metallic coils, which occlude larger arteries such as the internal iliacs. Complications from embolization are uncommon, affecting about 5–10% of patients, and mainly comprise infection and fever. However, as with almost any technique, rare but fatal complications can occur; a death from septicaemia following embolization of fibroids in a nonpregnant woman has been reported.[41] There is a necessary exposure of the mother (and fetus if placement of catheters is done pre-delivery) to 10–15 rad of radiation.[32] The use of the technique is, of course, limited by the availability of the specialized imaging equipment required (including a radiology table), and the relative shortage of suitably trained interventional radiologists, who must also be on standby to arrive at short notice for emergency procedures. Even in units with appropriate equipment and staff, it will be difficult to institute such therapy in less than 45 min.

Uterine artery ligation

Uterine artery ligation is performed by passing a ligature around the uterine artery, usually at, or just below, the level of a lower segment incision that has (or could have been) performed. The medial bite should include some myometrium, and the lateral bite should be clear of the lateral uterine vein, passing through a clear window in the broad ligament. The obvious danger is inclusion of the ureter, which should be identified separately from the uterine artery so that it can be positively excluded (however, simple ligation of the ureter is not a life-threatening complication, unlike haemorrhage, and can nearly always be rectified later). Uterine artery ligation has been advocated as a useful manoeuvre by O'Leary, who in 1995 reported a series of 265

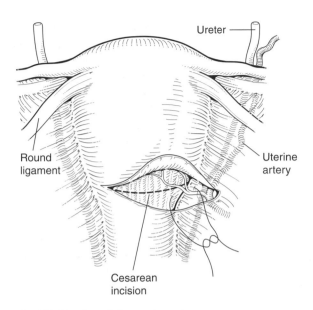

Fig. 6.16 Ligation of the uterine artery.

cases where it had been performed.[42] There were only 10 cases where the technique was deemed inadequate. Uterine artery ligation may well be performed inadvertently, and more often than is commonly realized, when extensions of uterine lower segment incisions are being sutured, and so it seems unlikely that there are any serious long-term sequelae. It is certainly a reasonable procedure to perform before resorting to hysterectomy for uterine atony, if uterine compression sutures are not sufficient (Fig. 6.16).

Internal iliac ligation

In desperation, blood flow to the pelvis can be reduced by ligation of the internal iliac artery (also known as the hypogastric artery). This requires incision of the peritoneum on the lateral sidewall of the pelvis. Ligation must be done distal to the origin of the posterior branch, which if ligated, can result in compromised blood flow to the gluteal muscles. The reported success of the procedure ranges from 43 to 90%.[43–46] However, the procedure is not taught to most trainees in obstetrics and gynaecology in the UK, and it is therefore necessary, in most cases, to involve a vascular surgeon or gynaecological oncologist

in the operation. If bleeding has not responded to uterine compression sutures and/or ligation of the uterine artery, then the obstetric surgeon will have to consider carefully whether any further delay in performing a hysterectomy is appropriate.

Caesarean hysterectomy

The Confidential Enquiry into Maternal Death in almost every triennium records deaths from obstetric haemorrhage in cases where resort to hysterectomy was unduly delayed by attempts to conserve the uterus.[47,48] Hysterectomy can be a life-saving procedure, and it should be considered as soon as it is apparent that haemorrhage may pose a threat to the woman's life, and/or the conservative measures described above are not available or are not working. The threshold will clearly be lowest in older women of high parity with medical reasons why another pregnancy would not be advisable. The classical indications are (in order of frequency) uterine atony (43%), placenta accreta (30%), uterine rupture (13%), extension of a low transverse incision (10%), and leiomyomata preventing uterine closure and haemostasis (4%).[49] Cases of placenta accreta are associated, in about half the cases, with previous caesarean section. The risk of a low-lying anterior placenta being accreta increases with successive caesareans, rising from 4% in women with no scar to 60% with three or more prior caesareans.[50,51] The potential need for hysterectomy in cases of caesarean section for placenta praevia is the main reason why such cases should, wherever possible, be attended by a clinician of considerable experience (consultant level). Consideration should be given, in such cases as can be anticipated, to obtaining signed informed consent for hysterectomy prior to embarking on the caesarean section.

The history of caesarean hysterectomy has been well reviewed by Durfee.[52] The first reported fully documented case of caesarean hysterectomy with survival of the patient was by Eduardo Porro in 1876. However, over the next 20 years, the mortality rate in published series was often over 80%. In the UK, Godson (who pioneered the lower-segment incision for caesarean section) and Lawson Tait introduced a series of modifications that improved survival. By 1900 Reed of Chicago published the primary indications for the procedure, which were:

- dead fetus with infected uterus
- secondary atresia of the vagina
- carcinoma of the cervix
- uterine atony, leading to intractable haemorrhage
- ruptured uterus.

By 1922, deaths had fallen to less than 5% and the procedure was even being advocated for sterilization. However, with the introduction of antibiotics, and more active management of labour, sepsis became a very rare indication. Tubal ligation replaced hysterectomy for sterilization. The major indication for hysterectomy in current practice is haemorrhage that cannot be controlled by the conservative methods described above.

Once it is decided that hysterectomy is necessary, it is usually simplest to start with a subtotal procedure. This is particularly appropriate if the mother has been in labour, and the cervix is fully dilated. It can often be difficult to identify the junction between the cervix and the vagina until the body of the uterus has been removed. An attempt to remove the whole uterus in one go, especially when the cervix is fully dilated, is more likely to cause damage to the bladder, and leave remnants of the cervix in any case.

The ovaries and distal Fallopian tubes are first separated from the body of the uterus using two large, straight clamps (such as Kelly's clamps) and cutting the broad ligament, Fallopian tube and round ligament, proximal to the clamp. Some authors recommend taking the round ligament and ovarian pedicle separately, as this reduces the size of the pedicles (making them easier to tie) and also allows more obvious access to the broad ligament, which makes identification of the uterine artery (and ureter if necessary) easier. Some authors suggest that the relatively avascular midpart of the broad ligament can be divided directly, but it is probably safer to apply a series of straight clamps down the side of the uterus to just below the level of a lower segment incision (as usually used to deliver the baby).

Each clamp should be inside the previous one (i.e. nearer to the body of the uterus). As each pedicle is taken, it should be transfixed at either end and then tied and cut. This allows the peritoneum to fall laterally, taking the ureter with it and helping to keep it out of harm's way. The final vascular pedicle clamp (again, a Kelly or Gwilliam) should be applied from each side, through the anterior uterine incision where the baby was delivered, to include the uterine artery and a small bite of the wall of the lower segment of the uterus. Once again, this should be cut, transfixed and tied. A further clamp can then be placed across the lower segment, into the lower segment incision and including the posterior wall of the lower segment, but this is not essential. The body of the uterus can then be removed by cutting above this final pair of clamps. If the bleeding was due to an atonic uterus, removal of the body of the uterus will already have led to the cessation of most of the bleeding. If the placenta was low lying, then bleeding below the clamps will probably be continuing. It is then best to control the lower segment edge bleeding by the application of Allis or Ochsner clamps. The lower segment below the clamps can now be inspected easily, and most of the bleeding will probably be controllable by direct pressure while the next step is considered. This will usually be to identify the cervix, so that a clamp can be applied at each side, over the broad ligament, to the point where the cervix joins the vagina. This clamp is usually angled at 45° between the lateral and midline planes, so as to avoid the ureter. The remaining lower segment and cervix can then be removed. Haemostasis at the edge of the vagina is most easily obtained by oversewing the edges (for example, with a locking absorbable suture) and leaving the vagina open. This enables ongoing inspection of haemostasis, and also allows drainage of any continuing ooze into the vagina postoperatively. It is not necessary to remove the entire cervix; the objective throughout is to stop the bleeding. If that has been achieved, then continuing attempts to remove the remainder of the cervix may provoke further bleeding, the ligatures may slip, or the ureter may be damaged. If the hysterectomy was straightforward, and good haemostasis has been achieved, then it may be appropriate to approximate the two edges of the vagina, thus closing the vault.

A number of useful 'tips' have been suggested by Plauche.[53] Damage to the bladder can occur, especially if the bladder is adherent to the lower segment because of a previous caesarean section. The bladder should be inspected carefully for any holes, to avoid subsequent urinary peritonitis. The balloon of a Foley catheter in the bladder can be manipulated from the outside of the bladder, and pulled up against the bladder fundus and posterior wall, which usually makes any holes much more obvious (the balloon can be seen through the hole). Such defects should be closed with fine absorbable suture, in two layers, with invagination of the second layer. The first layer should be a continuous suture, and the second can be either continuous or interrupted. If haemostasis has been achieved but there is concern that the ureters have been occluded, it is usually better to close up and perform an intravenous urogram in the following few days, rather than risk restarting bleeding by further surgery. An occluded ureter will cause the kidney to stop working, but renal function returns remarkably quickly once ureteric patency is re-established. This can be done at relative leisure by a specialist urological team, once the immediate danger of acute haemorrhage has receded. A damaged ureter that leaks urine is a more serious immediate problem and once control of haemorrhage has been obtained, the involvement of a urologist is advisable. They will either place a stent into the ureter from inside the abdomen, using a short longitudinal incision, or pass a ureteric catheter up the ureter from inside the bladder.

Other small points, which may all be helpful in some circumstances, are: the use of wet packs to keep the bowel away from the bleeding areas (facilitates access); delivering the uterus out of the abdomen, to improve access and slow bleeding by causing traction and pressure on its lateral attachments; and use of a large Robert's tube drain through the vagina in cases of persistent slow ooze (to prevent haematoma formation).

If there is continuing ooze, and any bleeding points cannot be readily identified and ligated or oversewn, direct pressure with a pack is often the quickest way to arrest the flow. This also allows time for any resuscitation of the patient that needs to be done, and for additional help (e.g. from a vascular surgeon) to be sought. It cannot be emphasized enough that teamwork is essential in modern practice, and the objective is to save the patient's life, not the surgeon's reputation for solo excellence. In addition, continuing pressure for up to 10 minutes (which can seem half a lifetime) often reduces, or occasionally even abolishes, further bleeding. Clotting status can be checked and corrected if necessary. Pelvic tamponade with a balloon, or similar device such as the Logothetopulos pack,[19,54] or leaving a pack in situ, can also be considered. Ligating the internal iliac artery or embolization may succeed where all else has failed.

REFERENCES

1. Park E H, Sachs B P 1999 Postpartum hemorrhage and other problems of the third stage. In: James D K, Steer P J, Weiner C P, Gonik B (eds) High risk pregnancy – management options. W B Saunders, London, pp 1231–1246

2. Duthie S J, Ven D, Yung G L et al 1991 Discrepancy between laboratory determination and visual estimation of blood loss during normal delivery. European Journal of Obstetrics, Gynecology, and Reproductive Biology 38:119–124

3. Razvi K, Chua S, Arulkumaran S, Ratnam S S 1996 A comparison between visual estimation and laboratory determination of blood loss during the third stage of labour. Australian and New Zealand Journal of Obstetrics and Gynaecology 36:152–154

4. Drife J 1997 Management of primary postpartum haemorrhage. British Journal of Obstetrics and Gynaecology 104:275–277

5. Prendiville W J, Elbourne D, McDonald S 2000 Active versus expectant management in the third stage of labour (Cochrane Review). In: The Cochrane Library Issue 4. Update Software, Oxford

6. McDonald S J, Prendiville W J, Blair E 1993 Randomised controlled trial of oxytocin alone versus oxytocin and ergometrine in active management of third stage of labour. British Medical Journal 307:1167–1171

7. Soriano D, Dulitzki M, Schiff E et al 1996 A prospective cohort study of oxytocin plus ergometrine compared with oxytocin alone for prevention of postpartum haemorrhage. British Journal of Obstetrics and Gynaecology 103:1068–1073

8. McDonald S, Prendiville W J, Elbourne D 2000 Prophylactic syntometrine versus oxytocin for delivery of the placenta (Cochrane Review). In: The Cochrane Library Issue 4. Update Software, Oxford

9. Bigrigg A, Chui D, Chissell S, Read M D 1991 Use of intra-myometrial 15-methyl prostaglandin F2 alpha to control atonic postpartum haemorrhage following vaginal delivery and failure of conventional therapy. British Journal of Obstetrics and Gynaecology 98:734–736

10. Chua S, Chew S L, Yeoh C L et al 1995 A randomized controlled study of prostaglandin 15-methyl F2 alpha compared with syntometrine for prophylactic use in the third stage of labour. Australian and New Zealand Journal of Obstetrics and Gynaecology 35:413–416

11. el-Refaey H, O'Brien P, Morafa W et al 1997 Use of oral misoprostol in the prevention of postpartum haemorrhage. British Journal of Obstetrics and Gynaecology 104:336–339

12. Surbek D V, Fehr P M, Hosli I, Holzgreve W 1999 Oral misoprostol for third stage of labor: a randomized placebo-controlled trial. Obstetrics and Gynecology 94:255–258

13. Bamigboye A A, Hofmeyr G J, Merrell D A 1998 Rectal misoprostol in the prevention of postpartum hemorrhage: a placebo-controlled trial. American Journal of Obstetrics and Gynecology 179:1043–1046

14. Adekanmi O A, Purmessur S, Edwards G, Barrington J W 2001 Intrauterine misoprostol for the treatment of severe recurrent atonic secondary postpartum haemorrhage. British Journal of Obstetrics and Gynaecology 108:541–542

15. O'Sullivan J V 1945 Acute inversion of the uterus. British Medical Journal 2:282–283

16. Ogueh O, Ayida G 1997 Acute uterine inversion: a new technique of hydrostatic replacement. British Journal of Obstetrics and Gynaecology 104:951–952

17. Hester J D 1975 Postpartum hemorrhage and reevaluation of uterine packing. Obstetrics and Gynecology 45:501–504

18. Maier R C 1993 Control of postpartum hemorrhage with uterine packing. American Journal of Obstetrics and Gynecology 169:317–321

19. Robie G F, Morgan M A, Payne G G J, Wasemiller-Smith L 1990 Logothetopulos pack for the management of uncontrollable postpartum hemorrhage. American Journal of Perinatology 7:327–328

20. Marcovici I, Scoccia B 1999 Postpartum hemorrhage and intrauterine balloon tamponade. A report of three cases. Journal of Reproductive Medicine 44:122–126

21. Bakri Y N, Amri A, Abdul J F 2001 Tamponade-balloon for obstetrical bleeding. International Journal of Gynaecology and Obstetrics 74:139–142

22. Johanson R, Kumar M, Obhrai M, Young P 2001 Management of massive postpartum haemorrhage: use of a hydrostatic balloon catheter to avoid laparotomy. British Journal of Obstetrics and Gynaecology 108:420–422

23. B-Lynch C, Coker A, Lawal A H et al 1997 The B-Lynch surgical technique for the control of massive postpartum haemorrhage: an alternative to hysterectomy? Five cases reported. British Journal of Obstetrics and Gynaecology 104:372–375

24. Dacus JV, Busowski MT, Busowski JD et al 2000 Surgical treatment of uterine atony employing the B-Lynch technique. Journal of Maternal–Fetal Medicine 9:194–196

25. Ferguson J E, Bourgeois F J, Underwood P B et al 2000 B-Lynch suture for postpartum hemorrhage. Obstetrics and Gynecology 95:1020–1022

26. Lewis G, Drife J O 1998 Why mothers die. Report on confidential enquiries into maternal deaths in the United Kingdom, 1994–96. London Department of Health, Department of Health Welsh Office, Scottish Office Department of Health, Department of Health and Social Services, Northern Ireland

27. Brown B J, Heaston D K, Poulson A M et al 1979 Uncontrollable postpartum bleeding: a new approach to hemostasis through angiographic arterial embolization. Obstetrics and Gynecology 54:361–365

28. Duvauferrier R, Priou G, Tasson D et al 1984 Emergency uterine embolization in postpartum hemorrhage secondary to coagulopathy. Journal of Radiology 65:285–288

29. Feinberg B B, Resnik E, Hurt W G et al 1987 Angiographic embolization in the management of late postpartum hemorrhage. A case report. Journal of Reproductive Medicine 32:929–931

30. Greenwood L H, Glickman M G, Schwartz P E et al 1987 Obstetric and nonmalignant gynecologic bleeding: treatment with angiographic embolization. Radiology 164:155–159

31. Oei P L, Chua S, Tan L et al 1998 Arterial embolization for bleeding following hysterectomy for intractable postpartum hemorrhage. International Journal of Gynaecology and Obstetrics 62:83–86

32. Hansch E, Chitkara U, McAlpine J et al 1999 Pelvic arterial embolization for control of obstetric hemorrhage: a five-year experience. American Journal of Obstetrics and Gynecology 180:1454–1460

33. Pelage J P, Le D O, Jacob D et al 1999 Selective arterial embolization of the uterine arteries in the management of intractable post-partum hemorrhage. Acta Obstetrica et Gynecologica Scandinavica 78:698–703

34. Descargues G, Clavier E, Lemercier E, Sibert L 2000 Placenta percreta with bladder invasion managed by arterial embolization and manual removal after cesarean. Obstetrics and Gynecology 96:840

35. Murakami R, Ichikawa T, Kumazaki T et al 2000 Transcatheter arterial embolization for postpartum massive hemorrhage: a case report. Clinical Imaging 24:368–370

36. Lingam K, Hood V, Carty M J 2000 Angiographic embolisation in the management of pelvic haemorrhage. British Journal of Obstetrics and Gynaecology 107:1176–1178

37. Deux J F, Bazot M, Le Blanche A F et al 2001 Is selective embolization of uterine arteries a safe alternative to hysterectomy in patients with postpartum hemorrhage? American Journal of Roentgenology 177:145–149

38. Badawy S Z, Etman A, Singh M et al 2001 Uterine artery

embolization: the role in obstetrics and gynecology. Clinical Imaging 25:288–295

39. Dubois J, Garel L, Grignon A et al 1997 Placenta percreta: balloon occlusion and embolization of the internal iliac arteries to reduce intraoperative blood losses. American Journal of Obstetrics and Gynecology 176:723–726

40. Levine A B, Kuhlman K, Bonn J 1999 Placenta accreta: comparison of cases managed with and without pelvic artery balloon catheters. Journal of Maternal–Fetal Medicine 8:173–176

41. Vashisht A, Studd J, Carey A, Burn P 1999 Fatal septicaemia after fibroid embolisation. Lancet 354:307–308

42. O'Leary J A 1995 Uterine artery ligation in the control of postcesarean hemorrhage. Journal of Reproductive Medicine 40:189–193

43. Thavarasah A S, Sivalingam N, Almohdzar S A 1989 Internal iliac and ovarian artery ligation in the control of pelvic haemorrhage. Australian and New Zealand Journal of Obstetric Gynaecology 29:22–25

44. Likeman R K 1992 The boldest procedure possible for checking the bleeding—a new look at an old operation, and a series of 13 cases from an Australian hospital. Australian and New Zealand Journal of Obstetrics and Gynaecology 32:256–262

45. Nandanwar Y S, Jhalam L, Mayadeo N, Guttal D R 1993 Ligation of internal iliac arteries for control of pelvic haemorrhage. Journal of Postgraduate Medicine 39:194–196

46. Das B N, Biswas A K 1998 Ligation of internal iliac arteries in pelvic haemorrhage. Journal of Obstetric Gynaecological Research 24:251–254

47. Anonymous 1991 Report on confidential enquiries into maternal deaths in the United Kingdom 1985–87. HMSO, London

48. Anonymous 1998 Report on confidential enquiries into maternal deaths in the United Kingdom 1994–1996. The Stationery Office, London

49. Clark S L, Yeh S Y, Phelan J P et al 1984 Emergency hysterectomy for obstetric hemorrhage. Obstetrics and Gynecology 64:376–380

50. Clark S L, Koonings P P, Phelan J P 1985 Placenta previa/accreta and prior cesarean section. Obstetrics and Gynecology 66:89–92

51. Zaki Z M, Bahar A M, Ali M E et al 1998 Risk factors and morbidity in patients with placenta previa accreta compared to placenta previa non-accreta. Acta Obstetrica et Gynecologica Scandinavica 77:391–394

52. Durfee R B 1969 Evolution of cesarean hysterectomy. In: Mickal A (ed) Clinical obstetrics and gynecology. Harper and Row Publishers, New York, pp 575–589

53. Plauche W C 2002 Cesarean hysterectomy: indications, technique, and complications. Clinical Obstetrics and Gynecology 29:318–328

54. Hallak M, Dildy G A, Hurley T J, Moise K J Jr 1991 Transvaginal pressure pack for life-threatening pelvic hemorrhage secondary to placenta accreta. Obstetrics and Gynecology 78:938–940

Gynaecological techniques

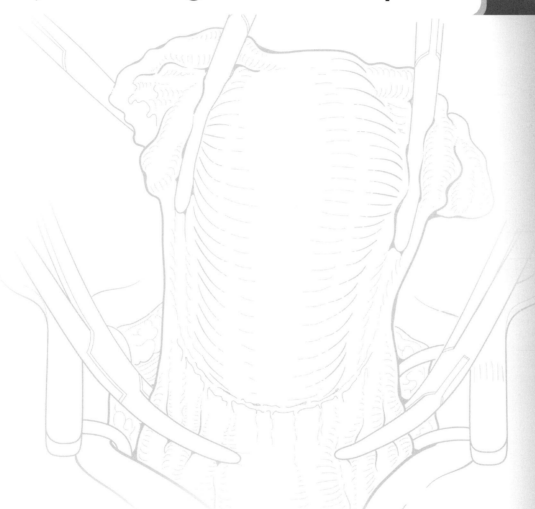

The abdominal approach to pelvic surgery

David Oram

Introduction

Writing in the preface to the ninth edition of *Bonney's gynaecological surgery*, its editor John Monaghan[1] advocates that 'operations should flow with a style and natural pace, rather like a well choreographed dance'. Speed, accuracy and safety in surgery, however, is a product of experience and it is incumbent on doctors in training to avail themselves of every opportunity to watch, assist and operate under supervision. It is extremely important in the training years for a surgeon to grasp the chance to watch as many senior surgeons as possible operate. There are enormous variations in style, technique and even demeanour that need to be appreciated, and it is a great privilege for the young doctor to be able to 'pick the gems'. The trick then is to incorporate them into their own technique and to assess what works for them. The end result should be a composite which is open to further refinement as experience develops.

Of equal importance is the need for senior surgeons to teach, and teach constantly in the operating theatre. This is more important now than ever. The concept of a consultant-based rather than a consultant-led service has inevitably led to doctors in training performing fewer operations themselves. This, combined with the fact that the duration of training is now shorter than it was, is a potential recipe for the production of undertrained inexperienced surgeons. In this context, the frequently expressed complaint that 'once you become a consultant, you never see your colleagues operate' should no longer be allowed to prevail.

This chapter is designed to provide the trainee surgeon with a series of surgical tips, and examines how they may be applied to a standard gynaecological procedure, namely abdominal hysterectomy. Although the author fully acknowledges that there is more than one way to perform any surgical procedure, and that, with experience, surgeons will develop personal prejudices, the chapter, in accordance with the editor's wishes, is deliberately didactic. Notwithstanding this, it is to be hoped that the reader will discover a few useful hints that can be included in their personal amalgam of surgical technique previously mentioned.

General principles

Always use the 'KISS' principle

The KISS principle or 'Keep It Simple Stupid' is important. Overelaboration in surgery should be avoided; it inevitably leads to an increase in overall operating time and this should be eschewed. Some of the best surgeons have utilized video-recordings to analyse their technique, and are inevitably surprised by the number of unnecessary hand movements and time-wasting manoeuvres that they make. Ligatures need only be held in certain defined instances. Do not develop three pedicles when two will suffice, as this runs the risk of increased tissue damage and often clutters up the operating field with extra instruments. The surgeon should constantly strive to discover the simplest and safest way to achieve the operative goal, and these two factors are frequently not mutually exclusive.

It's all about tissue planes

Surgery is indeed all about tissue planes, and gaining access to them usually requires a degree

of boldness. The inexperienced surgeon quite correctly will be cautious and with this inevitably comes a degree of timidity. Such tentative technique may lead to attempts at blunt dissection with fingers or gauze before the correct tissue plane is entered, and the result is often increased bleeding and occasionally organ damage. This is never more evident than when opening the uterovesical fold of peritoneum in order to mobilize the bladder at hysterectomy. Timidity leads to this incision being made too high, and the bladder being pushed down digitally or with a swab before the correct tissue plane has been identified and entered. Bleeding from the plexus of bladder veins, and sometimes damage to the organ itself, are the consequence. Overconfidence in surgery is to be discouraged as much as timidity; the outcome, of haemorrhage and organ damage, is usually identical. The surgeon should aspire to a confidence in dissection that displays not only a knowledge of anatomy that permits boldness, but also an awareness of the pitfalls inherent in cavalier technique.

Cut under tension

Linked to the points made above and below is the concept of cutting tissues when they are put under tension. This facilitates entry into the correct surgical plane, and requires help from the surgical assistant in order to achieve the desired result.

Organize assistants

Surgery is learnt in three phases: learning to assist, learning to perform the operative procedure, and learning to organize the assistants. There is a tendency to under-utilize assistants, and a regular sight in an operating theatre is to watch a surgeon struggling, trying to retract and dissect at the same time while the assistant stands idly by. The experienced surgeon recognizes the importance of working as a team and involves the assistants not only to retract and cut ligatures but also to pick up tissues to facilitate cutting under tension and thereby aiding dissection. In longer surgical procedures, assistants can be deployed to carry out routine phases of the operation while the lead surgeon assists and relaxes for a short period.

Remember to use your feet

Operating in the pelvis with the patient in the Trendelenberg position can be uncomfortable and physically demanding. It is important to move one's body not only to relieve discomfort but also to optimize access and view. It is also important to stand back once in a while and visually take in an overall picture of the regional anatomy so that it prevails in the mind's eye. It is a mistake for the surgeon to remain crouched over the incision with eyes focused exclusively on the points of the dissecting scissors. Such a practice is analogous to driving a car with eyes focused on the rear bumper of the car in front, oblivious to the overall pattern and behaviour of the traffic flow.

Ensure adequate exposure

Inadequate exposure of the operative field will inevitably cause the surgeon to struggle. On being called to assist a junior colleague in difficulty, a consistent first move by the more experienced surgeon is to enlarge the incision and thereby improve both exposure and access. A lower midline incision can be enlarged by extending it around the umbilicus if necessary, while improved access through a transverse incision can be gained by dividing the rectus abdominis muscle on one or both sides and ligating the inferior epigastric artery.

Plan the appropriate incision—in advance

In order to avoid falling into the trap of inadequate exposure and impaired access, careful thought needs to be given to the type and size of the incision required prior to the operative procedure. Factors that will influence this decision include the nature of the pathology, the size of the patient and the mobility and size of the tissue to be removed. In contrast to what has already been said, in a thin patient with benign pathology and mobile tissues there is no need to make too large an incision—a small transverse suprapubic approach will often suffice. With smaller incisions, perioperative morbidity is less, recovery time is quicker and, furthermore, cosmetic awareness *is* important. However, this ceases to be a priority consideration in cases of malignancy or even suspected malignancy, or when large or relatively fixed masses are to be dealt with, when a vertical incision is mandatory. It is worth remembering that even in grossly obese patients, the most efficient way to gain access to the peritoneal cavity might be by a transverse incision below the pannus, where the abdominal wall is at its thinnest. This is a situation not infrequently encountered in endometrial cancer patients.

Give nature a chance

There is nothing that fills one with more foreboding about what is to come than to watch a surgeon make the initial hesitant incision, barely severing the skin, and then put the knife down and immediately reach for the diathermy forceps. The next few minutes of the operation are spent fruitlessly dealing with minor capillary bleeding points before the knife is retrieved, a tentative incision is made into the subcutaneous fat, and the diathermy procedure is repeated! Many of these tiny superficial bleeders will stop spontaneously if allowed to do so. Vessels will go into spasm and clots will form provided time is given and the tissues are left relatively undisturbed. In real terms, what this means is that the tissues should not be rubbed by having swabs dragged across them. Swabs should be used to dab only and then removed gently. The same is true for diffuse oozing from a tumour bed or peritoneal surfaces where an ovarian cyst might have been adherent, or the raw surface in the pelvis following a hysterectomy. In these circumstances, beware the bored but helpful SHO wielding the sucker! Injudicious use of the sucker is to be discouraged every bit as much as dragging swabs. Diffuse bleeding can often be controlled by direct and sustained pressure using an abdominal pack (2 minutes on the clock). During this time the assistant should arm himself with a swab on a stick and a Robert's forceps. The pack should then be removed slowly, gently and progressively. Any persisting bleeding points can then be identified, secured and controlled with the assistant's help. Suction should be used in a purposeful and directed manner to reveal a specific bleeding point or points, which can then be ligated or cauterized, it should not be wiggled haphazardly over raw surfaces, thereby disturbing the natural clotting process.

Think ahead

Working every operating list with the same experienced scrub nurse/sister, who knows your surgical style and idiosyncrasies, is a rare event for many surgeons these days. It is, however, a privilege to work with someone who is poised, watching the surgery, armed with a selection of instruments, and who places the appropriate instrument firmly in your palm sometimes without you needing to ask for it, and certainly without you having to look up from the operative field. When surgery flows with this sort of teamwork, it can be a truly beautiful, even emotional, thing to observe. The reality is that different personnel are involved in different operating lists and the surgery is only able to flow in an uninterrupted fashion if the surgeon plans ahead. It is always worth checking that instruments and sutures of choice are available before the operation starts. Intra-operatively it is worth telling the scrub nurse a minute or two in advance what instruments/sutures/drains, etc. are to be needed imminently. It is only with this degree of forward planning that surgery will fulfil the choreographic requirements alluded to in the opening sentence of this chapter.

It would now be appropriate to examine how some of these principles may be applied to the performance of an abdominal hysterectomy.

Total abdominal hysterectomy and bilateral salpingo-oophorectomy

Incision

Having planned in advance, and discussed with the patient, a decision has been taken to perform a transverse suprapubic incision. The overall size and the exact position of the skin incision is determined on the operating table and is dependent on local anatomy but, in general terms, it should be made approximately two finger breadths above the symphysis pubis and, if possible, below the upper limit of the pubic hairline. This can be modified depending on the presence, for example, of skin creases. It needs to be symmetrical and it is better to cut a straight line rather than to attempt a 'smile'(Fig. 7.1). A bold incision is made through the skin and this is carried on through the subcutaneous fat only in the midline until the rectus sheath is reached. The sheath is then also incised transversely for 3 cm on either side of the midline. In doing this the median raphe and the underlying pyramidalis muscle are exposed (Fig. 7.2). The

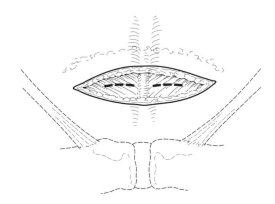

Fig. 7.1 Transverse suprapubic skin incision, rectus sheath to be opened as shown.

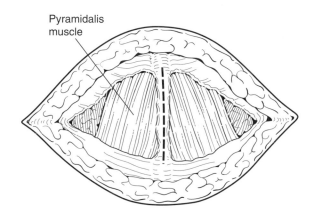

Fig. 7.2 Rectus sheath opened, pyramidalis exposed.

index and middle fingers of the left hand are then hooked under the superior aspect of the cut sheath and the tissues pulled upwards so that they are under tension. The knife is still being held in the right hand and a firm incision is made through the median raphe and the upper aspect of pyramidalis muscle until these fall away to expose the underlying peritoneum. The knife may now be placed in a kidney dish and the incision enlarged by a digital stretch using the index fingers of both hands in both a north–south and east–west direction, taking care laterally not to damage the inferior epigastric vessels which run below the rectus abdominis muscles (Fig. 7.3). The peritoneum is now fully exposed and can be incised in its upper part. This can be achieved safely by a single penetration with a blunt artery forceps or, more traditionally, elevating it away from the bowel with two artery forceps and then making an incision between them with a scalpel. The window in the perito-neum thus made can now be enlarged using curved Mayo scissors. Move your feet, bend your head and incise the peritoneum in a cephalad direction first and then repeat the exercise inferi-orly looking for the end of the translucent area which marks the fundus of the bladder. It will be noted that this modified Cohen technique of opening the abdomen is quick, it is simple, it does not require an extensive undercutting of the rectus sheath and it is associated with relatively little bleeding. At this point, if any vessels require diathermy coagulation, they can be dealt with.

Procedure

On opening the peritoneal cavity, the abdominal contents can be inspected and the patient placed in the Trendelenberg position, and the small and large bowel packed away with moist abdominal packs. A self-retaining retractor, such as a Balfour or a Gosset, is now used to retract the wound edges. A good tip is to use two such retractors placed at right angles to each other, a practice that usually provides excellent exposure of the pelvic organs (Fig. 7.4). The uterus is now grasped by the surgeon's left hand and drawn upwards, and the structures in the left adnexa identified. In particular, the round ligament is noted, running from the cornu of the uterus to the pelvic side wall. In uncomplicated hysterectomies this is of little significance, but when the anatomy is

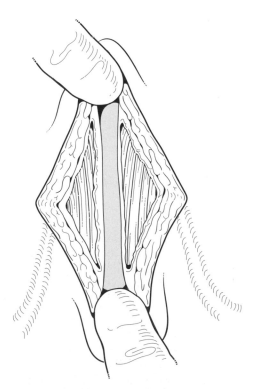

Fig. 7.3 Digital splitting to expose peritoneum.

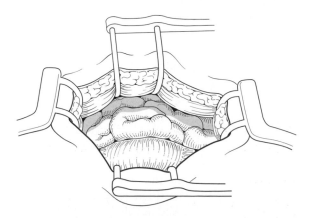

Fig. 7.4 Balfour retractors at 90°.

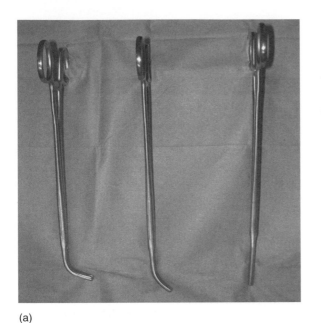

(a)

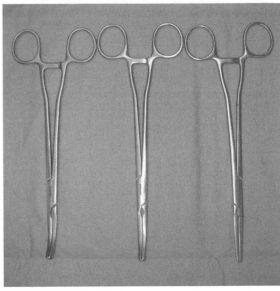

(b)

Fig. 7.5 (a) (b) Straight, semi-curved and fully curved Zeppelin clamps.

distorted by tumours or adhesions or endometriosis the identification of the round ligament is extremely important. In these circumstances, the round ligament is your friend and is a reliable anatomical landmark that will lead you into the correct tissue plane between the leaves of the broad ligament, which, in turn, will allow identification of the ureter, which is important in such difficult operative circumstances.

In a normal hysterectomy, the assistant is requested to draw the structures of the left adnexa laterally, including the round ligament, the Fallopian tube and ovary, and the suspensory ligament of the ovary at the back of the broad ligament. All three of these structures are then grasped by the surgeon, adjacent to the uterus, using a long, straight, heavy tissue forceps (clamp). There are several eponymous versions, such as Howkins, Gwilliams and McCullochs' clamps, but the author prefers currently to use straight Zeppelin clamps for this procedure (Fig. 7.5a, b). Clamp placement is important, and by moving the feet and bending the head a translucent area in the back of the broad ligament can be identified and the tips of the clamp should be aimed at this (Fig. 7.6). A small curved artery forceps is now used to grasp the

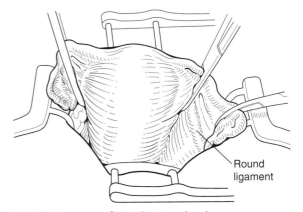

Fig. 7.6 Placement of straight Zeppelin clamps.

round ligament at its mid point and, with instructions to the assistant to elevate the tissue, the surgeon may now boldly and quite safely transect the round ligament under tension with a single bite of the scissors (Fig. 7.7). This definitive incision will lead directly into the broad ligament, the two leaves of which can be separated by splaying the points of the scissors, thereby displaying the areolar tissue contained within. At this point it is the author's preference to use the scissors to open the anterior leaf of the broad ligament infero-medially until the

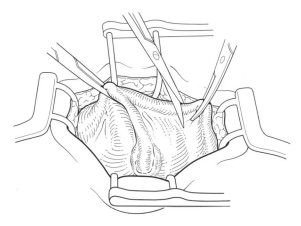

Fig. 7.7 Incising round ligament.

bladder fold of peritoneum is reached. By drawing the Fallopian tube and ovary medially, the infundibulo-pelvic ligament is now placed on the stretch. The posterior leaf of the broad ligament can be incised either digitally or using the scissors, and the pedicle thus formed is now ready to be transected. For this purpose a semi-curved Zeppelin clamp can be used (Fig. 7.8). It should be placed reasonably close to the ovary at a time when these structures are being drawn medially so that there is no possibility of catching the ureter at this point. There is no need to place extra clamps in the wound to deal with back bleeding, and the two pedicles thus formed can be transfixed and ligated using o-Vicryl® sutures and the ends can be cut, unless it is anticipated that further retroperitoneal exploration is necessary, in which case the round ligament

suture can be held in a small artery forceps. This procedure is repeated on the other side.

Although not part of routine practice, if there is any need to identify the path of the ureter in the pelvis, this can now be achieved easily by gently exploring the base of the broad ligament digitally. Both index fingers should be used to separate the areolar tissue gently in a controlled fashion, in a north–south direction medial to the iliac vessels, and in so doing the ureter will appear on the medial side of the surgeon's fingers and the great vessels of the pelvic side wall on the lateral. The technique is usually bloodless, but any small-vessel bleeding encountered can usually be left to nature to deal with, or controlled by localized pressure. The bladder is now deflected inferiorly, the uterovesical fold of peritoneum is elevated using a Robert's forceps placed in the midline—the correct positioning of this clamp is crucial. If it is placed too high or too low, the wrong tissue plane will be entered, the dissection will be hampered, bleeding might ensue, or the bladder itself might be damaged. It is correctly positioned when the assistant is able to 'tent up' the fundus of the bladder (Fig. 7.9). If the surgeon has any doubt as to where the bladder edge starts, it can be palpated digitally, but ordinarily this is not required and a bold incision can now be made through the peritoneum. If the correct tissue plane is entered, the bladder will start to fall away from the front of

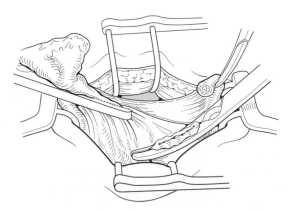

Fig. 7.8 Clamping the infundibulo-pelvic ligament.

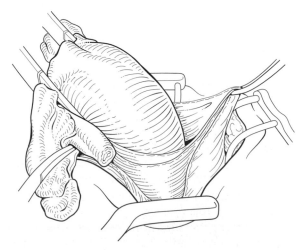

Fig. 7.9 Elevating the utero-vesical fold.

the uterus, and can be further encouraged to do so by gently stroking it inferiorly with the back of the scissors still held in the surgeon's hand. This gives visual reassurance that initial bladder mobilization is occurring; the procedure can be completed with the index finger, either on its own or with a gauze swab rolled around it. The bladder deflection is complete when the bottom of the cervix can be identified and the longitudinal fibres of the vagina become visible. Using the technique described, it is important to achieve adequate bladder deflection, particularly in the region of the vault angles, but it is important not to stray too far laterally as bleeding from bladder veins can be encountered in this area.

The uterine artery pedicles can now be taken, and for this the author chooses to use quite heavy angled Chelsea hysterectomy clamps, and these are placed relatively low at the cervico-uterine junction and can be swivelled to incorporate the upper parts of the uterosacral ligaments posteriorly (Fig. 7.10a, b). It is quite safe to place these clamps at this level, provided the bladder has been thoroughly mobilized previously. The clamps are placed transversely and abut on to the firm tissue of the uterus on either

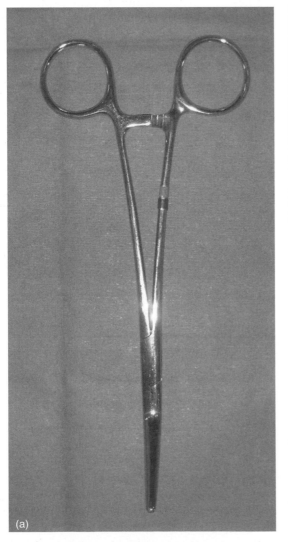

(a)

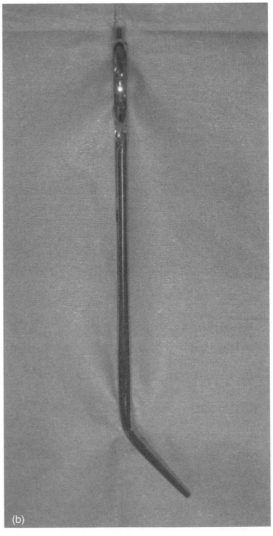

(b)

Fig. 7.10 Angled Chelsea hysterectomy clamps.

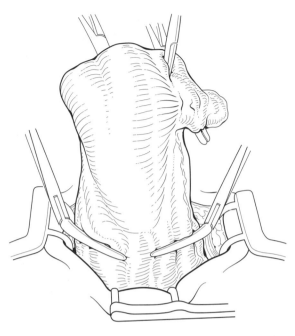

Fig. 7.11 Placement of uterine pedicle clamps (posterior).

side (Figs 7.11 and 7.12). They are then freed using a scalpel until their tips can be swivelled. At this point the author, while acknowledging that it is an unorthodox or idiosyncratic manoeuvre, chooses to hold the uterus forward and run the

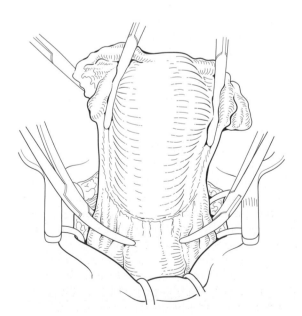

Fig. 7.12 Placement of uterine pedicle clamps (anterior).

knife over the uterosacral ligaments posteriorly, which allows further upward mobilization of the uterus, allowing, in turn, the placement of the next set of clamps below the cervix and above the bladder. The placement is transversely across the vagina, obviating the need to open the vagina itself. The clamps chosen for this are once again angled Chelsea hysterectomy clamps, which can often be placed with their points touching. The vagina can then be transected above these clamps with the scalpel, and the uterus, tubes and ovaries removed. There are now four angled clamps in the incision, and these can be trans-fixed using o-Vicryl® sutures once again. It is the author's practice to transfix the vaginal vault angle clamps at the front and back of the clamp and to hold the sutures, once tied, with small artery forceps, which will allow traction for a final inspection of the vaginal vault. The central part of the vagina can now be closed, either with a mattress suture or a continuous suture, depending on the size of the opening. Some surgeons prefer to leave the central part of the vault open for drainage, in which case the vaginal vault edge can be oversewn to ensure haemostasis. The operative procedure is now complete. However, haemostasis must be secured, and at this point a short pause with pressure being placed on a pelvic pack is probably a judicious move. After a little time this can be slowly and gently removed and, if necessary, any defined bleeding points can be dealt with either by diathermy or directed suturing.

Closure

There is no need to close either the pelvic peritoneum or the parietal peritoneum and the rectus sheath can be closed using a continuous suture of 1-Vicryl®. A suction drain can be placed beneath the rectus sheath and brought out through the skin at a point inferior to the incision, if that is the surgeon's choice, and the skin closure can be effected using a subcuticular suture of something like Monocryl®.

There are, of course, many variations of this operative procedure, but the technique described is simple and is reproducible time after time. It is for surgeons in training to consider it, practise it under supervision and to decide whether it is to their liking or not. Thereafter perhaps parts, if not all, of the moves described may be incorporated into their individual technique.

Operative variations

The problem of the long cervix

Difficulties with the above technique can be encountered either because the cervix is unduly long or because the surgeon has placed the uterine clamps at too high a level. This prevents the placement of the vaginal vault clamps below the cervix. In this circumstance the development of an extra pedicle is required. This is best achieved using straight or semicurved clamps placed vertically along either side of the cervix. These clamps must always be placed medial to the uterine pedicle, thereby ensuring that the ureters will not be caught. It is also important to ensure that the bladder is displaced well below the tips of the clamps before the contained tissue is incised, usually with a scalpel. Following this manoeuvre the cervix will now be accessible and the hysterectomy can be completed as described above. It should be emphasized that the development of this extra pedicle is only rarely required, and with correct clamp placement the three-pedicle technique usually suffices.

Opening the vagina

Some surgeons prefer to open the vagina and transect it under direct vision. Once again it must be ensured that the bladder is mobilized inferiorly, and perhaps protected by a Deaver or a Harrington bladder retractor. The longitudinal fibres of the vagina below the cervix can usually be identified easily, and the anterior vaginal wall can be grasped with Littlewood's forceps in the midline. It is then tented up and incised boldly with a heavy scissors. The aperture thus made can be enlarged by withdrawing the scissors with the points spread. Fully curved Zeppelin clamps can then be applied across the vaginal vault by placing the anterior prong of the clamp inside the vagina and swivelling the clamp in order to allow the posterior prong to grasp the posterior vaginal vault wall. The pedicle thus formed can be transected, the uterus removed and the vaginal vault dealt with as previously described.

The midline incision

In certain clinical circumstances a lower midline incision is the incision of choice. This might be the case if a previous scar exists, or in the presence of large fibroids, and always if ovarian malignancy is suspected. The identification of the midline is often aided by the presence of a faint linea nigra, and the incision can be made, in the case of a right-handed surgeon standing on the patient's right, from below the umbilicus to the level of the pubic bone. The incision is then continued through the subcuticular fat in the midline until the rectus sheath is reached. It is important at this point to discourage the assistant from retracting the wound edge, as this causes distortion and access in the midline is hampered. The operating surgeon should stand back a little, survey the incision, make a judgement as to the position of the midline, and incise the sheath longitudinally in its upper part with a scalpel. If there has been no drifting off the midline, the next tissue to be visualized would be the peritoneum itself or the extraperitoneal fat lying between the two rectus abdominis muscles. If the midline has been lost, the muscle itself will appear. In this circumstance the midline can be regained by grasping the edge of the sheath with two Kocher's forceps placed a few centimetres apart and elevating them, thereby placing the sheath under tension (virtually the only use for these forceps in the whole of gynaecological surgery). While holding the sheath under tension, a scalpel can be gently stroked between the sheath and the underlying muscle until separation is achieved and the peritoneum of the midline becomes visible. The peritoneum should be opened in the upper part of the incision, using either the blunt entrance previously described or by the more traditional method of tenting the peritoneum using artery forceps and incising with a scalpel. The aperture thus made is then enlarged in a cephalad and caudal direction under direct vision with Mayo scissors.

Closure

The generally accepted method of closing a midline incision is a mass closure with a looped non-absorbable suture, such as nylon or PDS®. It is important to take good bites of tissue on either side of the wound, incorporating the rectus sheath, the rectus abdominis muscle and the peritoneum. Sometimes it is helpful to use two separate sutures, starting at the top and the bottom of the wound and tying the knot where they meet in the centre. The knot can either be buried or else the ends cut short so that it is less of a focus of irritation, particularly in the thin patient. The skin can be closed with a subcuticular suture such as Monocryl® or Prolene®, with staples or, less commonly, with interrupted sutures.

Paramedian incisions are not generally employed in current gynaecological surgical practice.

Preoperative measures

Know your patient

It is vitally important to take time to get to know your patient preoperatively. An understanding of her concerns, whether they be centred on the surgery itself, hospitalization in general, a fear of anaesthesia or anxiety regarding the welfare of her family while she is away, is crucial in providing her with comprehensive care. To achieve this, time must be taken at the first consultation, the pre-admission clinic, and the preoperative ward round, to allow for the fullest communication in both directions. Nothing is more important than the patient herself and her well-being. She should be treated with overt kindness and consideration, even if on occasions the circumstances are testing because of the personality involved. It must be remembered that fear and anxiety can present as hostility and anger, characteristics that dissipate rapidly when the relief of the postoperative period is attained.

Consent

Good communication is everything. The patient needs to be given a thorough explanation of the planned operative procedure, including possible intra-operative variations, e.g. laparoscopic surgery proceeding to open surgery; myomectomy proceeding to hysterectomy. The author finds the use of simple diagrams helpful in such preoperative discussions. For many procedures, including hysterectomy, information booklets are available and can be provided. Once again, time must be taken to examine surgical options, e.g. conserving or removing ovaries at the time of hysterectomy. The patient herself might require time to consider issues, such as total or subtotal hysterectomy. The pros and cons of these issues should be explained clearly, and an opportunity for her to discuss possible management options with her husband or partner, or family doctor, must be allowed.

In many ways it is more difficult to be a good doctor now than it was a decade ago. Largely because of the buzz words 'non-directive counselling'. No-one would advocate a 'doctor knows best' attitude, but some patients require help with decision making, and the clinician who is allowed time to get to know the patient will recognize this and respond appropriately. The introduction of clinical governance and emphasis on the identification of bad doctors are laudable, but good doctors should not be constrained in advising and caring for their patient on an individual basis. The concept of informed consent is fully outlined in documents produced by the Department of Health,[2] the Royal College of Obstetricians and Gynaecologists and Chapter 2 of this volume. Fine judgement is often required, again on an individual basis, as to where to draw the line between ensuring that the patient is comprehensively informed about the impending surgical procedure and preventing her becoming terrified by the recitation of a list of all possible complications. It cannot be overemphasized that the time taken to show kindness to patients and to communicate thoroughly preoperatively may prevent all sorts of problems postoperatively.

Appropriate investigations

It is the responsibility of the operative surgeon to ensure that the patient has been adequately assessed preoperatively. Investigations such as haematological and biochemical assessment, cardiological and imaging tests, and blood cross-matching should be undertaken on an individual basis. The results should be known and available prior to commencing surgery.

Deep vein thrombosis prophylaxis

Protocols will vary between hospitals, but the use of subcuticular heparin, elasticated stockings, pneumatic pressure stockings and low molecular weight dextran may all be employed.

Intra-operative measures

Management of complications

The maxim that must be strictly adhered to here is that any surgeon encountering intra-operative difficulties, of whatever nature, should never be afraid to seek help from colleagues.

Bleeding

The basic principles of compression and correcting clotting in diffuse bleeding situations have been addressed earlier in this chapter, and their importance cannot be emphasized too strongly. In this context, a continuous calm dialogue with the anaesthetist is essential. An excellent anecdotal review of this subject was published in the *British Journal of Obstetrics and Gynaecology* in 1998 by Rennie and Cardozo[3] and is worth reading so that message is reinforced.

In the case of a solitary bleeding source such as a slipped pedicle or a laceration to a great vessel in the pelvis, it is important to locate the source of the haemorrhage as accurately as possible. It is easy for the inexperienced surgeon to panic and attempt 'blind' suturing. This rarely helps, frequently makes matters worse, and can cause further damage. Take time to isolate the source of the haemorrhage and control the bleeding point by occluding it with tissue forceps or compression, and then gently suture, cauterize or ligaclip, if possible under direct vision. Ligaclips are useful in this context but they should never be used injudiciously, as, once placed, if they fail to control the bleeding point, they are in the way of further attempts with other clips or sutures.

Viscus damage

Bladder damage

Damage to the bladder wall so that the bladder is entered is usually incurred at the time of mobilization from the lower uterus and cervix during a hysterectomy. The complication is usually recognized at the time. Uncomplicated tears in the fundus of the bladder should be repaired immediately. A check should be made to ensure that the ureteric orifices are not involved, and then the defect can be repaired, usually in a double layer of Vicryl® sutures. An indwelling catheter and antibiotic cover post-operatively for a minimum of 5 days should be employed. Such injuries generally heal well and there are no long-term sequelae. If, however, there is ureteric involvement in the injury, the inexperienced gynaecological surgeon would best be advised to involve the expertise of a senior or urological colleague.

Bowel injury

Damage to both small and large bowel can occur when dense adhesions, secondary to previous surgery, infection or endometriosis, are encountered. If unexpected pathology such as this is encountered, the trainee surgeon should anticipate possible dissection difficulties and ensure adequate senior supervision before any problems occur. Occasionally, even in the most experienced hands, the bowel lumen is opened inadvertently. Again, this is usually recognized at the time of surgery. Small tears in the small bowel with no vascular compromise can simply be closed transversely to avoid luminal stenosis, in two layers using fine Vicryl®. More extensive damage might require segmental resection and either end-to-end or side-to-side anastomosis, achieved by single-layer suturing or a stapling technique. Open damage to the large bowel often requires more difficult intra-operative decision making. Uncomplicated tears in healthy non-irradiated bowel, particularly if the patient has had a preoperative bowel prep, can once again be closed in two layers. In more complicated injuries, any primary repair or resection and re-anastomosis should be protected by a defunc-tioning stoma, which can be closed at a later date. Adequate peritoneal toilet should be prac-tised and antibiotic cover given. The use of drains in this context has diminished in recent years.

Antibiotic cover

There is now good data to indicate that it is advantageous to administer a single dose of a broad-spectrum antibiotic during the intra-operative period, as this tends to have a beneficial effect in reducing morbidity in the postoperative period.

Postoperative measures

First 24 hours

Leave an indwelling catheter in the bladder. It generally does not bother the patient during this time. Indeed, she is usually grateful that she does not have to make trips to the bathroom, manipulating intravenous lines and drains. It also contributes to the assessment of post-operative fluid balance and, in some instances, prevents long-term bladder problems that de-velop secondary to postoperative retention and overdistension.

Traditionally, the introduction of postopera-tive feeding has followed the pattern of sips of fluid only until bowel sounds are present, free fluids only until flatus is passed, and solid food thereafter. The author still persists with this convention but acknowledges that many gastro-intestinal surgeons now permit a far more liberal regimen. The bowel has usually been mani-pulated and packed away during the course of an abdominal hysterectomy, which justifies a cautious approach. Furthermore, it is rare for a patient to have much of an appetite on the first postoperative day, nausea is a far more frequently encountered problem than hunger.

Modern analgesic drugs and techniques are now highly sophisticated and good pain relief should be available for all patients. In many instances patient-controlled analgesia (PCA) is the preferred option, but postoperative anal-gesia should be individualized and planned in conjunction with, and under the direction of, anaesthetic colleagues.

Breathing techniques, calf exercises and the importance of early mobilization will have been explained to the patient preoperatively and the involvement of a physiotherapist to encourage these events is important in the immediate postoperative phase.

Day 2 until discharge on day 7

Transient pyrexia in the first 24 hours post-operatively is often due to a degree of atelectasis and does not require specific therapy. Persisting pyrexia can occur secondary to chest infection, urinary tract infection or wound infection, and it is wise to have a low threshold for commencing antibiotics once the appropriate investigations have been completed.

Paralytic ileus is a worrying event, strangely, more for the attending clinician than for the patient herself in many cases. It is fundamentally important for the clinician to keep his or her nerve in this situation, particularly if the ileus is slow to resolve. It is well to remember that, especially in non-malignant cases, it virtually always will. It is very often sufficient merely to restrict oral feeding and fluids, and there is no initial rush to insert a nasogastric tube, which is an uncomfortable experience for the patient and can often be avoided, particularly if she is not vomiting repeatedly. In the majority of instances it is sufficient to ensure that electrolyte balance is maintained and then merely *wait*.

REFERENCES

1. Monaghan J M (ed) 1986 Bonney's gynaecological surgery, 9th edn. Bailliere Tindall, London
2. Department of Health 2001 Reference guide to consent for examination or treatment. HMSO, London
3. Rennie J, Cardozo L 1998 The Seven Surgeons of King's: A fable by Aesop. British Journal of Obstetrics and Gynaecology 105:1241

The vaginal approach to pelvic surgery

Patrick Hogston

Introduction

Vaginal surgery can achieve the removal of a diseased or dysfunctional uterus, as well as being part of the restoration of structure and function in cases of pelvic organ prolapse. With the reduction in need for hysterectomy for dysfunctional bleeding, due to alternative therapies, it would appear that, at the beginning of the 21st century, surgery for uterovaginal prolapse will become a major part of elective gynaecological surgery. Although one study has suggested that abdominal surgery may give fewer cases of re-operation, the majority of patients will benefit from a vaginal approach using appropriate techniques and suture material. Such surgery should be reconstructive, to restore structure and function, and not destructive. Simply making the vagina smaller is neither the goal nor the purpose of vaginal reconstructive surgery.

Somewhat difficult to learn, and equally difficult to teach, there is concern that the art and skill of vaginal surgery may be lost altogether. Rather than developing an excuse to perform an operation abdominally, the surgeon should develop the reason to perform vaginally—no visible scar, less pain, and a faster recovery and return to normal activities. In some instances, the place of laparoscopy may allow for a vaginal approach, but this still needs to be defined.

History

The first professionally performed vaginal hysterectomy for prolapse was performed by Choppin in New Orleans, USA in 1861. Most operations for prolapse for the next 50 years did not involve hysterectomy, rather some means of constricting the vagina. Progress was made by the description of the Manchester operation of anterior–posterior repair, perineorrhaphy and amputation of the cervix in 1908, some 20 years after it had first been performed. The cervical amputation was largely superseded after 1934 by vaginal hysterectomy, after Heaney's description of a technique still in use today. He also inspired the more widespread use of vaginal hysterectomy for benign disease, which was also reported from centres in Europe.

Pelvic anatomy for the vaginal surgeon

Most doctors learn their anatomy from texts that rely on the study of elderly, often malnourished, female cadavers, which bear little resemblance to the findings at surgery in the healthy younger woman. They rely on a small number of dissections and give little credence to the huge variations in normal found by the surgeon. This leads to the use of unnatural and unphysiological concepts in pelvic reconstruction. Furthermore the findings in the anaesthetized patient are quite different from those in the unanaesthetized, and in the lithotomy position different from those standing upright. Trainee gynaecological surgeons thus need to re-examine and redefine the normal anatomy of the living. Vaginal surgery may be extirpative when only hysterectomy is performed, but more usually reconstructive when something is also required to return abnormal organ relationships to a more usual state. It must be recognized, of course, that many changes leading to prolapse are due to permanent damage to nerves, connective tissue and muscles, and that some correction is compensatory rather than truly reconstructive.

Support of the vagina

There are six different, but interrelated, systems responsible for the support of the vagina. They can be injured or damaged either separately or together, but must be identified individually if restorative surgery is to be achieved successfully. The systems are:

- the bony pelvis to which the soft tissues attach
- the cardinal and uterosacral ligament complex
- the subperitoneal connective tissue
- the urogenital diaphragm, including pubourethral ligaments and endopelvic fascia
- the pelvic diaphragm, pubococcygeus and the levator plate
- the perineum and perineal body.

For many years there were heated debates as to whether the major support to the vagina was suspension from above or support from below by the pelvic floor. Mengert's classic contributions showed that prolapse of the uterus did not occur as long as the upper two-thirds of the parametrial tissues were intact, thus confirming the importance of suspension. However, Bonney[1] emphasized the importance of the pelvic floor in supporting the lower part of the vagina, and these concepts have been developed further by DeLancey.[2] Cadaver dissections consistently show the vagina to be a straight tube extending postero-superiorly to the sacral promontory. Studies in the living provide an impressive demonstration of something quite different. The upper vagina is almost horizontal, pulled into the sacral hollow by the uterosacral ligaments and also compressed against the levator plate (Fig. 8.1). When the uterosacral ligaments fail, the apex of the vagina, with or without the uterus in place, will descend. It has always been taught that this failure is due to attenuation and stretching, and thus that the ligaments should be shortened and reattached to the vagina at hysterectomy. However, it may be that in some, if not all, cases the ligament tears in a similar fashion to ligaments of the knee with traumatic injury. If this is the case, the ligament will be detached from the cervix or vaginal vault and will remain attached to the sacrum. The ligament must be specifically identified in order to reattach it to the vault and give the necessary postoperative support. This will be discussed further below.

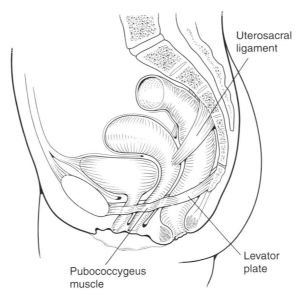

Fig. 8.1 The vaginal axis in the standing position. The vagina is pulled into the sacral hollow by the uterosacral ligaments. It then is compressed by intra-abdominal pressure against the levator plate formed by the fusion of the fibres of pubococcygeus behind the rectum.

Cardinal and uterosacral ligament complex

These ligaments attach to the postero-lateral aspect of the cervix at the level of the internal os and to the lateral vaginal fornices. The ligament runs postero-superiorly and fans out to attach to the sacral fascia opposite the sacro-iliac joint. As well as support, they convey sympathetic and parasympathetic nerves, blood vessels and lymphatics to and from the cervix.

Endopelvic fascia

The vagina is surrounded by endopelvic fascia, which fuses laterally and is then attached to the pelvic sidewall. Anteriorly, the bladder is supported by a layer ill-defined by anatomists but usually easily identified surgically as the pubocervical or pubovesicocervical fascia. It is attached bilaterally to the arcus tendineus fascia pelvis, a line running from the mid pubic symphysis to the ischial spine. In addition, the urethra is suspended by the posterior pubo-urethral ligaments, which themselves attach to the pubic symphysis (Fig. 8.2). Prolapse of the

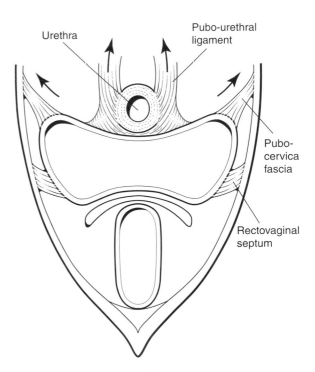

Fig. 8.2 The urethra is suspended by the pubourethral ligaments (central arrows) and supported by the attachments that connect the vagina to the pelvic sidewall (lateral arrows).

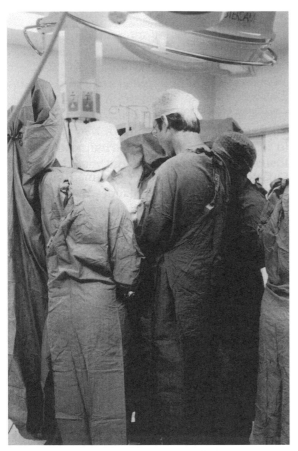

Fig. 8.10 Standing for vaginal surgery allows the surgeon and both assistants better access to the operative field.

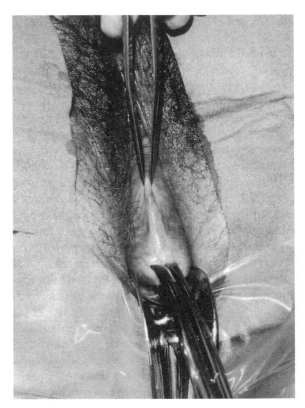

Fig. 8.11 Elevation of the anterior vaginal wall demonstrates the site of the pubocervical ligament.

re-sharpening, so often a scalpel is used, but scissors do give better control and judgement for many surgeons. With the cervix held on traction by tenaculae, the gap between the rugae of the anterior vaginal wall and the smooth cervix is more obvious. Elevation of the anterior vaginal wall will demonstrate the pubocervical ligament and the anterior incision should be at this junction (Fig. 8.11). This may be at some distance from the external os (even 10–15 cm) in women with prolapse and an elongated cervix. The depth of the incision is also critical to entering the correct plane between the bladder and cervix, and therefore needs to be through the full thickness of the vaginal mucosa.

Posteriorly the incision should be at the base of the cul-de-sac. In cases of prolapse, the sac of peritoneum behind the cervix is usually more obvious. There is a characteristic transverse crease where the cervix and vagina fuse and the pouch is 1–2 cm posterior to it. Bleeding tends to be greater the closer the incision is to the external os, whereas the risk of injury to the bladder and rectum will be greater the higher the incision. Care in using landmarks and experience dictates a compromise, both reducing bleeding and avoiding inadvertent injury.

Vaginal dissection and bladder reflection

After incising the vagina, the tenaculae are removed and reapplied to the cut edge to pull the vaginal skin over the cervix. This will help to ensure the dissection is continued in the correct plane. The full thickness of the vaginal skin should be reflected back for a short distance around the cervix. If the cervix is very elongated, this dissection will be more extensive, particularly as the anterior peritoneum may be at a considerable distance from the incision. It is important to fully reflect the bladder from the cervix, and this requires the division of the supravaginal septum. It is preferable to use sharp dissection with the scissors, points down to the cervix, to both cut and push the tissues, rather than using an opened swab, which often leads to unnecessary bleeding and even tearing of the bladder wall. It often helps to identify the bladder by its looseness and the position of the catheter balloon, and the anterior wall is picked up and placed on some tension. This then facilitates the division of the supravaginal septum. It is not necessary to open the peritoneum at this stage and it is usually easier once the uterosacral ligaments have been secured.

Opening the posterior peritoneum

Posteriorly, the peritoneum must be entered before proceeding. The peritoneum should be easily identifiable if the incision has been at the correct level, and can be entered (Fig. 8.12). Some peeling of the vaginal skin from the underlying tissue may be required, particularly with a long cervix. The posterior vaginal skin should be pulled taut and the peritoneum should be visible. If the cul-de-sac is not entered, repeated blind attempts should be avoided as damage to the rectum may result. In the rare case when the peritoneum cannot be entered it is best to start the hysterectomy extraperitoneally and clamp the uterosacral ligament pedicle. An alternative is to cut the posterior lip of the cervix vertically in the midline with heavy scissors, starting at the external os and continuing until the peritoneum is reached and opened from the cervical side. This keeps the incision close to the cervix and well away from the rectum, thus avoiding any damage.

Once opened the cul-de-sac should be explored with a finger to ensure no undue adhesions, mass or scarring. Bleeding from the posterior wall can sometimes be a problem. A locking stitch of peritoneal edge to vagina can be used, although excision of some peritoneum may be necessary later in cases of prolapse.

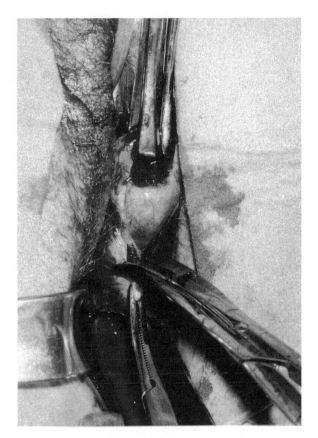

Fig. 8.12 Entry into the pouch of Douglas.

Uterosacral ligament pedicle

The next step is to clamp, cut and tie the uterosacral ligaments. Ideal clamps by Zeppelin™ are shown in Figure 8.13, with the smaller clamps ideal for vaginal hysterectomy. The larger clamps are used for the upper pedicle and for oophorectomy. When placing the clamp, it will be close to the cervix if no prolapse is present, but it is important to identify strong tissue in cases of prolapse. This tissue will then be used to support the vagina at the end of the operation. The ligament is then cut and tied. When suturing, additional space is provided if the cervix is pushed into the pelvis out of the way. When placing the stitches, use flexibility of wrist to follow the needle's curve to ensure smooth passage and avoid laceration of tissues; this is easier if you are standing and can move more freely. A technique of suture ligation such as that

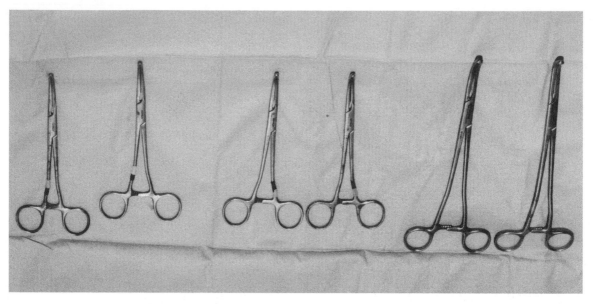

Fig. 8.13 Range of Zeppelin™ clamps suitable for vaginal hysterectomy.

shown in Figure 8.14a is required. A commonly used technique is illustrated in Figure 8.14b. This leaves a small part of the pedicle not ligated and is therefore not recommended. The knots should be tied by the non-dominant hand and the needle guarded at all times. Incorporation of vaginal wall into the uterosacral ligation stitch is useful for support (see later).

Anterior peritoneal entry

The anterior dissection was described above. The peritoneum may already be in view but, in many cases, it is best to take the uterosacral pedicles and then continue with the anterior dissection when some descent has taken place. The bladder is retracted and this pushes the ureter further away and ensures its safety (Fig. 8.15).

Sharp dissection can then be continued by meticulously snipping the fine fibres that bind the connective tissue capsule of the bladder to the cervix. In cases of previous caesarean section this can be easier than at abdominal hysterectomy. The vesico-uterine space will have been

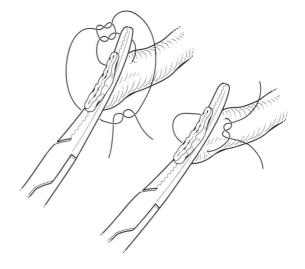

Fig. 8.14 (a) Suitable method of tying the pedicle. (b) A method commonly used but not advised (see text).

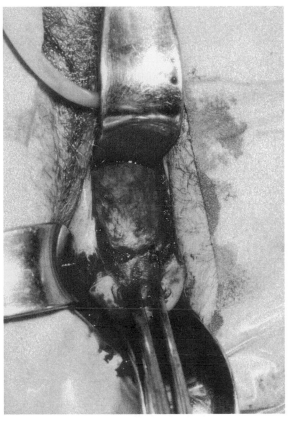

Fig. 8.15 Reflection of the bladder is completed and the peritoneum is in view.

entered as described above, by incising the supravaginal septum. The scar will be in view and can be grasped and the dissection performed above or below it as required. A narrow retractor can elevate the bladder and the uterovesical fold will come into view.

Difficulty in this area is often because the surgeon is too deep, and occurs particularly when the cautious trainee believes he is safer closer to the cervix and fails to divide the supravaginal septum. However, this is a common cause of excess bleeding and is only rectified when a more superficial plane is entered. Use the catheter balloon to delineate the bladder edge and then carefully dissect between the bladder and the cervix and not within the cervix itself. Other manoeuvres include passing a flexible sound through the opened posterior peritoneum around the fundus to identify the

peritoneum, or delivering the fundus posteriorly to allow access to the uterovesical fold.

If the bladder is entered don't panic. Continue the dissection with the bladder open, as the anatomy can be delineated. Once the bladder is free, close the defect, not before. The bladder should be closed in two layers with 2/0 absorbable sutures, and a catheter left in situ for 5–7 days, depending on the size of the laceration. The patient will need to be informed but reassured that the bladder heals very quickly.

It is often necessary to clamp the next portion of the cardinal ligament before reaching the anterior peritoneum. Cutting another pedicle close to the cervix results in further descent of the uterus and this brings the peritoneum with it.

The anterior peritoneum can now be opened, although some wait until after the uterine pedicle is taken. As each pedicle is taken, the cervix and uterus descends closer to the surgeon. It is seen as a glistening layer and, once opened, the retractor is placed into the anterior peritoneal cavity.

Uterine arteries

The next pedicle is taken. This will consist of upper cardinal ligament and the uterine vessels. One clamp only should be used, and both tips should be placed within the peritoneal cavity, i.e. peritoneum to peritoneum. This seals the vessels within the broad ligament. It is obvious that this pedicle must be tied securely as slippage and retraction can result in the need for laparotomy. Once tied, the suture should be cut and not held, lest it is pulled off. Having secured this pedicle, the uterus will normally deliver either anteriorly or posteriorly.

Removal of the uterus

If the uterus will not deliver, or there has not been progressive descent, one should reassess the situation. Is there an unidentified mass, broad ligament or fundal fibroid? Is the uterus bigger than initially thought due to adenomyosis? Are there unidentified adhesions? If the inexperienced has run into trouble—call for help, even if only telephone advice. The options will reflect confidence, experience and the technical ability of the surgeon, but clearly with the patient's best interests first—hence the need always to discuss the possibility of an abdominal incision preoperatively.

In the above situation, the next best option is usually to use a morcellation technique, initially by dividing the uterus (bisection). A further pedicle may be necessary, unless it is certain that the uterine arteries have been taken. When bisecting the uterus, protect the anterior and posterior vaginal walls with retractors and feel behind the uterus to exclude adhesions (Fig. 8.16). If fibroids are present, they can be removed individually to reduce the bulk of the uterus. The final infundibulo-pelvic ligament pedicle can now be clamped, cut and double tied.

Finally check all the pedicles to ensure they are dry and examine the ovaries if they are being retained.

Peritoneal closure

This has been very much part of standard vaginal hysterectomy. One reason was that the pedicles were exteriorized from the peritoneal cavity, so that if they slipped postoperatively any bleeding

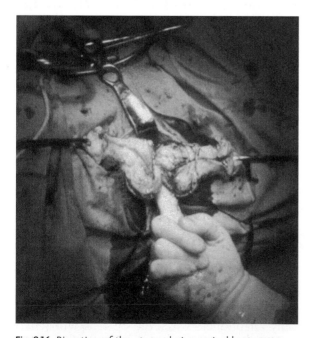

would be via the vagina and not silently into the abdomen. It is realized that closure of the peritoneum at abdominal hysterectomy is unnecessary and possibly increases risk of ureteric damage. The same applies in vaginal hysterectomy and closure can be very difficult. Furthermore, placing the stitches may result in bleeding which is more difficult to deal with. It is therefore preferable to ensure good knot tying, check the pedicles, and not close the peritoneum as a separate layer. It is possible to incorporate the peritoneum in the closure of the vaginal skin, which can be useful to reduce bleeding, especially from the posterior wall.

Support of the vaginal vault

The round ligaments play no part in the support of the uterus and hence using these ligaments to support the vault after hysterectomy has no anatomical basis. Furthermore, such a manoeuvre may pull the vault anteriorly when it needs to go posteriorly. Obliteration of cul-de-sac is standard and anatomically sensible, despite the lack of good evidence of its benefit.

Many traditional texts describe using the already tied uterosacral ligament pedicles to then support the vault, often by approximating them in the midline. These sutures should not be tied in the midline, as it puts unnatural strain on both the ligaments and the sutures, and the ligaments do not join in the midline in the normal woman. In cases without prolapse one should consider what happens at abdominal hysterectomy. Here the uterosacral ligaments are incorporated into the vaginal vault, since they are usually clamped with the vaginal angles and the suture ensures that the vagina remains attached to the ligament. In vaginal hysterectomy the uterosacral ligament may have been separated from the vagina prior to clamping, or was already separate before surgery, and therefore needs to be reattached. This can be done by ensuring that the vaginal closure stitch incorporates the uterosacral ligament. In cases of prolapse, one should not rely on rapidly absorbable sutures, and a separate delayed absorbable is suggested. The original description of McCall[6] used silk, and although support was good, there were problems

Fig. 8.16 Bisection of the uterus during vaginal hysterectomy.

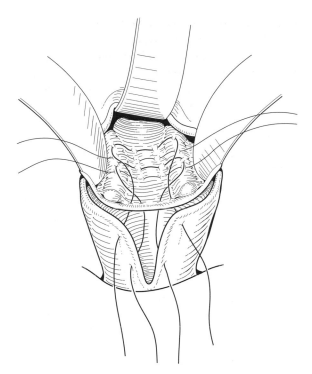

Fig. 8.17 Support of the vaginal vault using McCall's culdoplasty. A separate stitch incorporates the vaginal wall, peritoneum and the uterosacral ligaments.

with suture erosions. He described tying the sutures together to give a shelf of support (Fig. 8.17) and there is good evidence for this technique,[7] despite it not being truly anatomical.

Advanced and alternative techniques

Vaginal oophorectomy

Traditionally in the UK the ovaries are not removed at vaginal hysterectomy. When performed for prolapse in postmenopausal women, the ovaries are usually small and often difficult to access. In premenopausal women the consideration of oophorectomy should be discussed, as it can often be achieved safely. The technique may be salpingo-oophorectomy after clamping the infundibulo-pelvic ligament, or oophorectomy by clamping the ovarian ligament only. One side can be made easier by doing this while still attached to the uterus.

Morcellation

Occasionally other techniques to reduce the bulk of the uterus will make delivery easier. Bisection has been discussed, but myomectomy and simply cutting parts of the uterus away to decrease bulk will help.

Much of surgery is rediscovered from generation to generation, and no more so than in vaginal hysterectomy. Clamps were only used routinely from the early 20th century. In cases of limited access, clamps can be dispensed with until the uterine arteries are ready to be taken. Using infiltration, the uterosacral and cardinal ligaments can be cut with scissors or cutting diathermy, as they are not very vascular. They remain attached to the vaginal skin and hence are easily secured, if necessary, later. This allows the uterus to descend until the uterine arteries are accessible to clamps.

Reconstructive surgery

The support of the vaginal vault described above is one form of vaginal reconstruction, and this must be carried out when the hysterectomy is performed for prolapse. Good support of the vaginal vault is essential to cure the patient's symptoms, as vault descent is nearly always symptomatic. Women with symptomatic uterine prolapse usually have some degree of bladder descent, as the bladder is attached to the cervix. Support of the vault alone may be sufficient, but often an anterior repair is also required.

Cystocoele

The use of the term 'anterior repair' is often used synonymously with cystocoele repair. Nichols and Randall[3] describe two types of cystocoele—namely distension and displacement. The former refers to that due to ligament stretching, the latter due to disruption of the ligament attachments to the pelvic sidewall. Alternatively, distension cystocoele may refer to central defects and displacement due to lateral or paravaginal defects (see p. 114). In the former, the vaginal rugae are lost and the vaginal mucosa thin, whereas in the latter the rugae are maintained. Furthermore, in the latter case supporting the central prolapse will still reveal lack of support of the lateral sulci. Clearly, both types can occur together, although the prevalence of each has not been reported. In the UK paravaginal repairs are rarely undertaken, and there are few data to show how successful cystocoele repair is. Whether this has led to a higher failure rate than in the USA is not entirely clear. A central repair of a paravaginal defect may still compensate enough to give the patient symptomatic improvement, even if the anatomic defect has not been corrected. However, in cases of recurrent cystocoele it is essential to assess for a paravaginal defect.

When considering an anterior repair, it is important to consider the history, particularly the urinary symptoms (if any) and the examination findings of coexistent prolapse. The supports of the urethra are usually stronger than those of the bladder, and hence urethral prolapse is less common. However, when bladder prolapse is complete, the urethra becomes kinked at the junction with the bladder. This can mask the presence of stress incontinence (occult stress incontinence, see below).

Repair of an asymptomatic cystocoele is not indicated unless it is part of a vault repair. Vault prolapse, including uterine prolapse, is usually associated with cystocoele and it is traditional to repair it at the same time as the hysterectomy and vault support. While there are no surgical trials of repair versus no repair of cystocoele in these circumstances, there is no good reason to go against traditional teaching. The procedure is relatively simple, with minimal morbidity, and adds little more than 20 minutes or so in experienced hands. Patients with symptomatic, urodynamically proven, genuine stress incontinence may be treated at the same time. This can be by vaginal urethropexy and bladder neck support, colposuspension or tension-free vaginal tape (TVT).

Occult urinary stress incontinence

Occult urinary stress incontinence, or genuine stress incontinence (GSI), refers to a patient who is clinically dry but only because her stress incontinence is masked by urethral kinking that has resulted from a large prolapse. If this kinking

is simply eliminated at surgery by treatment of the prolapse, the stress incontinence will then become apparent. Such patients may demonstrate incontinence of urine if the prolapse is digitally reduced or held by a pessary. Urodynamic studies are difficult to perform in this situation, and hence a preoperative diagnosis is often difficult to make. Furthermore, there is little evidence to show whether such patients should have an anti-incontinence procedure at the same time as a repair, and, if so, which one. Not all patients with stress incontinence need, or want, an operation; anti-incontinence surgery has a definite complication rate and, if it fails, subsequent surgery has a higher failure rate. The only randomized study shows a similar rate of stress incontinence (approximately 8%) whether an anti-incontinence procedure is carried out or not, but a higher rate of complications if it is. There are no satisfactory studies to indicate what investigations should be carried out and how, nor if an operation is chosen, what that should be. On that basis, in the majority of cases no treatment for occult stress incontinence should be carried out at the time of a vaginal repair. Patients should be reassessed when back to normal activities. Such a two-stage approach is particularly feasible with the advent of tension-free vaginal tape (TVT), a day-case procedure.

Technique of cystocoele repair

In the majority of cases, a vaginal hysterectomy will have just been completed. It is therefore quite simple to continue the anterior wall incision to the level of the bladder neck. It is not necessary to continue this along the urethra unless there is a significant urethrocoele. Urethral dissection has been shown to adversely affect pudendal nerve function. There is no evidence to support urethral buttressing as a preventative measure, nor is it an effective treatment for stress incontinence.

With chronic cystocoeles, the vaginal wall may be oedematous and fibrosed, and bleeding can be significant. The surgeon should aim to enter the vesicovaginal space by sharp dissection at the earliest opportunity, as it is more difficult if the initial dissection is in the wrong plane. The anterior wall should be placed on tension using tissue forceps. The avascular space begins where the fusion of the vaginal wall and cervix ends. Thus, when a hysterectomy has been performed, the space will already have been found. If not done, the vaginal skin above the cervix should be grasped and an incision made. The full thickness of the vagina should be incised perpendicular to the axis of the cervix to expose the space. Allis clamps can then grasp the skin edge and the incision continued to the urethrovesical junction, where it ends. The flaps are dissected against a finger placed outside the vaginal skin to act as counter pressure. This separates the full thickness of the vagina from the bladder laterally. In cases of previous hysterectomy, it is important to do this posteriorly as well. The dissection may be as far as the pubic rami if the fascia is detached in a paravaginal defect. The musculoconnective tissue of the pubocervical fascia should then be apparent, as it has been dissected from the vaginal epithelium. Any separation must be done with care to avoid damage to the blood supply.

The first step in correction is to plicate the fibromuscular connective tissue of the bladder with 2/0 delayed absorbable sutures such as polydioxanone (PDS®) or polyglyconate (Maxon®). With large cystocoeles this can be done in two, or even three, layers and corrects the ballooning. The upper stitch should be at the level of the bladder neck and will correct any urethral funnelling. The pubocervical fascia should then be plicated or approximated using delayed absorbable sutures.

The vagina is then closed. If closing a hysterectomy as well, the McCall sutures are tied at the end of the procedure and the vault is elevated.

Urethral support

The urethra is suspended from the pubic bone by the anterior and posterior pubo-urethral ligaments. In severe cases of prolapse, the urethra may lose its support and many textbooks teach the routine use of pubo-urethral ligament plication to prevent postoperative stress incontinence. As indicated above, there are few data to support this manoeuvre and it is not recommended. In patients with symptomatic stress incontinence, the choice lies between pubo-urethral ligament

plication, colposuspension or TVT. It is generally accepted that vaginal repair techniques have a higher failure rate than retropubic bladder neck suspension, although the morbidity of the latter is considerably higher. TVT may be the answer, although it is important to have a bridge of skin between the urethra and the rest of the anterior wall to prevent slippage of the tape.

Paravaginal repair

This is included for completeness, but is not a widely accepted technique in the UK and should not be undertaken without suitable experience in vaginal surgery. It can also be performed by laparotomy or laparoscopy. A paravaginal defect occurs when the fascia has become detached from the white line (see above). Central plication of the fascia will not cure the anatomical defect. After completing the dissection, access to the retropubic space will be available and the pubis and ischial spine will be the landmarks. Four permanent sutures, such as Gore-Tex™ or polyamide, are inserted into the white line from the level of the retropubis, to the ischial spine, with one stitch at the urethrovesical junction. The sutures are then inserted into the fascia of the vaginal flap and the vagina closed. The sutures are then tied to approximate the vagina to the white line.

Use of mesh

In the case of recurrent hernias, general surgeons will use artificial material to good effect. In the case of vaginal prolapse, concern with rejection and excess fibrosis in women wishing to be sexually active have warned against its use. A new alternative of collagen-based biomaterial from the porcine small bowel is available and may act as a graft, allowing remodelling and eventual replacement by host tissue.

Rectocoele and defects of the perineal body

It is important to appreciate that the normal vaginal axis is almost vertical in the lower third   127 and almost horizontal in its upper two-thirds. It is not always easy to appreciate this in the anaesthetized patient in the lithotomy position. The uterosacral ligament suspends the upper vagina postero-superiorly into the hollow of the sacrum. This support is then continuous through the rectovaginal septum to the perineal body and levator plate. On examination in theatre, the vault and perineal body should move together—if not, part of this complex has broken.

The rectovaginal septum is an important structure, as described above. Many never recognize it because it forms the anterior border of the rectovaginal space, i.e. on the vaginal side, and many surgeons, once they have entered the space, only concentrate on the anterior wall of the rectum.

Defects in this septum can occur in a variety of locations and are usually, but not always, associated with defects in the perineal body. The most common type seen at surgery is thus in the lower vagina, associated with detachment from a damaged perineal body. However, lateral detachments can also occur and are recognized preoperatively when the mucosal rugae are maintained.

The perineal body is the cornerstone of vaginal support and is often damaged in women who complain of prolapse. In association with a weakened levator plate, the genital hiatus widens. This lack of support will make the development of future prolapse more likely.

Posterior repair and colpoperineorrhaphy

The terminology used is often somewhat confusing. Colporrhaphy refers to repair of the vaginal wall and can therefore be anterior or posterior. Perineorrhaphy refers to repair of the perineal body, and in cases where a posterior colporrhaphy is performed at the same time, the term (posterior) colpoperineorrhaphy is used. It is important to recognize that repair of rectocoele and repair of the perineum are separate operations, and although patients often need both, this is by no means universal. It should decided before the operation what is required, as under

anaesthesia, particularly regional, the laxity may seem more than it really is and lead to over-correction. Before scrubbing a careful examination will concentrate the surgeon's mind on to what procedure he or she is going to perform. Often a combined rectal examination will demonstrate how the only tissue between vagina and rectum is the anal sphincter and skin, and that the perineal body is totally destroyed. Extensive dissection will thus be required to identify perineal muscle and rectovaginal septum.

It is important to decide carefully on the incision before going ahead. Two tissue forceps, such as Littlewoods, should be placed on the mucocutaneous border and then approximated to give a three-finger introitus (Fig. 8.18). This will indicate how the introitus should look at the completion of the operation.

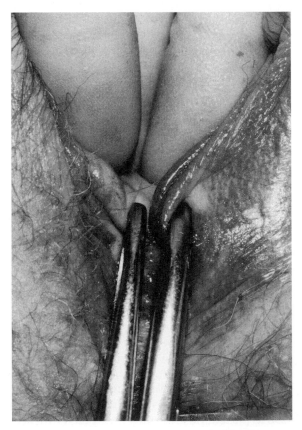

Fig. 8.18 Definition of the introitus as three fingers' diameter at the start of a posterior repair.

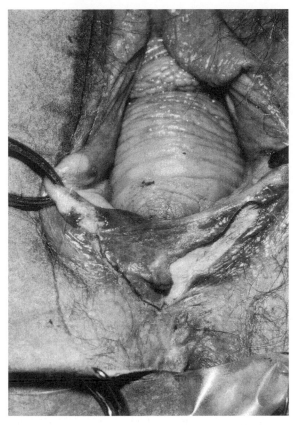

Fig. 8.19 Initial perineal incision. Note rugosity of rectocoele, suggesting a paravaginal defect.

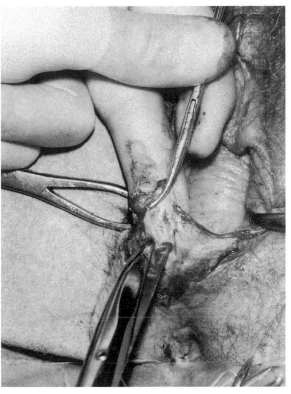

Fig. 8.20 Dissection against the surgeon's finger helps delineate the correct plane.

There are several different ways to make the incision and approach the dissection. In most cases, if perineorrhaphy is to be performed, an incision in the shape of an inverted isosceles triangle is made (Fig. 8.19). This should then be dissected as a flap, with a tissue forcep holding the skin. The surgeon can then dissect against this flap placed on tension and with his finger on the other side (Fig. 8.20). Using scissors, the internal surface of the posterior vaginal wall can be stripped of all tissue. Pressing the scissor tips against the counter pressure of the index finger of the other hand gives the surgeon more confidence to proceed steadily and avoids button-holing of the vaginal skin. Much of the dissection can proceed with the posterior vaginal wall intact, allowing a clean dissection. It also prevents

the surgeon from excising skin at the beginning of the operation. The alternatives described include finding the rectovaginal space and inserting the scissors underneath the vaginal skin to separate it from the vagina (Fig. 8.21). Care is required because if the plane is incorrectly identified at the outset, more dissection is carried out incorrectly than with the other techniques. The other alternative is to incise the posterior vaginal wall with a scalpel and then reflect back the vaginal skin, as shown, in similar fashion to that described above for the anterior wall (Fig. 8.22).

In cases of a low rectocoele, the dissection will not need to progress past the lower third of the vagina, as the defect in the rectovaginal septum will now be visible. If, however, there is a

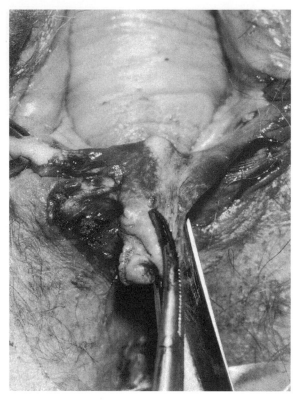

Fig. 8.21 Using Mayo scissors to tunnel under the vaginal skin.

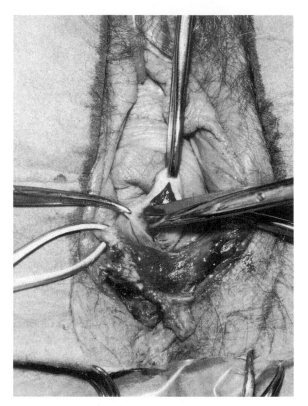

Fig. 8.22 An incision in the vaginal wall has been made and the skin reflected.

full-length rectocoele, or if sacrospinous fixation is going to be performed, then dissection will continue to the apex.

Rectal examination is advisable to demonstrate how close the rectum is, and should not be regarded as an admission of failure. It is a useful adjunct to defining where the surgeon is.

Excision of the vaginal mucosa

In cases of prolapse the vaginal mucosa is displaced and, although a minor amount of stretching may occur, it is wrong to excise large amounts of skin. This results in shortening of the vagina, a poor functional result and a risk of future prolapse due to distortion of the vaginal axis. A short vagina cannot be compressed against the levator plate, but rather tends to telescope and lead to inversion. Narrowing a wide introitus will lengthen the vagina, as this will convert width into length. In patients with a

shortened vagina, a way to gain vaginal length is by using a Z-plasty incision, whereby the incision is staggered and, when sutured, adds significant length (Fig. 8.23).

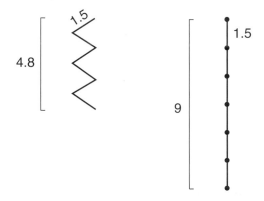

Fig. 8.23 An illustration of how a Z-incision will result in almost doubling of the length of the vagina.

Repair of rectocoele

By cleaning the vaginal mucosa of all tissue, it is possible to execute a thorough repair over the rectum. In many cases, ballooning of the rectal wall—a result of the rectocoele, and not the cause—may be reduced by one or more layers of 2/0 absorbable suture. The repair of the rectovaginal septum can be effected in two ways.[3]

Goff's classic posterior repair leaves the rectovaginal septum attached to the skin. This is only possible if the dissection has left the septum attached to the vagina. The surgeon excises a wedge of the posterior vaginal wall and then approximates the cut edges of the united skin and rectovaginal septum.

In Bullard's modification, the rectovaginal septum is separated and sutured as a separate

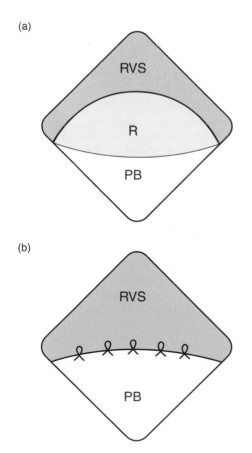

(a)

(b)

Fig. 8.24 (a) A low rectocoele (R) due to detachment of the rectovaginal septum (RVS) from the perineal body (PB). (b) Repair using interrupted sutures.

layer. This is particularly useful for low rectocoeles where the rectovaginal septum has become detached from the perineal body (Fig. 8.24). With lateral defects the dissection must continue laterally until the attachment of levator ani to the pelvic side wall is reached. The rectovaginal septum can then be reattached to the pelvic side wall.

In primary cases, with an isolated defect in the rectovaginal septum, delayed absorbable suture is reasonable, although many will still use rapidly absorbable sutures such as polyglycolic acid (Dexon®). In larger defects or when a concomitant sacrospinous fixation is required, then 0-calibre polyglyconate (Maxon®) or polydioxanone (PDS®) is recommended There are some data on the use of fine permanent sutures, but, until more data are available, permanent sutures should be reserved for recurrent cases.

For large posterior defects, start at the apex, depressing the rectum with the index finger of the other hand. The surgeon should ensure that the bite of tissue taken is sound by testing each time. One should not include levator muscle in these suture bites, as they do not belong in front of the vagina, except at the level of the perineal body. Regular checks to avoid excess narrowing of the vagina are recommended.

Perineorrhaphy

Historically this was performed so that the patient could retain a pessary. Damage to the perineum occurs at childbirth and persists either due to poor technique at primary repair or because the rapidly absorbable sutures commonly used do not allow sufficient healing. Sutures such as polyglycolic acid (Dexon®) lose their strength within 2 weeks, inadequate for sufficient healing of muscle and fascia.

The V-shaped incision allows better access to the perineal body. Often considerable scar tissue has to be mobilized by sharp dissection. The approaches to the dissection have been described above. In addition, the dissection can be done laterally against a finger in the lateral sulcus and the midline separation left until last. This is useful for recurrent cases when dissection is necessarily extensive. Bleeding can be troublesome in the area of scarring, and suction/irrigation can be useful. Higher up, bleeding is rarely a problem. Because of the relationship of the rectovaginal septum to the vagina, if separated fully the remaining vaginal skin will be thin.

Damage to bladder or bowel

During the course of the dissection, button-holing may occur. If in the midline, this can be incorporated in the incision, whereas laterally it can be sutured, or, if small, simply ignored.

Inadvertent rectal entry calls for adequate lavage to keep the area clean. The dissection should then be completed using this as a guide to prevent further entry. Only once the dissection has been complete should the defect be closed. This can be done in the traditional two layers of rapidly absorbable sutures to the mucosa and delayed absorbable sutures to the muscularis (Fig. 8.25).

Sacrospinous fixation

Although not a procedure for novice surgeons, an understanding of this will help them to recognize when such a procedure is necessary. Post-hysterectomy vault prolapse requires a technique to resuspend the apex of the vagina. If the utero-sacral ligaments can be identified, then a McCall's culdeplasty can be performed. In many cases, the ligament cannot be found as it has retracted back against the sacrum, or has atrophied. The sacrospinous ligament can be used to suspend the vault. After opening the posterior vaginal wall, the right pararectal pillar is opened to reach the pararectal space. The sacrospinous ligament is identified as a fan-shaped structure running backwards from the ischial spine. Two sutures are inserted into the ligament two fingerbreadths from the spine, thus avoiding the pudendal nerves and vessels running behind it. The sutures are then inserted into the vagina and tied after any rectocoele has been repaired and the upper vaginal wall closed. The vagina is then pulled into the hollow of the sacrum.

Postoperative care

General care of the postoperative patient is standard, but aspects of nursing care are critical. It is important to keep older patients warm, as this is cardio protective. Care ranges from sitting patients up early to improve pulmonary ventilation, to ensuring that spectacles and hearing aids are used as soon as possible to avoid sensory deprivation. Other aspects of nursing older patients include careful fluid balance and careful use of analgesics, as both narcotics and non-steroidal anti-inflammatory drugs have narrowed therapeutic ratios.

A catheter may not always be necessary in women who undergo hysterectomy in isolation. If a repair is performed at the same time, it is common to use a catheter, and an indwelling catheter for 24 or 48 hours should be sufficient. If a specific anti-incontinence procedure has been performed, many would opt for a suprapubic catheter. The alternative would be for a short period of an indwelling catheter followed by intermittent clean self-catheterization as required.

The use of a pack is common after repair surgery to act as a tamponade in view of the often extensive dissection undertaken. They are usually removed the next day. Patients find them very uncomfortable and adequate analgesia must be provided. There has never been a trial of using or not using a pack after repair surgery.

Early mobilization should be encouraged and one of the advantages of vaginal surgery is that such mobilization is much easier and discharge home quicker. With earlier discharge, it is important that patients know who to contact if they need advice or if they need to be seen again at short notice.

Fig. 8.25 What to do if you enter the bladder or bowel

- Don't panic
- Copious lavage if bowel opened
- Complete the dissection
- Close in two layers
- Use a catheter if bladder injury
- Document in the notes
- Inform patient the next day and discuss again prior to discharge

Conclusions

Vaginal surgery defines the gynaecologists separately from other branches of surgery. Trainees often lack exposure to vaginal surgery, due to an overall reduction in the prevalence of major gynaecological surgery, the reduction in training time and a traditional emphasis on abdominal surgery. However, with efficient training programmes and more structure to the teaching of vaginal surgery, opportunities should be readily available for those trainees wishing to learn.

REFERENCES

1. Bonney V 1924 The principles that should underlie all operations for prolapse. Journal of Obstetrics and Gynaecology of the British Empire 41:669–683
2. DeLancey J O L 1992 Anatomic aspects of vaginal eversion after hysterectomy. American Journal of Obstetrics and Gynecology 166:1717–1728
3. Nichols D H, Randall C L 1994 Vaginal surgery, 4th edn. Williams and Wilkins, Baltimore
4. Hofmeister F J, Wilfgram R C 1962 Methods of demonstrating measurement relationships between vaginal hysterectomy ligatures and the ureters. Americal Journal of Obstetrics and Gynecology 83:938–942
5. Kammerer-Doak D N, Rogers R, Maybach J J et al 2001 Vasopressin as an etiologic agent for infection in gynaecologic surgery: a randomised double-blind placebo controlled trial. American Journal of Obstetrics and Gynecology 185:1344–1348
6. McCall M L 1957 Posterior culdeplasty: surgical correction of enterocoele during vaginal hysterectomy: a preliminary report. American Journal of Obstetrics and Gynecology 10:595–597
7. Webb M J, Aronson M P, Ferguson L K et al 1998 Post hysterectomy vaginal vault prolapse: primary repair in 693 patients. Obstetrics and Gynaecology 92:281–285

FURTHER READING

Grody M H T 1995 Benign postreproductive gynaecologic surgery. McGraw Hill, New York

Hogston P 2001 Suture choice in general gynaecological surgery. The Obstetrician and Gynaecologist 3:127–131

Hogston P 2002 Uterovaginal prolapse. In: Pemberton J, Swash M, Henry M M (eds) The pelvic floor. W B Saunders, London, pp 251–264

Sheth S, Studd J 2002 Vaginal hysterectomy. Martin Dunitz, London

Ulmstein U, Henriksson L, Johnson P, Varhos G 1996 An ambulatory surgical procedure under local anaesthesia for treatment of female urinary incontinence. International Urogynecology Journal 7:133–137

Minimal access surgery: the laparoscope

CHAPTER

9

Janice Rymer

Diagnostic laparoscopy

Diagnostic laparoscopy has been used by gynaecologists for decades, but it is only recently that more complicated procedures have been undertaken through the laparoscope. The benefits to the patients are: smaller scars, less pain, fewer intra-abdominal adhesions and quicker convalescence. Health care providers are also attracted to minimal access surgery (MAS) because of increased potential for day-case procedures or short-stay surgery. However, it does mean that the health case providers have to provide major capital investment for equipment and training. Shifting to MAS also has significant effects on the roles of day-surgery staff and carers in the community.

The major reason why laparoscopic procedures moved forward so swiftly was the micro-miniaturization of television cameras. Prior to this, gynaecologists looked directly down the eyepiece of the laparoscope, which meant they only had one hand with which to manipulate instruments. Positioning for this technique was also very awkward. Now that a lightweight chip camera displays the video on a video monitor, the surgeon has two hands free to perform more sophisticated operations. Unfortunately, some zealots have proceeded without concentrating on safety, which is paramount, particularly with new procedures.

Indications

Diagnostic laparoscopy is an important tool in the evaluation of acute or chronic pelvic pain (Figs 9.1, 9.2). Ectopic pregnancy, pelvic inflammatory disease, endometriosis, adnexal torsion

135

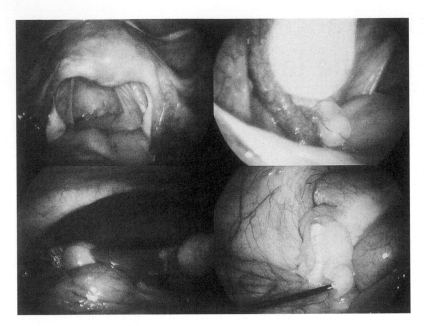

Fig. 9.1 At a diagnostic laparoscopy it is essential to inspect all surfaces carefully. The uterus, tubes and ovaries must be manipulated so that all surfaces are seen. The liver and appendix should also be inspected.

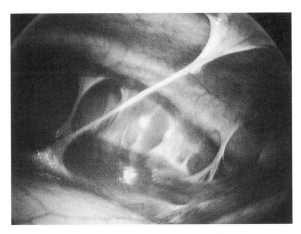

Fig. 9.2 The liver showing perihepatic adhesions indicating pelvic inflammatory disease (FitzHugh Curtis syndrome).

and other intrapelvic pathology can be diagnosed in a timely manner with the use of the laparoscope, and in many of these diseased states therapeutic procedures can be performed at the same time. Operations suitable for the laparoscopic approach are:

- tubal sterilization
- assisted reproduction procedures
- ovarian drilling
- adhesiolysis
- endometriosis, ablation or excision (Fig. 9.3)
- uterosacral ligament transection
- tuboplasty, fimbrioplasty, neosalpingostomy
- salpingotomy
- salpingectomy (for ectopic pregnancies)
- ovarian cystectomy
- salpingo-oophorectomy
- myomectomy
- hysterectomy with combined vaginal approach
- colposuspension and sacrocolpopexy (Fig. 9.4)
- presacral neurectomy
- pelvic lymphadenectomy
- radical hysterectomy
- pelvic floor repair.

Safety depends on:

- appropriate patient selection
- good visibility
- gentle instrument and tissue handling
- effective control of bleeding
- good equipment.

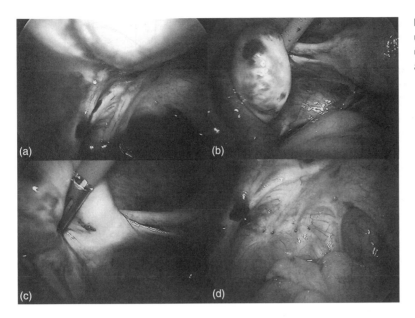

Fig. 9.3 Endometriosis (a) on the underside of the ovary, (b) on the uterus, (c) on the uterosacral ligaments and (d) in the pouch of Douglas.

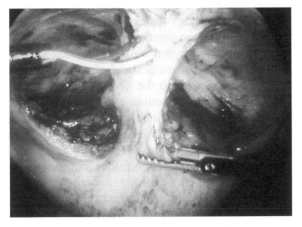

Fig. 9.4 Laparoscopic colposuspension showing dissection through the peritoneum into the Cave of Retzius.

Preoperative measures

Most units will arrange for the patient to have a pre-admission appointment, where it is essential that the following are ascertained:

- Is the operation the correct operation? Depending on the length of waiting lists, the situation may have changed for the patient and the operation may no longer be appropriate.
- Is the patient fit for day-case anaesthesia? Most units have quite specific requirements for deciding who is, and who is not, suitable for day-case anaesthesia and surgery.
- Is the patient in the best physical condition for the planned operation? This is a good opportunity for health counselling, and in particular targeting smoking and obesity.

The pre-admission visit should also highlight any features that might make surgery or recovery difficult—at this stage it is important to ensure that the patient appreciates that an open procedure may be necessary.

Contra-indications to laparoscopy

Contra-indications to diagnostic and operative laparoscopy include: bowel obstruction, ileus, peritonitis, intraperitoneal haemorrhage, diaphragmatic hernia and severe cardiorespiratory disease. The first three contra-indications have the unacceptably high risk of bowel perforation in patients with distended bowel. Although

137

filmy adhesions. Traction placed on an adhesion during stabilization of the involved structures can cause separation. Virtually any sort of laparoscopic instruments can be used. If bleeding occurs, the method should be stopped and electrosurgery or laser used instead.

Sharp dissection is used for thicker adhesive bands and for adhesions involving the bowel (Fig. 9.7). Microbipolar forceps are used if bleeding occurs.

The suction-irrigator can be used for blunt dissection and also as a form of aquadissection (Fig. 9.8). The hydraulic pressure is used to create tissue planes by the path of least resistance. Once an opening is made, the fluid can expand the space rapidly and safely. It can also separate filmy adhesions.

Electrosurgery is used in laparoscopy for coagulation and dissection. With a fine needle, adhesions can be lysed. The unpredictable nature of current arcing makes unipolar coagulation unwise around the bowel and ureter.

It is essential that all surgeons fully understand the principles of diathermy and are completely familiar with the settings of their machines. In unipolar diathermy the surgeon uses an active electrode with a small surface area tip to concentrate a powerful current, producing heat, at the operative site. The large return electrode plate, which completes the circuit, spreads the current over a wide area so it is less concentrated and it produces little heat (the power density is low). Therefore the current must return

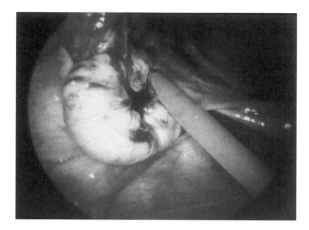

Fig. 9.8 Suction irrigation being used on an endometrioma.

to the ground electrode through the entire body, thereby risking arcing. With bipolar diathermy, the current goes between the jaws of the forceps, a lower voltage is used and there is decreased surrounding thermal damage to the tissue; thus bipolar diathermy is much safer (Fig. 9.9).

Laser dissection can be positioned with accuracy. It is useful as cutting and coagulation can be done in one single step.

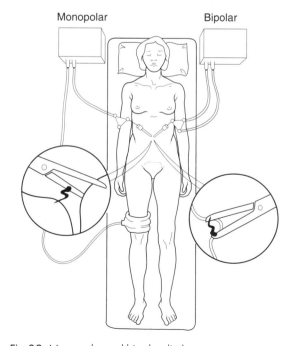

Fig. 9.9 Monopolar and bipolar diathermy.

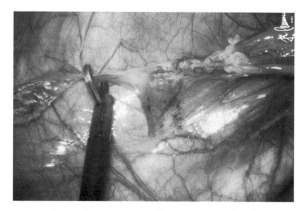

Fig. 9.7 Sharp dissection of adhesions on the left lateral pelvic wall.

At the end of the procedure all ports must be removed under direct laparoscopic vision, to ensure that there is no bleeding from the trocar insertion site. The final port should be removed slowly with the laparoscope inside the port, to ensure that there is no bleeding. The ports must be closed with sutures, glue or Steri-strips®. If the port is larger than 5 mm, the sheath should be formally closed. Hernias may develop if this is not done.

Complications

Probably the most common complication is equipment failure and it is essential that surgeons know their equipment.

A recently reported rate of complications for both diagnostic and operative laparoscopy was 3.2/1000. Factors that influence the rate of complications include: the presence of severe adhesions, endometriosis, complexity of the procedure and the competence of the surgeon. To date, the incidence of conversion to laparotomies as a result of complications is rare (0.23%). The best management of complications is prevention.

Pneumoperitoneum

Extraperitoneal insufflation occurs when the Veress needle fails to enter the peritoneal cavity. When recognized, the gas is allowed to escape and the needle reinserted. The emphysema resolves spontaneously. If severe, mediastinal emphysema can be seen, and there it will be difficult to ventilate the patient. Emphysema of the omentum is self-limiting, but makes visualization of the abdomen and pelvic structures difficult. Rarely, a penetrating injury to a blood vessel is not recognized and may lead to gas embolism and death.

Vessel injury

The Veress needle or trocar may traumatize omental, mesenteric or any major abdominal and pelvic blood vessels. Thin, small patients are at higher risk. Elevating the anterior abdominal wall and directing the needle or trocar towards the pelvic area may avoid most of these serious complications. Small vessel injury can be treated with coagulation. Major vessel injury requires repair. Mesenteric artery injury can lead to bowel ischaemia and subsequent resection. The pneumoperitoneum raises abdominal pressure and may tamponade blood vessels, masking a vessel bleed. The patient could go into shock when the pressure is released at the end of the operation. The epigastric vessels can be injured with the placement of ancillary trocars. Laparotomy is required if haemostasis is not successful.

Bowel injury

The risk of gastric injury rises due to gastric distension after intubation. If intubation is difficult, a nasogastric tube may be inserted to decompress the stomach before insertion of the Veress needle.

Injury to the intestines can occur during insertion of the Veress needles, the trocars, or at the time of operative laparoscopy. Injuries are more common in patients who have had previous abdominal surgery or pelvic adhesive disease. Bowel perforation with the Veress needle often goes undetected as the perforation usually seals off spontaneously. If the laparoscope perforates the bowel, it should be left in place to limit peritoneal soiling and facilitate identification of the injured site.

Extensive bowel dissection can lead to a postoperative ileus, which will resolve in a few days. Symptoms include nausea, vomiting and abdominal distension. Thermal injury can be caused by direct contact of electrical, thermal or laser energy with an organ or tissue.

Bladder and ureteral injury

The bladder can be damaged during trocar insertion. It is important to have an empty bladder prior to surgery to decrease the risk of perforation. Lacerations smaller than 5 mm may heal spontaneously if the bladder is drained continuously for 4–5 days postoperatively. Larger injuries require suturing.

Injury to the ureter is uncommon. It is particularly susceptible to injury if adhesions or endometriosis involve the pelvic sidewall.

Trocar hernias

These are rare. The 'Z' track method can lessen the risk of herniation.

Anaesthetic and postoperative complications

The most common complications seen in the recovery room are related to the respiratory and cardiovascular systems, nausea and vomiting.

Hypoxaemia is the most important respiratory complication occurring after anaesthesia and surgery. Causes include central respiratory depression, alveolar hypoventilation, ventilation and perfusion mismatch, etc. Therefore it is important that the pulse oximeter be used routinely in all patients. If hypoxaemia is persistent, blood gas analysis should be performed.

Hypotension is the most common cardiovascular complication. Causes include hypovolaemia, vasodilatation, cardiac dysrhythmias, etc. Renal function is an important indicator of cardiovascular function and patients are usually not allowed home until they have passed urine successfully.

Other complications in the recovery room include muscle pains due to suxamethonium, especially in young women who are ambulant soon after recovery. The pain resolves in a few days. Headaches and nausea are common after general anaesthesia. Intubation during surgery can cause trauma to the lips, teeth, pharynx and larynx, leading to a sore throat during recovery.

Pain management after surgery is an important factor to consider, as inadequate analgesia is often a contributing factor in all the common postoperative complications. Infection can also occur after surgery, but proper techniques during surgery and the use of prophylactic antibiotics will usually prevent it.

Complications during and after surgery can be avoided with:

- state-of-the-art equipment (particularly camera, monitor and insufflator);
- thorough preoperative evaluation, consultation and proper patient selection, bearing in mind the absolute and relative contra-indications to laparoscopy;
- familiarity with normal and distorted anatomy;
- meticulous dissection and vaporization;
- familiarity with instruments;
- adequate training of surgeons.

Ectopic pregnancy

The management of ectopic pregnancy has changed dramatically over the past few years. With the introduction of accurate serum beta human chorionic gonadotrophin (β-hCG) levels and transvaginal scanning, conservative management is more common. If women do require a diagnostic or therapeutic laparoscopy, they must be warned that there is a chance of a laparotomy, as with all minimal access procedures. The vast majority of ectopic pregnancies can be dealt with laparoscopically, although this technique would not be appropriate for a shocked patient with a major intra-abdominal bleed. Previous significant abdominal surgery may also preclude laparoscopic management.

Preoperatively, it is essential that a full blood count is taken and blood is available in case a transfusion is needed. The laparoscopic procedure is as above, with a 10 mm port subumbilically but with a 5 mm port in one fossa, and the pelvis is then inspected to identify the ectopic pregnancy, if present. On visualization of the pelvis, one can then decide whether to insert a further 5 mm trocar or one of 10–12 mm. RCOG guidelines now recommend that if an ectopic pregnancy is in the Fallopian tube, management depends on the status of the other tube. If the other tube is normal, then a salpingectomy should be performed. If the other tube is not normal, then a salpingostomy should be performed.

In performing a salpingectomy, the easiest procedure would be to use an endoloop. This is inserted through one of the ports and the whole of the tube is lassoed. The suture is tied tight and a further endoloop is placed just above the first. Using scissors, the tube is then divided and can either be placed in an endocatch or removed through the 10–12 mm port. The pedicle is checked for haemostasis and the pelvis is irrigated. If there is any oozing from any dissection, then a solution, e.g. Adept®, can be left in the pelvis to prevent formation of adhesions.

For a linear salpingostomy, an incision is made over the ectopic pregnancy and, using hydro-dissection, the ectopic is flushed out. Bipolar diathermy is used for any bleeding points, and the ectopic is removed again via an 'endocatch' or through the large port. It is prudent to leave fluid in the pelvis to allow flotation and to decrease adhesion formation.

If there is blood in the peritoneal cavity on entry, this should be suctioned and the situation assessed. If one is unable to control active bleeding, then the decision should be made to proceed to laparotomy.

After laparoscopic management of ectopic pregnancy it is important to ensure that serum β-hCG levels drop.

If the inferior epigastric artery is divided during introduction of the trocar, leave the trocar in situ as this will tamponade vessels. One can then insert a Foley catheter through the trocar, blow the balloon up, and then pull the balloon tightly up against the anterior abdominal wall and fix the catheter above the skin with an artery forceps, so that tension is applied to the inferior epigastric. Another method would be to diathermy the inferior epigastric from the other port, or one could under-run the artery using a figure-of-eight suture around the trocar site.

Conclusion

Laparoscopic procedures in gynaecology have had a dramatic impact on clinical practice and are achieving an increasingly important role in patient management. The advantages of laparoscopic surgery include a shorter hospital stay (often day surgery), thus increasing the number of patients treated and cutting waiting lists/time, and it is cost-effective. Intra-operatively it offers a shorter operating time and reduced blood loss. Postoperatively, the small incisions cause less tissue trauma, with faster wound healing and decreased recovery time. Less analgesia is needed as there is less postoperative pain. The patient is able to ambulate earlier and postoperative complications associated with prolonged bed-rest, e.g. atelectasis and deep vein thrombosis, are avoided. The patient can also return to eating and drinking earlier. The main theory of the potential benefits of laparoscopic surgery is avoidance of tissue handling that is necessary at laparotomy. Tissue damage with instruments during laparoscopy is reduced, resulting in reduced postoperative adhesion formation and fewer complications. Accumulating data also suggest that minimally invasive surgery provides immunological and oncological advantages compared to open surgery. The down sides to minimal access surgery are that it requires high capital investment, with specialized training. To the patients, laparoscopic surgery means smaller incisions, less disruption of their bodies and a much quicker return to normal activities.

FURTHER READING

Desai S V, Joseph K 2003 Gynaecological endoscopic surgery: current concepts. Alpha Science, Mumbai, India

Lower A, Sutton C, Grudzinskas G 1996 Introduction to Gynaecology Endoscopy. Isis Medical Media, Oxford

Minimal access surgery: the hysteroscope

Christopher Sutton

Diagnostic hysteroscopy

Ever since ancient times *Homo sapiens* seems to have had a desire to peer inside body cavities, and probably the earliest description of an endoscopic examination was from the school of Hippocrates[1] (460–375 BC) on the island of Kos, that described a rectal speculum similar to instruments used today.

The pioneer of modern endoscopy was Bozzini,[2] who invented a hollow tube through which natural human cavities could be observed. He reflected the light from a candle via a mirror, directing the rays along a metal tube, allowing him to examine the interior of the urethra in 1805. When he presented his technique to the medical faculty of Vienna the poor man was censured for 'undue curiosity'.

The first cystoscope was invented by Desormeaux[3] in 1865 and consisted of a light source that incorporated a lamp burning alcohol and turpentine with a chimney to enhance the flame. Desormeaux presented this to the Imperial Academy of Medicine in Paris and was rewarded with a share of the Argenteuil Prize. He also suggested that this endoscope could be used to inspect the interior of the uterus.

However, the first successful hysteroscopy was reported by Pantaleoni[4] in 1869, when he described his examination of a 60-year-old woman with postmenopausal bleeding. He found an intrauterine polyp and managed to cauterize it with silver nitrate, so this was not only the first diagnostic hysteroscopy but the first demonstration of intrauterine surgery.

Urologists were more ready to take up these new endoscopic techniques than gynaecologists, and the early development of diagnostic hysteroscopy was slow. The main reason for this was the difficulty in distending the uterus, due to the thickness of its walls and the small size of the cavity, and the tendency of the endometrium to bleed on contact or when distended. Additionally, there were problems with the distally situated light bulbs, causing excessive heat production, and the poor quality of the lenses available at the time. Nevertheless, in 1907 Charles David[5] described the use of a cystoscope with an internal light and lens system to examine the uterine cavity, and Rubin[6] in 1925, was the first to use carbon dioxide as a distension medium. Unfortunately, some patients were adversely affected by the pneumoperitoneum which resulted from the carbon dioxide gas and the method was abandoned.

The first flexible fibre optic hysteroscopes were designed by Mohri[7] in Japan in 1971, but the quality of the image was poor compared with the superb images obtained with the rod lens system designed by Professor Harold H. Hopkins,[8] a Fellow of the Royal Society, from Reading University. This, together with the cold light source invented by Fourestiere[9] in Paris in 1943, has revolutionized visualization of the uterine cavity and allowed the extraordinary advances of the past 25 years.

The old established method of investigating women with abnormal uterine bleeding was by dilatation and curettage, which has been found to only sample half of the available endometrium.[10] Following this, Gimpelson[11] found that hysteroscopic examination of the uterus was much more accurate than dilatation and curettage in reaching a diagnosis. These findings were further confirmed by Hamou,[12] and Raju and Taylor,[13] who showed a very high correlation between hysteroscopic appearances and curettage samples. The general consensus nowadays is that the oft-performed operation of dilatation and curettage should be replaced by hysteroscopy and endometrial sampling, which can usually be performed as an outpatient procedure.

Safety

In order to visualize the endometrium, it is first necessary to distend the uterine cavity. Edstrom

and Fernstrom[14] first used 32% Dextran 70, which has a molecular weight of 70 000 and is a thick, viscous fluid which is electrolyte free, non-conductive and biodegradable. It is optically clear and immiscible with blood, and therefore gives a very good view. Unfortunately, it is hydrophilic and if it accidentally enters the circulation its high molecular weight pulls with it at least six times its own volume of fluid, and cases of fluid overload and pulmonary oedema have been reported.[15,16] Additionally, cases of disseminated intravascular coagulopathy (DIC), adult respiratory distress syndrome (ARDS) and fatal anaphylactic reactions have also been described, and it has been withdrawn from the market in the UK, but is still available and used in some countries.

Although carbon dioxide was the first gas used for uterine distension, there were some fatalities from gas embolism, and bubbles of gas have been detected moving in the pelvic vessels during simultaneous hysteroscopy and laparoscopy.[17] The risk of embolism is proportional to the flow of infused gas.[18] Lindemann[19] demonstrated, in a series of experiments in dogs, that flow rates below 200 mL/min were associated with minimal changes in pulse rate and breathing, whereas flow rates above 400 mL/min were associated with tachypnoea and arrhythmias, and rates of 1000 mL/min were associated with death within 60 s. The maximum flow rate for hysteroscopy must be fixed at not more than 100 mL/min and, indeed, a flow rate of 40 mL/min is usually adequate. It is absolutely essential that all endoscopists are aware of this, and equipment designed for laparoscopy, which permits flow rates of 3000–4000 mL/min, must never be used for hysteroscopy. It is the policy in our hospital that laparoscopic CO_2 infusion equipment must never be stored in the same room as the equipment designed and used for hysteroscopy. As long as this precaution is taken, then CO_2 is extremely safe as a distension medium, is particularly suitable in the outpatient or office setting and is probably the one in general use universally. When used at the correct pressure, it tends to flatten the endometrium and gives excellent visibility. It has virtually the same refractive index as air and excellent photographs can be obtained with this medium. A continuous flow is necessary to replace any gas lost through the tubes. Its main disadvantage is that there is a tendency for gas bubbles to form, particularly when the CO_2 gas mixes with blood, and this can obscure vision. This can usually be prevented by good technique;[18] blood and mucus should be removed carefully from the cervical os with a dry swab and the hysteroscope should be slowly advanced under direct vision, creating a series of gas bubbles just ahead of the tip of the hysteroscope. It should be introduced under careful visualization, usually on a television screen, so that it is kept in the centre of the endocervical canal and introduced into the uterine cavity without touching or damaging the endocervical mucosa, which is the usual source of the bleeding.

Another disadvantage of CO_2 gas as a distension medium, is that occasionally the gas bubbles can create artefacts, which lead to a misleading diagnosis of intrauterine adhesions or synechiae. A simple trick to avoid this is to have a 20 or 30 mL syringe of warm saline solution attached to the input channel of the hysteroscope; using this to flush out the bubbles, one can get a clear view. As an alternative distension medium, some hysteroscopists use saline solution connected to an infusion bag that is squeezed to give sufficient pressure to distend the uterus, but this is considerably messier than CO_2 infusion equipment, which is specially designed for outpatient use.

As long as the intrauterine pressure does not exceed 40–50 mmHg, and the flow rate does not exceed 60 mL/min, then CO_2 distension is extremely safe, and since the procedure only takes a few minutes, the amount of carbon dioxide entering the abdominal cavity is only a few hundred millilitres and is absorbed rapidly.

Preoperative measures

The most important person in an abnormal uterine bleeding (AUB), or outpatient hysteroscopy clinic, is the nurse. Patients are understandably nervous at the idea of such an intrusive examination, and are usually advised to come with a relative or friend to keep them company and to drive them home afterwards, but obviously not to be present during the examination. Usually, patients are sent a fact sheet describing the procedure at the time that they are given an appointment, and the first job of the nurse is to welcome the patient in a fairly pleasant setting, a little like the sitting room at home, to explain the procedure and to answer any questions and to allay any anxieties. The importance of a kind, sympathetic and friendly nurse cannot be overemphasized, and the success or otherwise of the clinic depends very much on this as, of course, it does on the attitude of the doctor.

Outpatient hysteroscopy is not a particularly difficult procedure, and since the findings can be documented on videotape or still photographs, many centres are now training nurse hysteroscopists. The British Society for Gynaecological Endoscopy is actively encouraging this and is running several courses each year to train nurse hysteroscopists. However, at the present time most hysteroscopies will be performed by consultant gynaecologists, or gynaecologists in training.

The hysteroscopy clearly has to be performed in a semi-sterile (clinically clean) room, but nevertheless some attempts should be made to make the clinical setting less cold, via the introduction of some paintings on the wall or even, as at the Royal Surrey County Hospital, on the ceiling, because the patient is going to be looking at this during the major part of the examination.

The patient is invited to sit in a chair, and we find that it is much more patient friendly for the chair to tilt up by an electric mechanism, putting the patient in the correct position without the need for raising her legs up on lithotomy poles. Above all, the examination couch should be comfortable and care must be taken that the patient's hips are not hyperflexed. The procedure can be viewed on a video monitor and the patient should be asked whether or not she would like to watch the procedure, because some patients find it genuinely interesting and informative, but other patients find it a little unnerving, and their wishes must be respected. The monitor can perfectly easily be turned away so that the operator can view it, or if the patient wishes to view the procedure, then it can be turned so that both parties can view the procedure simultaneously.

Instrumentation

A diagnostic hysteroscope consists of an optical telescope with a diameter of about 3.5 mm, surrounded by a sheath (Fig. 10.1), which increases the diameter to 4 mm and allows the circulation of the distension fluid or CO_2. There are different angles of view varying from 0° to 12° or 30°, depending on the preference of the operator Fig. 10.2), but for simple diagnostic hysteroscopy a 0° or 12° view is the most suitable, allowing easier orientation within the uterine cavity yet still allowing biopsy forceps and the resectoscope loop to remain in the field of view.

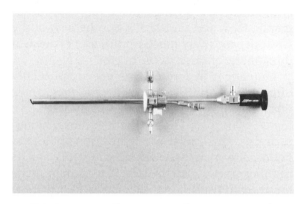

Fig. 10.1 Continuous flow operating hysteroscope with additional channel for biopsy forceps or laser fibre.

Some hysteroscopes have a separate channel for biopsy forceps or scissors, or for the introduction of a small, flexible laser fibre.

Rigid hysteroscopes usually incorporate the Hopkins rod lens system and give a bright, undistorted image which is as clear at the periphery of the fields of view as at the centre. This allows for superb optical visualization, but has the disadvantage at the moment, that dilatation of the cervix is necessary, usually up to about 5 mm to incorporate the outer sheath, although each year the diameter of these rigid hysteroscopes seems to get smaller. To avoid dilatation of the cervix, some hysteroscopists prefer a flexible hysteroscope similar to a gastroscope. This probably allows easier visualization of the cornual orifice

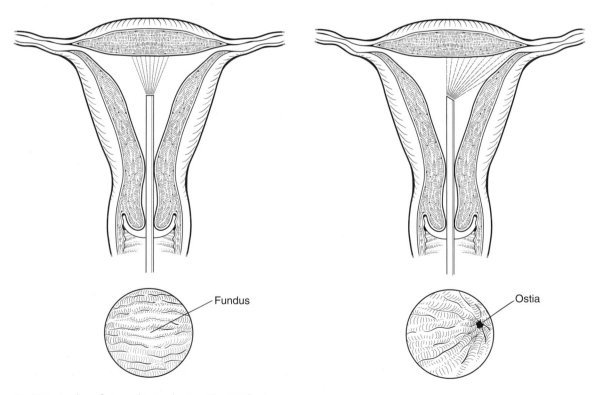

Fig. 10.2 Angles of view obtained using 0° or 30° hysteroscopes.

but, unfortunately, it produces a grid effect due to the flexible nature of the optical fibres, and this produces rather a grainy view which is far inferior to that obtained with a rigid hysteroscope. In my opinion they have no real advantage over rigid hysteroscopes; they are considerably more expensive and cannot be autoclaved.

Light source

The cold light source developed by Forestiere means that the light is away from the patient and is transmitted via optical cables, avoiding the dissipation of heat inside the uterine cavity. It is very important to handle these cables carefully, otherwise the fibres can break and after a period of time there is considerable loss of light intensity. With all optical fibre light sources it is also important to make sure that the light source is not switched on and lying unconnected on the patient or the drapes covering the patient, because the heat generated is, in fact, quite considerable before the light source is attached to the endoscope, and burns and even ignition of the drapes have been reported. A low-power source of about 150 W is adequate for simple diagnostic hysteroscopy, but if a video camera is used, a higher-intensity zenon or halogen light of at least 250 W is essential, and with this increased intensity the above precautions are even more important.

Documentation

The past decade has seen extraordinary developments in the technology of lightweight three-chip video cameras and the development of digital imaging. This allows the image to be displayed on a television monitor and allows recording of high-quality images on videotape or allows them to be stored digitally.

Recommended operative technique

Outpatient hysteroscopy can be performed on most patients once they have had adequate reassurance from the clinic nurse and the doctor.

It is not suitable for nervous patients and there may be difficulties with cervical stenosis in nulliparous women or women past the menopause. Some patients do require a paracervical block with 0.5% bupivacaine (Marcain®), but it is often sufficient to introduce a small Q-tip moistened with a solution of local anaesthetic into the endocervical canal and to allow 3 or 4 minutes to elapse before continuing with the procedure. It is also advantageous to encourage patients to take asprin or a non-steroidal anti-inflammatory agent about half an hour before coming to the hysteroscopy clinic.

Before inserting the hysteroscope, a bimanual examination should be performed to determine whether the uterus is anteverted or retroverted and also to gauge the reaction of the patient. Some hysteroscopists inject a small bleb of local anaesthetic into the anterior lip of the cervix before applying a single-toothed tenaculum, but in most patients this is not strictly necessary. This allows for traction on the cervix while a small intrauterine sound is passed to measure the length of the uterine cavity and to determine the degree of anteflexion and anteversion or retroversion. The cervical canal is gently dilated to the necessary diameter of the endoscope, but this should be done very carefully and gently to avoid bleeding which would obscure the view. In most parous women cervical dilatation is not necessary; it is usually possible to pass a small rigid hysteroscope without dilatation and this is probably best performed in the week following menstruation, when the endometrium is thin and there is very little bleeding. Unfortunately, the administrative problems of the National Health Service make this quite difficult to arrange, and this is particularly the case in patients who present with irregular menstruation or intermenstrual bleeding.

The hysteroscope is introduced as described above in order not to induce any unnecessary bleeding which would interfere with vision. Immediately following menstruation the endometrium is usually quite flat and atrophic, and similar to the appearance obtained in the endometrium of a postmenopausal woman. It is usually possible to visualize the cornual orifices by manipulation of the rigid hysteroscope, and, certainly, with the twisting mechanism of the flexible endoscope they are even easier to visualize. When the endoscope is close to the cornual orifice it can be visualized under magnification, and the gas pressure rising inside the uterus will, in the absence of any diseased state, allow it to open and close, with slight leakage of CO_2 or fluid into the abdominal cavity. Attention should then be directed to the fundus of the uterus to make sure that there is no asymmetry and no evidence of a septum. Although one would expect a bicornuate uterus to be absolutely obvious on hysteroscopy, it sometimes happens that the septum extends almost to the endocervical canal and, if the telescope is passed to one side of the septum, the diagnosis can easily be missed.

In the luteal phase of the cycle the endometrium is much more vascular and oedematous, and it is possible to indent the stroma using pressure on the telescope. This is particularly obvious in patients with various types of hyperplasia, but this should not be done deliberately, in view of the fact that it will almost certainly make the endometrium bleed. When the distal end of the telescope is placed close to the endometrium, it is possible to visualize the vascular pattern, to look at the gland openings, and sometimes to detect certain pathological features, such as adenomyosis, endometrial hyperplasia and endometrial cancer. If these latter findings are suspected, it is wise to take a directed biopsy through the operating sheath of the hysteroscope, but if no focal lesion is seen, then biopsy can be performed using a thick suction curette or a sample obtained with the Pipelle endometrial sampler.

Pathological findings

Polyps

Endometrial polyps are usually fairly obvious and should be removed by the biopsy forceps under direct hysteroscopic vision or by using a small electrosurgical loop (Figs 10.3, 10.4 and 10.5). Late luteal phase endometrium is thick and has a polypoidal appearance which can often be thought to be abnormal, and it is important to record the time of the menstrual cycle

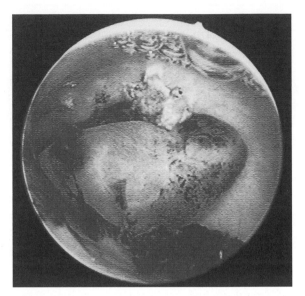

Fig. 10.3 Submucous fibroid.

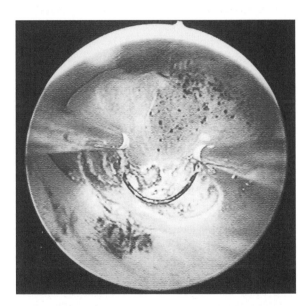

Fig. 10.4 Bed of submucous fibroid in Figure 10.3 after removal by resectoscope loop.

when the examination is taking place. Some adenomatous polyps are associated with atypical endometrial hyperplasia or cystic endometrial hyperplasia, and histological examination will differentiate between these various conditions. The rationale behind removing endometrial

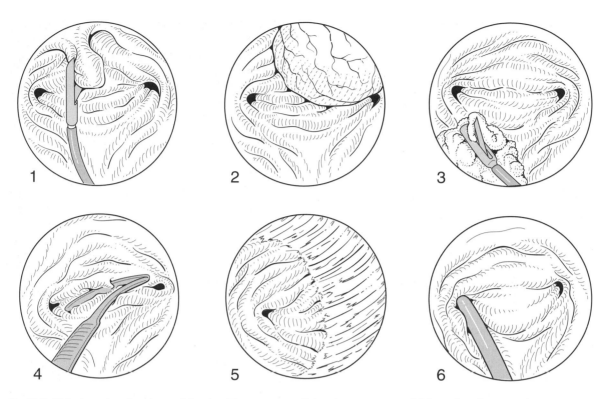

Fig. 10.5 (1) Pedunculated endometrial polyp. The narrow pedicle is being transected. (2) sessile submucous leiomyoma (3) Hysteroscopic biopsy of focal endometrical lesion. (4) Misplaced IUD partially embedded. (5) Partial occlusion of the uterine cavity by a thick adhesion; only the right tubal opening is visible. (6) tubal cannulation.

polyps is that very rarely there can be malignant changes in the base. Additionally it is possible for a polyp to become necrotic and ulcerated at the tip. As it will then give rise to intermenstrual bleeding, it should be removed. If there are multiple polyps, or if there is difficulty in removing them, it might be prudent to admit the patient for removal of these polyps with the resectoscope under general anaesthesia, which can nearly always be done as a day case. It is interesting how often these polyps can be missed by blind curettage, and it is educational to look inside the uterus before and after a curettage or an attempt to remove polyps by sponge forceps; in nearly all cases much of the pathology will have been left behind. If they are multiple, and particularly if there are submucous fibroids, they are much better removed accurately and precisely using a loop electrode similar to the one used for endometrial resection.

Submucous fibroids

Submucous fibroids can be recognized on diagnostic hysteroscopy, and are sometimes discovered on a hysterosalpingogram, particularly on a contact hysterosonogram. They are classified loosely on the basis of how much of the fibroid is projecting into the endometrial cavity and how much is within the myometrium (Fig. 10.6). Before planning treatment for women with these fibroids we generally obtain a three-dimensional ultrasound scan, which gives a diagram of the size and relative position of these fibromyomas. They usually have a whitish appearance and are relatively avascular, although occasionally they do have large blood vessels coursing over the surface. Occasionally they are associated with adenomyosis or endometrial hyperplasia and, rarely, they can coexist with endometrial carcinoma. Clinically they can present with

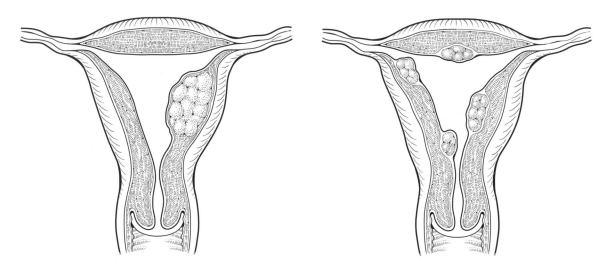

Fig. 10.6 Submucosal fibroids where the greater portion is located in the myometrium.

menorrhagia, and occasionally with colicky dys-menorrhoea as the uterus tries to expel them, and occasionally succeeds. There are descriptions from the Middle Ages of women passing eggs, usually described as wren's eggs. It is salutary to remember that such a description was usually associated with an accusation of witchcraft, and many women were put to death for admitting to such a phenomenon, which nowadays would be recognized as the passage of a calcified fibroid.

Small, often multiple, submucous fibroids are easy to recognize. Paradoxically, a woman can have a very large fibroid filling the uterine cavity, which can very easily be missed as the hyster-oscope passes between the fibroid wall and the endometrium on the other side; this is surpris-ingly easy to do. The fibroid should be examined from different angles by rotating the telescope to check whether or not there is a pedicle, and also to check that there is sufficient room between the fibroid surface and the other wall of the uterus in order to insert instruments to resect the fibroid or to use the neodymium:yttrium–aluminium–garnet (Nd:YAG) laser to transect the base of the pedicle. If there is an appreciable amount of the fibroid projecting into the myometrium, as demonstrated on the three-dimensional ultrasound scan, it is safer to administer a course of gonadotrophin-releasing hormone (GnRH) analogues for 2 or 3 months

to decrease the size of the fibroid and reduce the vasculature. It is also a wise precaution to perform resection of a fibroid with an appreci-able intramural component under laparoscopic vision on another television monitor, to make sure that one is not resecting too deeply into the myometrium, which can easily result in a large perforation.

Endometrial carcinoma

Endometrial neoplasia causes abnormal uterine bleeding as its first symptom in over 90% of cases, and normally presents as postmenopausal bleeding. However, it is important to realize that it can present before the menopause, parti-cularly in patients suffering from polycystic ovarian syndrome, diabetes, obesity and patients who have been on a prolonged course of high-dose tamoxifen. Most Abnormal Uterine Bleeding Clinics have been set up, not only to provide a rational course of therapeutic steps to relieve menorrhagia, but also to rule out endometrial cancer or, at least, detect it at a relatively early stage and, in fact, 75% of endometrial carcinoma cases are diagnosed as Stage I. Hysteroscopy allows the diagnosis to be confirmed and a direct punch biopsy under hysteroscopic visualization to be obtained for histological confirmation. It also allows the surgeon to delineate the limits of the tumour and, particularly, to decide whether it is invading the endocervical canal (carcinoma corporis et colis), which would require a completely different form of treatment, with lymphatic spread more in line with that of carcinoma of the cervix and, depending on the age of the patient, requires radical hysterectomy and lymphadenectomy with or without radiotherapy. Endometrial carcinoma is often preceded by different types of endometrial hyperplasia which can have characteristic appearances on hysteroscopy.

Cystic glandular hyperplasia usually presents as metropathia haemorrhagica and has a relatively low risk of malignancy (approximately 10–15%).[20] Cystic glandular hyperplasia often has a specific hysteroscopic appearance of widened glandular ostia with cystic glandular formation approximately 1 mm in diameter. The stroma is soft and boggy due to an increased endometrial thickness and it can easily be compressed by pushing the hysteroscope against it, leaving a series of deep indentations.

Adenomatous hyperplasia can give rise to various appearances, when the superficial vascularization takes on an arborescent pattern with vessel branches of different sizes and sometimes a 'corkscrew' appearance of the vasculature, occasionally with straight vessels similar to the appearance of microinvasive carcinoma of the cervix at colposcopy. The differentiation between adenomatous hyperplasia, especially the atypical variety, and endometrial cancer can be extremely difficult. The final diagnosis must always rest on histology, and multiple biopsies are essential.

Endometrial neoplasia is usually fairly obvious, but the tissue quite often bleeds profusely and sometimes the view inside the uterine cavity is obscured. In its early stage, adenocarcinoma shows irregular, polylobular, delicate excrescences which are partly necrotic or bleeding, and the vascularization is irregular or anarchic with no discernible arborizing pattern. For further information on the various appearances of endometrial hyperplasia and carcinoma the reader is referred to specialized texts. Probably the best are Mencaglia et al (1999) or the excellent manual of gynaecological hysteroscopy written by Mencaglia and Hamou (see 'Further reading' for details).

Lost intrauterine devices

Sometimes an intrauterine device is misplaced and one arm of the coil burrows into the myometrium and, with this twisting on its axis, the thread is often brought up within the uterine cavity. Attempts to remove these blindly or with coil retrieval devices are often difficult and uncomfortable for the patient, but the coil or any fractured remnants of it can usually be clearly seen on hysteroscopy, allowing removal to be achieved much more simply. It is sometimes necessary to perform abdominal and pelvic ultrasound in cases where the intrauterine device has migrated completely through the uterine wall, and in these cases the device usually has to be retrieved laparoscopically.

Retained products of conception

Pregnancy is a contra-indication to hysteroscopy; enquiries should always be made about the possibility of pregnancy and the last menstrual period should always be recorded. After an incomplete miscarriage, retained products are usually removed by suction curettage, but some women continue to bleed from a small placental polyp or some retained products of conception, which are abnormally adherent to the uterine wall. These can usually be located by ultrasound, but often it is necessary to perform a hysteroscopy to identify a placental or fetal remnant, and once it is localized it is much easier to remove it.

Other roles

Another useful role of hysteroscopy is to identify uterine septae or adhesions, which might be contributing to infertility or recurrent pregnancy loss. Large avascular septae can be excised using the hook electrode or a neodymium YAG (Nd:YAG) laser, but care must be taken not to penetrate too deeply and also to avoid a bicornuate uterus, which may not require any treatment at all. We perform most of our hysteroscopic metroplasties under laparoscopic control to evaluate the outside shape of the uterus and to avoid perforation, which could have potentially serious sequelae if the energy source is still activated, damaging the bowel or large blood vessels.

Endometrial resection

For many years gynaecologists have been working in adjacent operating theatres to our urological colleagues and have watched the operation of transurethral resection of the prostate with a detached fascination, but did not have the foresight or perspicacity to translate the modus operandi to endoscopic removal of the endometrium. The first reported use of electrosurgical resection was by Robert Neuwirth from New York, who used it to remove symptomatic submucous fibroids.[21] The first description of endometrial resection was by DeCherney and his colleagues.[22] They ablated the endometrium in a small series of patients with intractable bleeding who, for one reason or another, were unsuitable for abdominal or vaginal hysterectomy.

Indications and patient selection

Although it has been estimated that up to 58% of women currently being treated by hysterectomy for menstrual dysfunction may be suitable for endometrial resection or ablation,[23] this does require very careful patient selection. The selection criteria for endometrial ablation are set out in Fig. 10.7.

Endometrial resection or ablation is an invasive procedure with a very definite complication rate, and some of these complications can be serious or indeed fatal. It should therefore never be embarked on lightly and women must be absolutely certain that they have completed their family and preferably have had tubal occlusion, since pregnancies can occur following this procedure but they are often associated with complications, some of which may be serious or even life threatening.

The patient should be complaining of severe menorrhagia, sufficient to seriously affect her

Fig. 10.7 Selection criteria for endometrial ablation

- Severe menorrhagia based on subjective assessment.
- Failure of adequate medical therapy.
- Family complete or no wish to conceive in future.
- Next logical step would be hysterectomy.
- No sign of hyperplasia or endometrial carcinoma on transvaginal ultrasound and pipelle endometrial sampling.
- No other gynaecological pathology, particularly adenomyosis or pelvic infection.
- No contra-indicating medical condition.

It is important to perform an ultrasound scan to assess the thickness and regularity of the endometrium, but also to rule out any ovarian pathology. It is not necessary to do a preoperative hysteroscopic assessment unless the endometrium is to be ablated by the Nd:YAG laser, rollerball diathermy or second-generation endometrial ablation devices.

lifestyle and should give a history of heavy menstrual blood loss, usually with the passage of fairly large clots, and having to use both internal and external protection and usually having to change this every hour or so when the flow is at its worst. Most patients will also give a history of flooding, and this usually occurs when they pass urine and most of this blood is flushed down the toilet, thus rendering many estimates of menstrual blood loss by observation of tampon staining an inaccurate assessment of the true loss.

Patients should have been given a fair trial with medical therapy, particularly prostaglandin synthetase inhibitors and tranexamic acid.[24] Apart from patients with ovulatory disorders causing their menorrhagia, progestogen therapy has never been established as an efficacious treatment, although it is widely used.[24] Many of the younger patients can be encouraged to take the oral contraceptive or a similar preparation, which will reduce menstrual blood loss in most patients, even though they may not need to use it for contraception. There is little doubt that endometrial resection is less effective in the younger age group and it is worth persevering with medical therapy or possibly going directly to hysterectomy, since endometrial resection tends to be more effective in patients in their mid-forties and older. For younger patients the levonorgestrel-releasing intrauterine device

(Mirena®) should be offered, and patients must be warned to expect irregular bleeding over the first few months following insertion.

Endometrial ablation should only be advised when the next logical step would be to advise a hysterectomy and all other methods have failed. The uterus should be smaller than a uterus at 14 weeks' gestation, with a cavity of 12 cm or less. Some authorities would suggest a slightly lower upper limit of 12 weeks and 10 cm in length.[25] If the patient has large intramural fibroids distorting the cavity, the procedure will be more difficult and the result less good, but submucous fibroids less than 5 cm in diameter can be removed at the same time as the endometrial resection. Larger fibroids should be reduced in size by a 3-month course of GnRH analogues, which will also decrease their vascularity.

The patients should be assessed preoperatively by a transvaginal ultrasound and an endometrial biopsy, preferably associated with an outpatient hysteroscopy. Patients with prolapse would be better advised to have a vaginal hysterectomy and repair of the prolapse, and patients with other conditions such as endometriosis will also require therapy directed towards that disease. Many patients with painful, heavy periods will, not surprisingly, fail to have pain relief unless they have some form of procedure directed at this, such as a uterine nerve ablation performed laparoscopically at the same time[26] and if endometriosis is contributing to the dysmenorrhoea, that can also be vaporized or ablated via the laparoscope.[27] It is of interest that premenstrual tension often improves following endometrial ablation, but this must not be the primary indication for treatment.

Although adenomyosis is not a contraindication to endometrial resection, there is little doubt that these patients do not do as well and often end up with quite severe cyclical pain, eventually requiring hysterectomy. Unfortunately, adenomyosis can only be diagnosed accurately retrospectively after hysterectomy, but it can be clinically suspected by the association of severe dysmenorrhoea and a tender uterus on bimanual examination, particularly if performed during menstruation. Additional evidence pointing to a diagnosis of adenomyosis is the dusky red and blotchy uterus seen at laparoscopy, the characteristic appearance of gland openings at hysteroscopy and the changes in the junctional zone, best seen on a magnetic resonance imaging (MRI) scan.

Preoperative considerations

A certain amount of time is required to explain the procedure and its complications to these patients, and I often find it helpful to draw a diagram to explain exactly what is intended at the time of admission for surgery. It must be stressed that there is a very definite failure rate of the order of 10%, and that only about a third of the patients will become amenorrhoeic, and they are mainly the women over 45. It is also important to explain that there are complications of haemorrhage, which might require balloon tamponade, or that of intra-operative perforation, which may necessitate laparotomy or even emergency hysterectomy, although this is fortunately rare.

It is vital to make the patient understand that this is not a contraceptive procedure and if she has not been sterilized then she must take precautions to avoid pregnancy. She should be offered the possibility of tubal occlusion by laparoscopy at the same time.

Patients should be warned that they will initially have a heavy period after leaving hospital and this will become a serosanguinous discharge which can last a few days or even several weeks. They must also be warned that they could have two or three heavy periods during the healing phase. It takes 6 months for the scar tissue to finally form inside the uterus and it is only at that time that the result can be realistically assessed. There is no point in seeing patients for final assessment before that time.

Endometrial thinning

It is helpful to have a thin or absent endometrium at the time of the procedure and this can occasionally be arranged if the operation can coincide with a patient's menstrual period, but many of these patients have irregular periods and the logistics of this are by no means easy. The endometrium can be removed by a suction catheter in a similar way to performing a termination of pregnancy, but this often does not give as good a result as one would anticipate, and also induces a great deal of bleeding.

There is little doubt that the best results are obtained if the endometrium can be thinned by the use of danazol, 200 mg twice daily for 6 weeks prior to the procedure, starting with the onset of the next menstruation, or by giving luteinizing hormone releasing hormone (LHRH) analogues such as Zoladex® (Astra Zeneca, Wilmslow, Cheshire, UK), 3.6 mg as a subcutaneous injection, or Synarel® (Upjohn, Haywards Heath, UK), as a nasal spray in each nostril morning and night for 6 weeks. The advantage of the injection is that compliance is assured, which may not be the case with the nasal spray once the patient realizes that it can induce quite severe hot flushes as well as headaches. Danazol is notorious for its many side-effects, but if the patients can be encouraged to avoid salt-containing food or beverages and to drink more pure water, the weight gain is usually minimal, and most patients tolerate the side-effects well for the short period of time that they are on this drug. We have found that the LHRH analogues do result in a thinner, less active and less vascular endometrium, but occasional unwanted side-effects, such as severe cervical stenosis, can also occur with the analogues and this is rarely seen with danazol[28].

Most of our patients are admitted for day-case surgery and are only in hospital for a few hours. They usually do not have any premedication unless they are unusually anxious, and are allowed to return home a few hours after surgery, provided they are accompanied by a responsible adult. In order to avoid unpleasant menstrual cramps after the procedure, 5 mL bupivacaine is injected as a paracervical block at the completion of surgery.

Since the operation is performed via the vagina and one is therefore working in a contaminated environment, and since the glycine or sorbitol solution, although sterile, is not intended for intravenous use (and yet this does occur if there is any extravasation of fluid

when the myometrial vessels are transacted), it is recommended that patients should have prophylactic antibiotics. We use either Kefzol® or Augmentin®. This is slightly controversial, and in over 900 cases when we did not use prophylactic antibiotics we only had one patient with endometritis, but nevertheless it has been reported and is associated with quite a severe morbidity, so this simple prophylactic step is now recommended.

Instrumentation

The Hysteroscope

To perform endometrial resection, a rigid 10-mm hysteroscope is used with a Hopkins rod lens system and a fibre optic cable to transmit light from a cold light source. The hysteroscopic resectoscope in common use, uses a continuous-flow outer sheath (Fig. 10.8) to allow optimum visibility, the key to any operative hysteroscopy procedure. Clear irrigating fluid, usually sorbitol or glycine, is circulated under rapid flow conditions to rinse the uterus of blood and tissue debris that would otherwise obscure the operator's vision. It is absolutely essential that isolated inflow and outflow channels run the whole length of the resectoscope, so that the fluid flows around the front of the telescope to maintain clear vision at all times. It is vital that the inflow and outflow tubing is correctly placed according

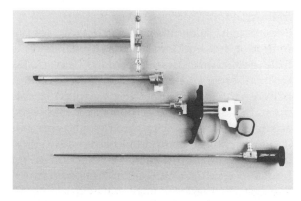

Fig. 10.8 Component parts of operating hysteroscope.

to the direction of the arrows, since the system is not designed for reverse flow and visualization is completely lost. The position of the outflow ports are extremely important. When the outflow holes are provided only on one surface, as with the Storz and Wolf models, the surgeon has to keep rotating the resectoscope, especially when working on the anterior wall, to keep the field of view clear of bubbles. The resectoscopes made by Olympus and Circon ACMI have sheaths with outer ports that encircle the sheath on the top and bottom surfaces, respectively. This design allows the bubbles that inevitably form during the procedure to be removed automatically and to rise to the top of the uterine cavity, making it unnecessary to have to perform shaking movements of the end of the resectoscope to clear bubbles from the operator's view.[29]

Another difference between the various hysteroscopes is in the angle of vision, which varies widely with the different manufacturers and runs the whole gamut from 0° (Olympus and Storz) to 12° (Circon ACMI), 25° (Wolf) and 30° (Storz and Circon ACMI). The choice is a matter of individual preference, but it is worth testing several different types before purchasing one.

Recommended operative technique

The patient is placed in the lithotomy position and the operating field cleansed and draped in the usual manner with non-flammable antiseptic solutions. The patient should be asked to void before coming down to the operating suite and, if this is the case, it is not usually necessary to catheterize patients for this procedure. The resectoscope is assembled with the rollerball in position. A careful check is made to ensure that there are no air bubbles in the inflow system, which must be flushed through until they are all removed. This is a vital step and at all stages of the procedure one member of the operating room staff should be specifically nominated to check when the fluid container is almost empty, to ensure a change over to another container to avoid the risk of contamination with air bubbles. It must be realized that during the procedure of endometrial resection, large myometrial blood vessels are transected and there is instant access to both the arterial and venous system. Thus, if a large air bubble gains access to the circulation an air embolism can occur, which can be rapidly fatal.[30-33] Many deaths have been recorded throughout the world from this complication, and it is the most common cause of sudden death during this procedure. All theatre personnel must be made aware of this possibility which can easily be avoided by diligence. The anaesthetist must also be aware of this rare complication and know the resuscitation steps to take immediately this is suspected.

The cervix is grasped by two vulsellum forceps attached to the anterior lip and the uterine cavity measured with the uterine sound to check that it does not exceed 12 cm. The cervix is carefully dilated to a diameter just in excess of the diameter of the resectoscope and, with the fluid running, the resectoscope is introduced in order to inspect the inside of the cavity on the television monitor, which is connected by a video camera attached to the eyepiece. The operator should initially orientate himself by checking on the position of the tubal orifices and should note for any other anatomical abnormalities, such as an intrauterine septum or submucous fibroid, that may have gone undetected in the preoperative work-up.

No energy source should be activated unless there is an absolutely clear view. If the view is obscured by blood or tissue debris, then the reason for this must be sought and rectified before proceeding to any electrosurgery. Either there is insufficient pressure or flow on the inflow side, due to kinking of the tube or incorrect diameter of the delivery tubes, or equally due to blockage of the outflow system by tissue debris. Once a clear view is obtained, the electrosurgical generator is activated and the current mode and strength are selected, the rollerball is placed in the cornual area and the foot pedal depressed as the rollerball is moved towards the operator. The rollerball should always be pulled towards the operator and never pushed forward while the current is on. The cornual region is the thinnest part of the uterus and can be only a few millimetres thick. Rollerball coagulation can easily damage tissue up to 3 mm in depth.[34] Once the cornual area is coagulated, with three or four radial strokes coming down towards the operator for about 1–2 cm, the rollerball is rolled across the fundus to the other cornual area, where a similar procedure takes place. When starting hysteroscopic electrosurgery, it is safer to test the tissue effect of the rollerball at a mid point in the fundal region where the uterus is at its thickest, to make sure that the power density of the electrical energy is not too fierce. Different electrosurgical generators have their own specific settings for 'cut' and 'coagulate', and it is important to use the power settings recommended by the manufacturer. Great caution should be exercised in the cornual region because of its thinness, and many cases have been recorded where coagulative necrosis has occurred and the cornual area has later perforated during the procedure, merely due to the hydrostatic pressure of the irrigating fluid on the weakened tissue.

Once careful coagulation of both cornua has been achieved, the rollerball (Fig. 10.9) is changed for a resectoscope loop (Fig. 10.10), which is extended to its full length and sunk into the myometrium to its full depth in the centre of the posterior fundal region and pulled back towards the end of the hysteroscope, at the same time withdrawing the hysteroscope, to remove an endometrial strip down to the level of the internal os. It is vital to raise the loop gradually to the surface as one approaches the internal os because deep resection at this level will almost certainly

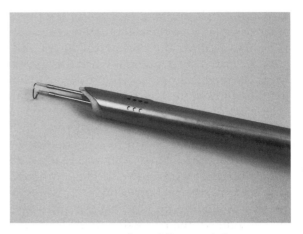

Fig. 10.10 Resectoscope loop, fully extended.

result in extremely heavy bleeding if branches of the lateral cervical arteries are unintentionally transected. At the end of each sweep the entire strip is removed on the end of the resectoscope loop and, as the resectoscope is withdrawn from the cervix, an assistant picks up the strip and places it on a gauze swab. The advantage of this technique is that there is no tissue debris left inside the uterus to obscure the operator's vision, and, by allowing the fluids to empty at the end of each sweep, there is no possibility of the development of fluid overload. We have used this technique on well over 1000 patients and have never had a single episode of fluid overload. It also has a further advantage of allowing the histologist to orientate the specimen to get an accurate measure of endometrial thickness and activity, and also to select any particular areas from which to take specimens.

The depth of penetration is, to a large extent, dependent on the size of loop used, and we have found that we get results that are just as good with a 7-mm loop compared with the more widely used 9-mm loop.[35] The cross-striations of the myometrial muscle can easily be recognized and differentiated from endometrium, and it is important to go down to that level, but on no account should the operator attempt a repeat pass, because the combined penetration would be much too deep and could result in perforation.

As soon as the hysteroscopic view becomes panoramic, the internal os has been reached and

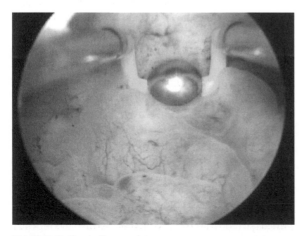

Fig. 10.9 Roller ball coagulator.

resection should not continue beneath this level, not only because of the already mentioned risk of damage to the lateral cervical arteries, but also because it does increase the risk of subsequent cervical stenosis, which would result in a painful haematometra.

This particular technique is the one employed by the author for the reasons given above, but other surgeons tend to chip away at the endometrium and can, of course, achieve the same result, but the disadvantage is in having to evacuate all the tissue debris periodically and also, because of the length of time that the irrigating fluid is kept inside the uterus, it is more likely that fluid overload will occur, especially during difficult and lengthy procedures. Therefore a careful watch must be kept on the input and the output. A nurse should be measuring this all the time and the surgeon must be warned if the deficit is over 1 litre. Consideration should be taken of possibly stopping the procedure or at least warning the anaesthetist to take precautions to observe for signs of fluid overload, and possibly administer diuretics. If the fluid deficit exceeds 1.5 litres, the surgery should be completed as quickly as possible, and if it exceeds 2 litres, then severe hyponatraemia and other metabolic disturbances are highly likely and surgery should be stopped immediately.

Some surgeons prefer to complete the procedure by superficially coagulating the area already resected, with the rollerball on a spray diathermy setting. This does allow any large vessels to be sealed by thermocoagulation and spray diathermy. By lowering the inflow pressure, these vessels can be easily identified, but in practice this can be merely alarming, and most of these vessels will seal off using the body's own haemostatic mechanisms. Only vessels that are spurting at the normal intrauterine pressure used for the operating procedure require to be sealed off with the rollerball, and, if this is not possible and the patient is bleeding heavily at the end of the procedure, a 30 mL balloon catheter should be inserted and the balloon inflated to allow tamponade of the bleeding blood vessels. This is rarely necessary and usually by the time the nursing staff have assembled the necessary equipment, the bleeding has stopped. However,

it is necessary on occasions and, if employed, the patient should not be discharged as a day case, but should stay in hospital overnight and the catheter removed the following morning. Prophylactic antibiotics should certainly be used in this situation. At the end of the procedure bupivacaine hydrochloride is injected as a paracervical block at 7 o'clock and 4 o'clock, taking care to check that a vessel has not been inadvertently entered, by withdrawing on the syringe before injecting the local anaesthetic.

The normal postoperative course

Most patients for endometrial resection are placed first on the operating list, then they can be seen by the surgeon at the end of the operating list and usually are fit to go home within the following few hours. They will have a fairly heavy period for a few days, which then settles down to become a watery pink discharge which can last for a week or can go on as long as 6 weeks. If it is more acceptable to the patient, it is perfectly acceptable to use tampons rather than relying on external sanitary pads.

Although the paracervical block with 0.5% Marcain® will reduce the incidence of postoperative menstrual cramps, some people do experience these when they get home and should be warned of this and told to take aspirin, Panadol® or non-steroidal anti-inflammatories, such as Ponstan®, Nurofen® or Brufen®.

There is considerable variability in advice as to when to resume normal activity. Adam Magos, one of the pioneers of this technique, recommends that patients should take 2 weeks off work in order to recover fully (personal communication), but in my experience I find that patients are perfectly able to resume full activity as soon as the anaesthetic effects have worn off, and I suggest that they can return to work in about 48 hours. Certainly our patients rarely have to take more than 1 week off work. Patients should also be warned that if they do develop a secondary infection (endometritis) some 10–14 days after the operation, which usually manifests as a heavy bright red bleed (more than a normal period) or an offensive discharge, then they should report immediately to their GP to be given a broad-spectrum antibiotic and metronidazole by mouth. It is important that this is clearly stated in the discharge letter to the GP (which should be posted at the latest on the day following the operation), so the GP knows exactly what to do should this rare occurrence arise. It is in fact very rare, since we use prophylactic antibiotics routinely as an i.v. bolus during the procedure.

When discharging the patient from hospital, it is also imperative to explain clearly that it is possible to have two, or even three, quite heavy menstrual periods during the following few months. This does not mean that the procedure has failed, because intrauterine scarring does take at least 6 months to form, and there is no value at all in seeing the patient in the follow-up clinic until 6 months has elapsed.

Complications

Electrosurgical endometrial resection suffers the disadvantage that it looks so easy to the uninitiated when viewing an expert performing it. It is, however, associated with more complications than any other procedure in the whole field of endoscopic surgery. For that reason it is necessary for a surgeon to go on a training course before embarking on these procedures, in order to learn the physics associated with electrosurgery and the hydrodynamics inherent in the fluid systems used to ensure a good clear view. Electrical energy should never be activated unless the surgeon can clearly see the field in which he is operating, and the rollerball or wire loop must always be pulled towards the operator and NEVER activated when it is pushed away from him. Perforation can be surprisingly difficult to recognize, especially when it is associated with bleeding, and if the radiofrequency energy is still activated, damage can occur to a wide variety of vessels and organs (Fig. 10.11).

The surgeon should be absolutely familiar with the hysteroscopic appearance of normal and abnormal uteri and should have done at least 50 diagnostic hysteroscopies before embarking on an operative procedure. He should then use various simulators and the uterine models made by Limbs and Things (Limbs and Things, Bristol,

Fig. 10.11 Complications of endometrial resection

1. Uterine perforation causing:
   - trauma to major blood vessels:
     — aorta
     — inferior vena cava
     — mesenteric artery
     — sacral artery
     — iliac artery
   - trauma to bowel resulting in peritonitis and/or septicaemia
   - trauma to bladder and/or ureter requiring laparotomy, ureteric stents
2. Haemorrhage requiring balloon tamponade, laparotomy, hysterectomy
3. Fluid overload
4. Endometritis and secondary haemorrhage
5. Intrauterine adhesions and haematometra
6. Unintended pregnancy
7. Burns

UK), which are excellent. It is possible to use both lasers and electrosurgery and the tissue effects simulated are very close to those encountered during actual surgery, although there is, of course, no bleeding. The next step is to use other simulators, such as a potato with a central cylinder bored out of it with an apple corer immersed in a solution of glycine. Following that, he should do a number of procedures with uteri that have been removed from a patient who has had a hysterectomy, and finally a series of patients who have given their consent for an endometrial resection to be performed before the uterus is removed at hysterectomy in order that the surgeon can learn this technique. The initial live cases should be done under the supervision of someone who is experienced in these techniques and it is better to begin with rollerball coagulation alone until experience is achieved. If at any stage of the procedure the view is obscured, then the procedure should be stopped until the situation is corrected. If at any time there is a fluid deficit of more than 1.5 litres, the surgery should either be finished rapidly or stopped; and if at any time the hysteroscopist sees a view similar to that obtained at laparoscopy, then a perforation has occurred, and the procedure should be immediately abandoned and either a laparoscopy or laparotomy undertaken. Laparoscopy will reveal the extent of the perforation and the amount of bleeding, but cannot reliably check the bowel for any sign of damage. Laparotomy will allow a careful inspection of bowel. If there is any injury, a wide excision of the area involved should be undertaken by a surgical colleague, because damage can occur up to 5 cm from the site of an electrical injury with monopolar radiofrequency energy. Even if a bowel perforation is not discovered, the patient must be kept in hospital for at least 3 days, and if she shows signs of increasing pain or develops a temperature or tachycardia, then laparotomy will be necessary to repair any bowel injury that is almost certain to be the cause of this.

Fluid overload

Fluid overload is very unlikely to occur with the technique described above, whereby the endometrium is removed in long continuous strips and after each pass the resectoscope is removed. There is no possibility of fluid overload occurring because the intrauterine fluid pressure is released each time the resectoscope is removed and there is very little chance of fluid entering the general circulation. Nevertheless, fluid overload is a very real risk in patients undergoing Nd:YAG laser photovaporization of the endometrium, because the hysteroscope is left inside the uterus throughout the procedure and large blood vessels are opened up, allowing direct entry of the irrigating fluid into the general circulation. In order to prevent serious complications from fluid overload, special infusion pumps (Fig. 10.12) must be used, which regulate the flow rate and the intrauterine pressure, ensuring a wide safety margin. Several different infusion pumps are available and they are all pressure, but not flow, limited. When a fixed intrauterine pressure of approximately 100 mmHg is set, the pump automatically turns itself off if this pressure is exceeded. Isotonic solutions, such as normal saline, are suitable for laser ablation, but strict attention to the volume of fluid infused and col-

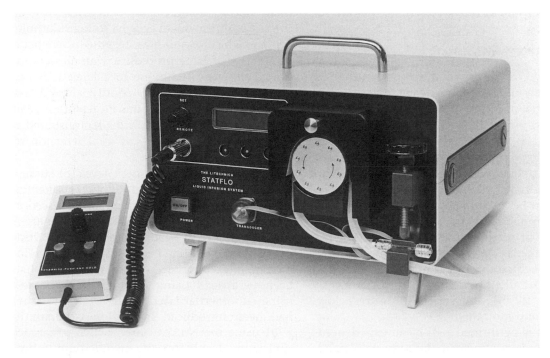

Fig. 10.12 Liquid infusion pump designed to vary flow rate to maintain intra-uterine pressure.

lected during the course of the procedure is necessary in order to recognize intravasation of fluid into the circulation at an early stage, because of the risk of pulmonary and cerebral oedema. With electroresection, it is necessary to use a non-electrolyte solution, such as 1.5% glycine. This amino acid is broken down to ammonium, with the potential risk of giving rise to high serum ammonium levels, which can result in the syndrome that has been recognized following transurethral resection of the prostate (TURP syndrome). This can result in water intoxification, hyponatraemia, hyperglycaemia, hyperammonaemia and subsequent cerebral toxicity, which can give rise to convulsions and death.

All of these problems can be avoided by removing the resectoscope at the completion of each resected strip of endometrium, and replacing the potentially dangerous glycine with sorbitol, which is broken down to much safer metabolites. With these precautions and a relatively short operating time of about 12 minutes, we have had no case of fluid overload in a series of about 1500 patients, but clearly one must be diligent, particularly if the rollerball is being used at the end of the procedure to seal off large and troublesome bleeding vessels.

Long-term results

Transcervical resection of the endometrium is an extremely useful treatment for patients with menorrhagia and also for patients with submucous fibroids. Although it looks simple to perform, it is in fact extremely difficult, and requires a learning curve of at least 50 operations before the operator can be said to be competent in its performance. Complications can occur very quickly, can be associated with severe morbidity and occasionally can be fatal. Although there was a spate of complications when the procedure was introduced, the establishment of training courses remedied this problem and the MISTLETOE study of all endometrial ablations in 1 year showed it to be very safe, with a very low morbidity and mortality.[36]

When it is performed well by an experienced operator it does appear to be safe, with good short-term results of about 90% effectiveness. We have found in a 5-year follow-up that the failure rate stabilizes after about 2.5 years, remaining constant at 83% when performed by a single experienced surgeon and 75% when performed by junior doctors in training.[37] This has also been shown in a long-term follow-up study from the Royal Free Hospital in London, which shows almost identical long-term success rates as our own study.[38] Thus, three-quarters of the patients can avoid hysterectomy by a simple day-case procedure and the majority of the patients are extremely satisfied with the result and grateful to have avoided a hysterectomy.

Conclusion

Although endometrial resection was first described in 1983 by DeCherney and Polan, using a urological resectoscope to remove the endometrium of women with intractable bleeding who were unfit for major surgery due to blood dyscrasias or extreme anaesthetic risk,[22] the technique was not really taken up in the USA. Jacques Hamou introduced a modified technique in Paris in 1985, but had to perform a partial endometrial resection, leaving some endometrial tissue above the internal os in order not to conflict with the dogma of the Roman Catholic Church, which would have regarded this operation as a sterilizing procedure. Hamou demonstrated this new technique to a large audience in Oxford in 1988 and, shortly after, Adam Magos, a senior lecturer with Professor Sir Alan Turnbull, working in Oxford, demonstrated a more extensive procedure of total resection of the endometrium.[39]

Subsequent reports of high levels of success in patient satisfaction led to an exponential increase in the use of endometrial resection and related techniques during the early 1990s. A survey in August of 1990 reported that 36 British centres had performed more than 4000 endometrial ablation procedures, of which 70% had been performed using resection and the rest using endometrial laser ablation.[40,41] The latter had been introduced by Milton Goldrath in 1981 using the Nd:YAG laser, which penetrates sufficiently deeply into the myometrium to produce satisfactory rates of oligo- and amenorrhoea. During the year from April 1993, more than 10 000 cases were performed in England and Wales alone, with 75% of all gynaecological units offering this service.[42]

This substantial change in the management of menorrhagia had taken place in the absence of good prospective research to establish the safety and long-term efficacy of these techniques. The early publications largely describe the personal series of experts in operative hysteroscopy, and reported excellent outcomes, though frequently with follow-up intervals of months rather than years. Subsequent reports began to emerge, describing increasing late failure rates of between 9 and 22%, and the need to resort to hysterectomy in many cases. It was suggested that the failure rate might be as high as 10% per annum,[43] with a report from one health region in England suggesting that introduction of endometrial ablation had merely led to an increase in the use of surgery for menorrhagia with no reduction in the rate of hysterectomy.[44] It appeared that the opportunity had been lost to mount large prospective studies comparing different treatments for menorrhagia, but happily common sense prevailed, and a number of good clinical randomized controlled trials providing grade A evidence were initiated, and reported in the last decade of the 20th century. The MISTLE-TOE study showed that transcervical resection of the endometrium (TCRE) is superior to medical treatment in terms of patient satisfaction (76 versus 27%; $P < 0.001$) and also, in finding treatment more satisfactory, willingness to have the treatment again. This study also showed a greater improvement in pain, bleeding, elevation of haemoglobin and improvement of quality of life.[45] It appeared from this study that, in those women with completed families, endometrial ablation is more effective than drug therapy. The above study compared endometrial ablation with antifibrinolytic, non-steroidal anti-inflammatory agents and combined oral contraceptives, but not with the levonorgestrel device, and it has been shown that in the long term this is more effective than other drug therapies and certainly the treatment of choice when fertility needs to be conserved. When fertility is not an issue, endometrial ablation, in skilled hands,

appears slightly more effective and with fewer side-effects and more prolonged effectiveness.[46,47]

There have been several randomized controlled trials comparing endometrial ablation with abdominal hysterectomy, conducted in Leeds,[48] Bristol,[49] Aberdeen[50] and London.[37] These showed that there were far fewer intra-operative and postoperative complications with endometrial ablation, and that operating time, recovery and hospital stay were clearly very much shorter with endometrial ablation procedures. Most of these studies were slightly unfair, in that they asked questions about patient satisfaction rate and quality of life 1 year after the procedure, when clearly the initial discomfort and increased complication rate of hysterectomy will largely be forgotten, whereas those with endometrial ablation, which is not designed to provide amenorrhoea in all patients, suffered from problems because at least 70% of them were still menstruating, even though the menstrual loss was much less than before. It is not really surprising therefore, that although patient satisfaction was high in both groups, it was greater at 1 year after hysterectomy, and there was more improvement in quality of life scores following hysterectomy. Another study by Alexander[51] showed that there was no difference in psychological outcome between the two techniques, but economic studies have suggested that although endometrial ablation is cheaper, 15% of patients will require a second treatment and about 20% will have a subsequent hysterectomy, so as time passes the total costs tend to converge.

There has only been one study comparing endometrial ablation to vaginal hysterectomy, which is known to be a much more patient friendly way of removing the uterus. There was no significant difference in patient satisfaction 2 years after these treatments, but the study was underpowered to detect significance at the level of difference observed.[52]

Summary

Endometrial ablation appears to be associated with less pain, shorter treatment time and quicker recovery after surgery, but in the long term hysterectomy is clearly more effective because it does produce complete amenorrhoea, and at 1 year there is better patient satisfaction because of this and the fact that the original discomfort and problems have been resolved by then in the majority of patients. Clearly, both procedures have their place in the surgical armamentarium and the preferred treatment will depend mainly on patient preference and operator experience. I have no doubt that endometrial ablation is an excellent procedure in correctly selected patients. Many of my patients have expressed considerable satisfaction and we have shown very good long-term results—with my patients we have cut down the hysterectomy rate for dysfunctional uterine bleeding by 85%. The few failures almost invariably have adenomyosis, which can usually be treated by an alternative minimally invasive therapy procedure, such as laparoscopic subtotal hysterectomy, which results in retention of the lower genital tract, much less postoperative urinary dysfunction, a short hospital stay and usually full recovery within 3 weeks.[53]

REFERENCES

1. Gordon A G, Taylor P J 1998 History and development of endoscopic surgery. In: Sutton C, Diamond M (eds) Endoscopic surgery for gynaecologists, 2nd edn. WB Saunders, London, Chapter 1, p 123

2. Bozzini P 1805 Der Lichtoeiter Odere Beschreibung Einer Eingachen Vorrichtung und Ihrer Anwendung zur Erleuchung Innerer Hohlen und Zwischeraume Deslebenden Animaleschen Korpses. Landes-Industrie-Tomtoi, Weimer

3. Desormeaux A J 1865 De l'endoscopie et de ses applications au diagnostic et au traitement des affections de l'uretre et de la vessie. Bailliere, Paris

4. Pantaleoni D C 1869 On endoscopic examination of the cavity of the womb. Medical Press Circular 8:26–27

5. David C 1907 De l'endoscopie de l'uterus ares avortement et dans es suites de couches a l'etat pathologique. Bulletin of Society of Obstetrics, Paris, December

6. Rubin I C 1925 Uterine endoscopy, endometroscopy with the aid of uterine insufflation. American Journal of Obstetrics and Gynecology 10(3):313–327

7. Mohri T 1971 Demonstration of the machida hysteroscope. In: Proceedings of the 7th World Congress on Fertility and Sterility, Tokyo and Kioto, October

8. Hopkins H 1953 On the defraction theory of optical images. Proceedings of the Royal Society A 217:408

9. Fourestiere M, Gladu A, Vulmiere J 1943 Laperitinioscopy. Presse Medicale 5:46–47

10. Stock R J, Kanbour A 1975 Pre-hysterectomy curettage. Obstetrics and Gynecology 45:537–538

11. Gimpelson R J 1984 Panoramic hysteroscopy with directed biopsies vs dilatation and curettage for accurate diagnosis. Journal of Reproductive Medicine 29:75–78

12. Hamou J 1986 Hysteroscopie et micro hysteroscopy. Masson, Paris

13. Raju K S, Taylor R W 1986 Routine hysteroscopy for patients with a high risk of uterine malignancy. British Journal of Obstetrics and Gynaecology 93:1259–1261

14. Edstrom K, Fernstrom I 1970 The diagnostic possibilities of a modified hysteroscopic technique. Acta Obstetrica et Gynecologica Scandinavica 49:327–330

15. Zebella E A 1985 Non cardiogenic pulmonary oedema secondary to intrauterine installation of 32% Dextran 70. Fertility and Sterility 43:479–480

16. Leake J F 1987 Non cardiogenic pulmonary oedema: a complication of operative hysteroscopy. Fertility and Sterility 48:497–499

17. Donnez J 1989 Instrumentation. In: Donnez J (ed) Laser operative laparoscopy and hysteroscopy. Nauwelaerts, Leuven, pp 207–221

18. Garry R 1998 Distension media and fluid systems. In: Sutton C, Diamond M (eds) Endoscopic surgery for gynaecologists, 2nd edn. WB Saunders, London, Chapter 53, pp 525–533.

19. Lindemann H J, Mohr J, Gallinat A et al 1973 Der Einluss von CO_2-gas. Wahrend der Hysteroscopie. Geburtshilfe und Frauenheilkunde 36:153–156

20. Monaghan J M 1999 Action in the event of malignant histology. In: Sutton C J G, Seth S S (eds) Menorrhagia. Isis Medical Media, Oxford, Chapter 18, p 207

21. Neuwirth R S l978 A new technique for and additional experience with hysteroscopic resection of submucous fibroids. American Journal of Obstetrics and Gynecology 131:91–94

22. DeCherney A H, Polan M L 1983 Hysteroscopic management of intrauterine lesion and intractable uterine bleeding. Obstetrics and Gynecology 61:392–397

23. Rutherford A J, Glass M R, Wells M 1991 Patient selection for endometrial resection. British Journal of Obstetrics and Gynaecology 98:228–230

24. Royal College of Obstetricians and Gynaecologists 1999 The initial management of menorrhagia. Evidence-based clinical guidelines 1. RCOG, London, pp 4–6

25. Broadbent J A M, Magos A L 1998 Transcervical resection of the endometrium. In Sutton C, Diamond M. Endoscopic surgery for gynaecologists. W B Saunders, London, Chapter 38, pp 294–306

26. Ewen S P, Sutton C J G 1995 A combined approach for painful heavy periods. Laparoscopic uterine nerve ablation and TCRE. Gynaecological Endoscopy 3:167–168

27. Sutton C J G, Ewen S P, Whitelaw N, Haines P 1994 Prospective, randomised, double blind controlled trial of laser laparoscopy in the treatment of pain associated

with minimal, mild and moderate endometriosis. Fertility and Sterility 62:696–700

28. Sutton C J G, Ewen S P 1994 Thinning the endometrium prior to endometrial ablation: is it worthwhile? British Journal of Obstetrics and Gynaecology 101(suppl 10):10–12

29. Brooks P G 1990 Resectoscopes for the gynaecologist. Contemporary Obstetrics/Gynaecology June:51–56

30. Corson S L, Brooks P G, Soderstrom R M 1996 Gynaecologic endoscopic gas embolism. Fertility and Sterility 65:529–533

31. Crozier T A, Luger A, Dravecz M et al 1991 Gas embolism with cardiac arrest during hysteroscopy. A case report on 3 patients. Anasthesiologie, Intensivmedizin, Notfallmedizin, Schmerztherapie 25:412–415

32. Perry P M, Baughman V L 1990 A complication of hysteroscopy: Air embolism. Anesthesiology 73:546–547

33. Brooks P G 1997 Venous air embolism during operative hysteroscopy. Journal of the American Association of Gynecologic Laparoscopists 4:399–402

34. Duffy S, Reid P C, Sharp F et al. 1991 Studies of uterine electrosurgery. Obstetrics and Gynecology 78:213–220

35. Ewen S P, Sutton C J G 1993 Complications of endometrial resection: is the smaller loop safer? Gynaecological Endoscopy 2(2):103–104

36. Overton C, Hargreaves J, Maresh M 1997 A national survey of the complications of endometrial destruction for menstrual disorders. The MISTLETOE study. British Journal of Obstetrics and Gynaecology 104:1351–1359

37. Pooley A, Ewen S P, Sutton C J G l998 Does trans-cervical resection of the endometrium really avoid a hysterectomy: life-table analysis of a large series. Journal of the American Association of Gynecological Laparoscopists 5:229–235

38. O'Connor H, Magos A 1997 The Medical Research Council randomised trial of endometrial resection versus hysterectomy in the management of menorrhagia. Lancet 349:897–901

39. Magos A L, Baumann R, Turnbull A C 1989 Transcervical resection of endometrium in women with menorrhagia. British Medical Journal 298:1209–1213

40. MacDonald R, Phipps J, Singer A 1992 Endometrial ablation: A safe procedure. Gynaecological Endoscopy 1:7–9

41. Goldrath M H, Fuller T A, Segal S 1981 Laser photovaporisation of endometrium for the treatment of menorrhagia. Americal Journal of Obstetrics and Gynecology 140:14–19

42. Maresh M, Overton C, McPherson K 1994 MISTLETOE update Royal College of Obstetricians and Gynaecologists. Medical Audit Unit (Pamphlet). RCOG Press, London

43. Lewis B V 1994 Guidelines for endometrial ablation. British Journal of Obstetrics and Gynaecology 101:470–473

44. Bridgeman S A 1996 Trends in endometrial ablation and hysterectomy for dysfunctional uterine bleeding in the Mersey region. Gynaecological Endoscopy 5:5–8

45. Cooper K G, Parkin D E, Garratt A M, Grant A M A 1997 A randomised comparison of medical and hysteroscopic management in women consulting a gynaecologist for treatment of heavy menstrual loss. British Journal of Obstetrics and Gynaecology 104:1360–1366

46. Crosignani P G, Vercellini P, Mosconi P et al 1997 Levo-norgestrel releasing intrauterine device versus hysteroscopic endometrial resection in the treatment of dysfunctional uterine bleeding. Obstetrics and Gynecology 90(pt 2):257–263

47. Kittelsen N, Istre O 1998 A randomised study comparing the levo-norgestrel intrauterine system (LNG IUS) and transcervical resection (TCRE) in the treatment of menorrhagia: preliminary results. Gynaecological Endoscopy 7(2):61–65

48. Gannon M J, Holt E M, Fairbank J et al 1991 A randomised controlled trial comparing endometrial resection and hysterectomy for the treatment of menorrhagia. British Medical Journal 303:1362–1364

49. Dwyer N, Hutton J, Stirrat G M 1993 Randomized controlled trial comparing endometrial resection with abdominal hysterectomy for the treatment of menorrhagia. British Journal of Obstetrics and Gynaecology 100:237–243

50. Pinion S B, Parkin D E, Abramovich D R et al 1994 Randomised trial of hysterectomy, endometrial laser ablation and transcervical endometrial resection for dysfunctional uterine bleeding. British Medical Journal 309:244–252

51. Alexander D A, Naji A A, Pinion S B et al 1996 Randomised trial comparing hysterectomy with endometrial ablation for dysfunctional uterine bleeding: psychiatric and psychosocial aspects. British Medical Journal 312:280–284

52. Crosignani P G, Vercellini P, Apolone G et al 1997 Endometrial resection versus vaginal hysterectomy for menorrhagia : long-term clinical and quality of life outcomes. American Journal of Obstetrics and Gynecology 177(1):95–101

53. Ewen S P, Sutton C J G 1994 Initial experience with supracervical hysterectomy and removal of the cervical transformation zone. British Journal of Obstetrics and Gynaecology 101(3):225–228

FURTHER READING

Mencaglia L, Hamou J Manual of gynaecological hysteroscopy. Available free of charge from Karl Stortz, D-78503 Tutlingen, Germany

Mencaglia L, Valle R, Lorraine J (eds) 1999 Endometrial carcinoma and precursors. Isis Books, Oxford

Minimal access surgery: image display and archiving

Christopher Sutton and Michael Scott

CHAPTER

11

Introduction

Photographic and video documentation is proving to be important in medicine for a variety of reasons:

1. Patient communication. Patients wish to fully understand their medical problem. They expect a comprehensive explanation of both diagnosis and appropriate treatment. Photographic images provide a convenient medium to help doctors explain this.

2. Follow-up. Images can remind the surgeon of the original problem and operation at a subsequent visit. Subsequent photographs can also be used to see if a medical condition is responding to treatment.

3. Doctor–doctor referral. Clear photographs of the medical problem enable referrals to be clearer and more concise. They may also reduce the need to repeat an investigation or operation.

4. Medico-legal claims. The number of medico-legal claims being brought against doctors is rapidly increasing. Video imaging can provide evidence that a surgeon has carried out an operation correctly; however, it may equally be used as evidence that the surgeon could have used a different technique.

5. Medical teaching. Photographs and video are used for a wide variety of teaching purposes.

The equipment

Light is produced using a light source, passes to the hysteroscope via a light lead and down the hysteroscope to the uterus (Fig. 11.1). The image is viewed through the hysteroscope. In order to

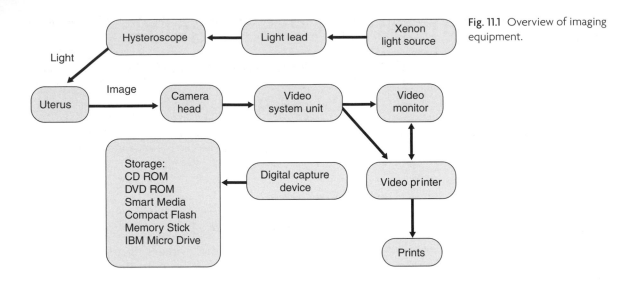

Fig. 11.1 Overview of imaging equipment.

project the image on to the monitor, a camera head is fitted on to the hysteroscope and the image sent to the video system unit. From here the image is displayed on a RGB monitor. Newer models allow the signal to pass to a digital capture unit to allow the production of digital image files. Prints are produced on a video printer using a freeze-frame facility on the camera.

Light source

All modern light sources use xenon because of its approximate colour temperature to daylight (5000–6200K). In combination with the camera and video control unit, automatic exposure compensation is obtained by adjusting light output or the aperture. This allows the operator to go from a wide to close-up view without having to adjust the exposure, thereby allowing seamless operating.

Light lead

A light lead carries a collection of fibreoptic bundles. It is important that they are handled carefully so as not to break any of the bundles. Breakage of bundles results in a reduction of light transmission to the uterus.

Hysteroscope

The hysteroscope must be clean and at body temperature to avoid fogging, in order to obtain good photographs.

Camera head

The first camera heads used for video-endoscopy used a three-colour tube system, but were large and heavy. Modern camera heads now use a CCD (charged couple device) to obtain the image (Fig. 11.2). These are smaller and lighter. A CCD is an integrated image sensor utilizing photo-

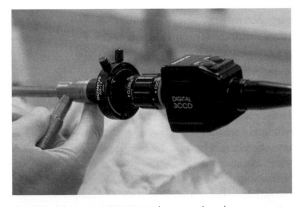

Fig. 11.2 Olympus 3CCD Digital camera head.

sensitive silicon. When light strikes the silicon, a current is generated in proportion to the light intensity falling on it. The number of photo-sensitive silicon elements determines the resolution, or number of pixels, that are produced. This is analogous to grains of silver halide on a photographic film.

The more modern cameras have a resolution of 410 000 pixels (NTSC) and 470 000 pixels (PAL). The way electrical charge is moved around the device is called charge coupling, hence the term CCD, charge coupled device.

A 3CCD camera has a separate CCD for each of the colours, red, green and blue (RGB), which when combined produce a full colour image. 3CCD cameras offer more accurate colour rendition than single-CCD cameras. They are, however, a lot more expensive and the question of just how accurate colour balance has to be during endoscopic procedures has led to more single-CCD cameras being made. These use a RGB imaging sequence to obtain a full colour image, i.e. every pixel sends a separate signal for red, green and blue light, which are then combined to produce a full colour image. With the improvements in signal to noise ratio and CCDs, these single-chip cameras produce excellent results. Newer models can be sterilized in an autoclave.

Video system unit

The video system unit, as we will refer to it here, is the name for the unit that receives the image signal from the camera head. In combination with the camera and light source, exposure can be controlled automatically to ensure continuous operating. White balance is also obtained using the video system unit by pointing the hysteroscope at a white swab and pressing the white balance. The video system unit processes the signal from the camera head which is then sent to a monitor or a digital capture unit, and is the backbone of the whole video system.

Monitor

High-quality RGB monitors should be used. They should be shielded from electromagnetic interference and have the capability of being used with PAL or NTSC video systems.

Thin-film transistor (TFT) and liquid crystal display (LCD) flat-screen displays may offer advantages over traditional monitors because of their light weight and compact shape. The colour quality, accuracy and viewing angle have improved enormously, and their application in medicine is increasing. Provided there are no problems with electromagnetic interference, they could become standard in the operating theatre. They offer the advantages of reduction in size, ease of portability and of being able to be placed and angled so the surgeon has a clear view.

Video printer

Video printers allow full-colour, photographic-quality prints from images freeze framed on the video system.

High-frequency interference

All electrosurgery and diathermy use high frequencies, which produce electrical and magnetic fields that interfere with video equipment. Most video and computer equipment is therefore electromagnetically shielded. As stated above, newer TFT and LCD screens are less susceptible to interference and are smaller and lighter.

Methods of documenting images

Images obtained through a hysteroscope can be either video or still photographs.

Still photographs

Currently the usual method of obtaining a still photographic print is by printing a still frame captured on the video monitor from a camera head attached to the hysteroscope (as shown in Fig. 11.1). Modern equipment that can capture images digitally is covered in the section below.

Still images can be also photographed directly through a hysteroscope, using a 35 mm camera, on to 35 mm photographic slide or print film.

Still images captured from video stills

The majority of hospitals use a video system where images are obtained through a hysteroscope on to a video monitor (see Fig. 11.1). When the appropriate image is on the monitor, the image is frozen and stored in the memory of a video printer. (Some systems send the image from the hysteroscope to the video printer and then to the monitor, but the end result is the same.) From here the image can be printed on special photographic paper. Up to four images can be printed on each sheet of paper, or a single image can take up the whole sheet (Fig. 11.3).

Although this is convenient, the image quality is limited by the number of lines on the screen (depending on whether it is PAL or NTSC), and electromagnetic interference or poor-quality cables can also affect quality.

Photographic film

Attaching a 35 mm camera via an adapter to the camera is still one of the easiest ways of producing quality photographs for documentation and

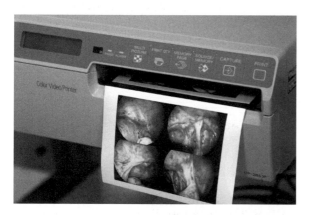

Fig. 11.3 The video printer is still the mainstay of photographic documentation in most hospitals. Here four separate video still frames have been printed.

teaching (Fig. 11.4). The cameras should have TTL (through the lens) metering and a way of compensating the exposure. It is often best to bracket the exposure ± two-thirds of a stop if using slide film, to ensure the best result. When using print film it is best to err on the side of overexposure as print film tolerates overexposure well. The ASA speed of the film depends on how good the light source is. Modern light sources provide a bright source of light so a daylight-balanced 200 ASA film suffices and gives good quality. If using older light sources, where the colour temperature of the light may be more yellow, one may have to think about using faster film, and even tungsten-balanced film, in order to get the correct white balance.

Converting photographs into digital images

The slide or negative produced can be scanned using a 35 mm scanner to produce a digital image in TIFF (tagged-image file format) or JPEG (Joint Photographic Experts Group) format. Alternatively a print can be scanned on a flat-bed scanner. These can be used for publications or computer on-screen productions.

Polaroid film and prints

Polaroid film has a relatively low ASA speed (sensitivity to light) so it has never been very practical to take photographs directly on to Polaroid film through a hysteroscope. It is, however, possible to make Polaroid images using a video freeze-frame unit. The advent of video printers has superseded this, so it is not considered in detail here.

Digital image capture device

The digital capture device (Fig. 11.5) is a recent introduction into medical practice. It converts

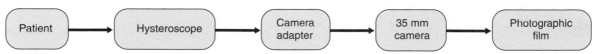

Fig. 11.4 Photographs can be taken through a hysteroscope using a 35 mm camera and adapter.

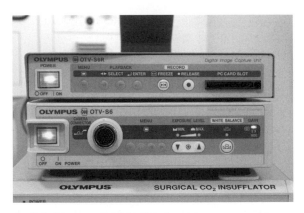

Fig. 11.5 Olympus OTV-S6 digital multi processor with OTV–S6R digital capture unit.

a digital signal produced by the video imaging unit into a digital file which is in a standardized digital photographic image format, e.g. JPEG image. This can then be printed through a video printer or stored on storage media, e.g. Smart Media, CD-ROM. Some digital capture devices allow the images to be written on to CD-ROMs, while others store the images on the memory cards used in digital cameras. The maximum number of images that can be stored depends on the size of the file of the photograph and the size of the memory card. The Smart Media card shown in Figure 11.6 is a 16 Mb size, although 128 Mb cards are now made. The use of different drivers in the software would allow the use of an IBM Microdrive, which is a similar physical size but can store up to 1 Gb of data! The current

size of a compressed photograph from the Olympus digital image capture device is 200 Kb. Thus it would be possible to store up to 5000 photographs on one 1 Gb IBM Microdrive. These could then be backed up on to a hard drive or CD- or DVD-ROM drive.

Advantages and disadvantages of still versus digital photographs

Photographic images
Advantages:

- Excellent quality—the image resolution only limited by lens and quality of film.

Disadvantages:

- Cannot get instantaneous results.
- Need to bracket exposures to ensure best results.
- Need to scan slides or negatives to get digital files for use in computer presentations.
- Time consuming to file and require space.

Digital capture unit/digital images
Advantages:

- You can see your results immediately.
- Easy to store and catalogue images.
- Photographs can be imported directly into computer presentations, e.g. Microsoft PowerPoint and Adobe PageMaker.

Disadvantages:

- Image quality is currently limited to around 410 000 pixels (NTSC) and 470 000 pixels (PAL).
- Outlay cost of a digital capture system.

Video image recording

VHS/SVHS

Video can be recorded via a normal coaxial cable and signal on to a VHS or SVHS video recorder.

Digital video (DV)

In order to record on to a DV tape, the video image signal must be in digital format. Therefore

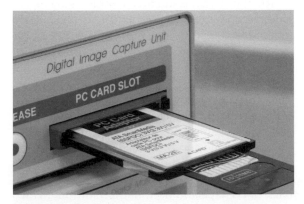

Fig. 11.6 Digital image capture unit showing PC card adaptor and 16 Mb Smart Media data storage card.

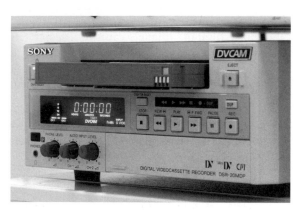

Fig. 11.7 Sony DVCAM digital video recording is possible on to DV or mini-DV tape, or directly on to a computer via an IE1394 Firewire link (see Fig. 11.8).

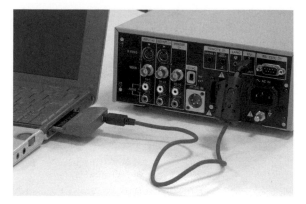

Fig. 11.8 Digital video capture can be performed directly on to a laptop via a PCMCIA DV capture card. Some laptop computers (like Apple Mac and the Sony shown) have an IE1394 Firewire slot, which obviates the need for a capture card.

there are two ways to record on to digital video (DV):

1. Analogue video signal from the camera or video imaging system can be converted to DV using a DV recorder or analogue to digital converter. There is a loss of quality compared to a pure digital signal from source.
2. The digital signal is produced at source (the camera) and sent directly to a digital video recorder. This is only possible with more recently introduced equipment such as the Olympus OTV-S6 digital multi processor which outputs a digital signal directly to an appropriate DV or mini-DV recorder (see Fig. 11.7). Dyonics have also produced a system where capture of digital stills or digital video can be stored immediately on CD-ROM.

There is also the possibility of recording straight on to the hard drive of a computer from the IE 1394 (Firewire) port of the DV recorder (see Fig. 11.8). The appropriate software must be installed on the computer. If the computer does not have a Firewire port, a DV capture card can be used in the PCMCIA slot, as shown in Figure 11.8.

Video imaging applications

Video can be used in its pure form and played back on a video recorder. This is the usual method for using VHS and SVHS video. Digital video has the advantage that it can be transferred to computer and edited. Still images and titles can also be added.

Recent advances in microprocessor speed have meant that even home computer users have the ability to edit video in real time. Software is a lot cheaper and easier to use. Video clips can be cut and edited so as to show only the most important parts of an operation for teaching purposes.

Computer standards for video editing

Just as there are video standards of PAL and NTSC, there are different standards of transferring digital video to computer for editing. The two standards for editing are QuickTime files and AVI files. Apple users have traditionally used QuickTime files for use in Adobe Premiere, and the latest version of Final Cut Pro and Quick Time are also still used on the IBM platform when using Adobe Premiere. MPEG2 and AVI files can be used in more simple editing programs on the IBM platform, e.g. MGI Videowave, and can be embedded into Microsoft PowerPoint presentations.

Once edited, the final video can be converted back to DV tape and used like a traditional video tape that has been edited and has had any titling and stills embedded. The video can also be compressed to MPEG files to reduce storage space, or stored using its original QuickTime or AVI file structure on to a hard drive or CD-/DVD-ROM drives.

For embedding video into Microsoft Power-Point, it is best to save the file as an AVI or MPEG2 file. For putting the video on a website, MPEG (1 and 2) is a better format as it is compressed to take up less space, and will therefore download from the Internet quicker.

Once video has been compressed using MPEG, the data has been compressed and effectively lost. It is inevitable that quality is not as good as that of the original AVI files.

The Dyonics system of recording digital video on CD-ROM captures the images digitally and then uses MPEG2 compression to make the files a more manageable size, which will also fit conveniently on to a CD-ROM. This means the video is conveniently organized on the CD-ROM in named files, allowing easy access and cataloguing of video clips. However, there is loss of original data because of MPEG compression, so the quality of playback is not as good as video recorded on to DV tape which is uncompressed.

The optimum system for recording quality video is by capturing on to DV tape. This can be compressed using MPEG for convenience and cataloguing, or used as a primary source to input video to computers for presentations, or for showing on a video recorder.

The future: three-dimensional endoscopy and video imaging

A three-dimensional image can be obtained through a video endoscope by using two CCDs at the end. Recent advances in the quality and reduction of size of CCDs has enabled an improvement in the quality of image to allow three-dimensional operating to the surgeon with special equipment. Although three-dimensional operating is advantageous in abdominal laparoscopic surgery, it offers less advantages when operating in the uterus. This is because a single operating hysteroscope is utilized and there is little room to pass a second operating instrument through the cervical os.

Storage of photographic media and digital photographs

Traditional storage of photographs has been in the notes of patients. Digital image files offer the advantage of being easy to catalogue, retrieve and incorporate into teaching material. Prints can still be obtained, if needed, by printing using a digital printer.

Some digital capture devices allow the labelling of images, facilitating image retrieval at a future date. Hardware and software packages are now available that allow the sorting and viewing of the different photographs by patient and date. These can be printed as Index Prints with all necessary details of surgeon, patient, date, time, etc.

It is best to store digital photographs as JPEG compressed images. This allows a 768×504 pixel (i.e. full screen) image to be compressed and take up only 50 Kb of disk space.

Potential problems storing digital photographs

The main problems with digital photographs are:

- maintaining confidentiality
- preventing substitution with another photograph or altering the original image
- storage.

To maintain confidentiality, photographs should only be kept on a secure computer system where users need passwords to log on. This is no different to current medical computer systems that store patients' records and laboratory results.

The problem of stopping photographs being touched up or altered from the original is a potentially more difficult problem. This has been overcome by a process of 'watermarking' photographs. This is a process of embedding a digital signal on top of the photograph which does not affect the image very much. When the photograph is viewed with special software it shows up whether it has been altered in any way.

With the advent of large-capacity hard drives, storing digital images is less of a problem. It is best to store photographs in a compressed format using the JPEG file format. These take up less space than raw image or TIFF files.

Summary

The technology now exists for the recording on videotape of all hysteroscopic operations. This can be on traditional VHS/SVHS systems or DV (digital video). Newer systems capture the video and compress it directly to MPEG digital files.

Using a digital capture device, all clinical photographs taken during hysteroscopy can be stored digitally as well as being printed using a video printer, as is current practice. These digital photographs offer the convenience of being stored on data storage cards or on the hard drive of a computer. The photographs can be catalogued, viewed and retrieved when necessary. Images can be printed as and when required. They are also in a suitable format to be incorporated directly into computer presentations for medical teaching purposes.

To maintain confidentiality, access to these digital images on computer systems must be restricted to authorized persons only.

General surgical principles in obstetrics and gynaecology

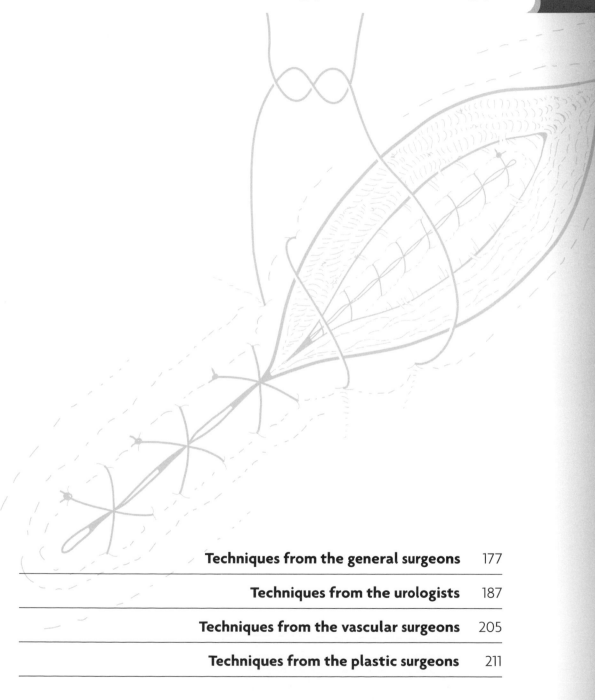

Techniques from the gastrointestinal surgeons

Simon Atkinson

CHAPTER

12

Operations that involve the bowel: general principles

The maintenance of gastrointestinal integrity in surgical procedures other than those involving the gut accounts for much of the low morbidity and mortality associated with such surgery. As soon as the integrity of the gastrointestinal tract is breached, there is considerable potential for septic complications, including abscess and fistula formation, systemic sepsis and multiple organ failure. This last complication, if involving three-organ failure, has a 70% mortality and remains the most serious complication. This is particularly so if there is unplanned or iatrogenic injury that goes unrecognized and subsequent definitive management is delayed.

Preoperative investigations and appropriate preparation and planning for potential gastrointestinal surgery can greatly reduce the risk of encountering these complications.

Preoperative investigation and staging

Possible involvement of the gastrointestinal tract should be suspected in any malignant disease of pelvic or perineal origin. Moreover, 'benign' disease, such as endometriosis or fibroids, can either extend into the gut or, by mass effect, make surgery technically difficult, increasing the risk of inadvertent bowel injury.

Preoperative staging should aim to assess whether gastrointestinal surgery is likely to be required. Clinical examination should include a thorough rectal and bi-manual examination, and possibly rigid sigmoidoscopy. Any symptoms suggesting colonic pathology should be assessed by either double-contrast barium enema or colonoscopy. The former has the advantage of demonstrating extrinsic deformation and any fistulation, the latter the advantage of direct visualization of the bowel wall and obtaining biopsies. Transvaginal ultrasound will provide good definition of local disease but is limited to the pelvis. Transrectal ultrasound may provide additional information about presacral disease. Transabdominal ultrasound has high sensitivity for liver metastases but is poor at intestinal pathology. Computed tomographic (CT) cross-sectional imaging is very sensitive in detecting solid pathology in the abdomen and, although less so, the pelvis, particularly if this is combined with intravenous, oral and rectal contrast. The bony pelvis may cause artefactual degradation of CT images and magnetic resonance imaging (MRI) can provide useful information, particularly about anal sphincteric anatomy and defects therein.

Laparoscopy can demonstrate gastrointestinal involvement by pelvic pathology and is a standard gynaecological investigation. However, it may be the case that pathology within the pelvis attracts attention to the detriment of careful examination of the gastrointestinal tract and associated organs. Gentle manipulation with atraumatic graspers will assess fixity of upper rectum, colon and small bowel. Visualization of the liver may reveal small metastases not seen on non-invasive imaging, and fine parietal and visceral peritoneal metastatic deposits may also be noted and biopsied. In addition, deposits of endometriosis may be found outwith the pelvis, adherent to the gastrointestinal tract.

Instruments

Surgical instruments used to operate on the bowel are broadly similar to those used in standard gynaecological practice. A major procedure involving intestinal surgery, unless laparoscopically assisted, requires good exposure via an adequate incision. Retraction of the abdominal wall is of crucial importance and a number of different retractors are in common use. Parti-

cularly useful are retraction systems that allow fixed positioning of a number of retractors. This may obviate the need for a second assistant and help when the first assistant is inexperienced. In addition, malleable retractors that can attach to these systems are excellent for holding bowel that has been packed away to aid exposure. Laparoscopic instrumentation is being increasingly used not only for gynaecological surgery but also for minimally invasive intestinal mobilization and laparoscopically assisted intestinal resection.

In handling the bowel, the fingers are often the most sensitive and gentle instruments. In open surgery, separation of bowel along tissue planes is best accomplished by a combination of finger dissection and sharp dissection using McIndoes or Metzenbaum scissors. Haemostatic forceps used for ligation of mesenteric vessels prior to intestinal resection should be as fine as possible, but still appropriate for the size of vessel to be ligated.

Intestinal anastomoses can be either sutured by hand or, increasingly, by disposable stapling devices. Hand-sewn techniques have the advantage of being applicable to different intestinal anastomoses, having good control over tissue apposition along the length of the anastomosis and low cost. Stapling devices can facilitate anastomoses that would otherwise be technically inaccessible, are thought to be quicker but are more expensive.

Sutures

Again, suture materials are broadly similar to those used in gynaecological surgery. Most suture materials used are soluble, with varying times to loss of tensile strength. Intestinal anastomoses are usually constructed with a 2/0 or 3/0 braided or monofilament suture. Monofilament sutures run well through tissues but may 'pursestring' an anastomosis if used in a continuous manner without 'locking' the suture. Closing the abdomen requires stronger sutures with longer strength maintenance times. A No. 1 monofilament suture of either permanent or dissolvable material is often used in a continuous mass abdominal closure.

Incisions

The widest access to all abdominal and pelvic viscera is obtained through the midline incision. When preoperative investigations suggest intestinal involvement, the midline incision has the major advantage of being able to be extended superiorly to gain access to the supracolic compartment. Paramedian incisions are now rarely used, largely because of the popularity of the midline mass closure with continuous monofilament sutures. Transverse lower abdominal incisions, such as the pfannenstiel, are only used when no access to any intestinal structure other than the sigmoid colon and rectum are likely to be required. However, a wide pfannenstiel incision can be used in prostatic and bladder surgery, and it is possible to perform an anterior resection of the rectum if such an incision is extended to the left.

Preoperative measures

All major surgery needs good preoperative assessment of cardiovascular and respiratory function. Much gynaecological surgery can be carried out through a transverse lower abdominal incision and may not have a marked effect on respiratory capacity in the immediate postoperative period. However, the midline incision, particularly if extended superiorly, can result in significant respiratory distress, usually because the pain of the incision reduces chest wall movement. This disadvantage of the higher incision may be reduced by good postoperative analgesia, including patient-controlled and epidural analgesia. Assessment includes any potential requirements for postoperative high dependency or intensive care. Preoperative preparation for surgery that may include intestinal resection also requires careful planning of potential anastomoses and, especially, consideration of the possibility that a stoma may be required. It may be prudent to forewarn either urological or gastrointestinal surgeons if their assistance may be required, and to confirm that instruments and sutures for gastrointestinal resection are available.

Full preparation of the colon should be undertaken whenever preoperative investigations reveal colonic involvement. It is important to avoid dehydration, particularly in the elderly and those unable to take adequate oral fluids. In these cases consideration should be given to bowel preparation as an in-patient, with intravenous fluid replacement.

Certain groups of patients for whom gastrointestinal surgery is contemplated can be considered as high risk. Systemic conditions such as diabetes mellitus and those requiring treatment with corticosteroids have increased risk of anastomotic and wound complications. Obesity and, conversely, malnutrition pose similar excess perioperative risks, as do organ-specific conditions such as ischaemic heart disease, chronic obstructive pulmonary disease and chronic renal failure. Preparation for such high-risk patients will include optimizing their co-morbid conditions by specialist medical review. Perioperative malnutrition is often difficult to address and little benefit has been demonstrated by hyperalimentation prior to surgery. Construction of a feeding gastrostomy or jejunostomy intraoperatively can provide good postoperative access to the gastrointestinal tract, and may be useful in the malnourished patient. However, there are potential complications in any breach of gastrointestinal integrity and the risk–benefit ratio for these procedures is not yet defined. Nasogastric feeding postoperatively is an alternative, but may be uncomfortable, results in increased incidence of infective respiratory complications and can cause oesophageal and nasopharyngeal trauma. In contrast, obesity with a body mass index of 35 or over is usually not amenable to preoperative reduction, even if adequate time is available prior to surgery. Postoperatively, adequate calories must still be provided for the obese patient to avoid significant catabolism. Obesity carries independent risks, particularly those of wound dehiscence, basal atelectasis and deep venous thromboses. Thrombo-prophylaxis against venous thromboembolic complications is standard for most pelvic procedures and should be maintained for gastrointestinal surgery. Commonly, either twice-daily unfractionated heparin or once-daily low molecular weight heparin are administered subcutaneously.

Counselling and informed consent are crucial parts of preoperative discussions with patients and their relatives. The indications for surgery, an explanation of the planned procedure itself and the likely postoperative course are standard practice. However, it is also important to explain the main risks and possible complications associated with the procedure. In particular, if it is in any way possible that an intestinal stoma may be required, be it a colostomy or an ileostomy, this must be discussed with the patient and, if appropriate, with their relatives prior to surgery. The consequences of either a temporary or permanent stoma are often best explained by nursing staff dedicated to 'stoma therapy', and they may be able to provide the most useful counselling to patients. They are also able to mark the site of the best position for a stoma in any particular patient. It is always poor practice for patients to have to undergo an unplanned construction of a stoma when it was predictable that such a stoma might be required. Even worse are cases where a stoma is an absolute indication during an operation but is avoided solely because the patient was not forewarned, and that absence of a stoma is eventually detrimental to the patient's clinical outcome.

Causes and sites of injury to the bowel

Planned intestinal resection and reconstruction carry risk of significant local and systemic sepsis if there is egress of intestinal contents. Unplanned injury to the intestinal tract compounds these risks considerably, and septic complications become certain if the injury goes unrecognized. The most common type of injury is a traumatic breach of the gastrointestinal wall by surgical dissection, particularly if the bowel wall is abnormally fixed. Such fixity includes adhesions from previous surgery or inflammation, radiation injury and involvement with malignant disease (Fig. 12.1).

A common site of intestinal adhesions is the peritoneum directly beneath previous abdominal incisions. Considerable care needs to be taken when incisions are made at sites of earlier

Fig.12.1 Factors increasing risk of gastrointestinal injury

- Previous abdominal and pelvic incisions
- Previous intraperitoneal surgery
- Extensive peritoneal adhesions
- Crohn's disease
- Diverticulitis
- Chronic intra-abdominal sepsis
- Sinuses and fistulae
- Previous radiotherapy to the abdomen or pelvis
- Extensive peritoneal malignant disease
- Inappropriate use of laparoscopy or minimally invasive surgery

surgery. Bowel can protrude through incisional hernias, and palpation of the previous incision when the abdominal muscles are contracted, or the patient is upright, may demonstrate defects in the anterior abdominal wall. Dissection of an earlier incision may expose bowel adherent to the linea alba, and injury can result if the wound edges are retracted forcefully. Extending an incision to areas where the peritoneum has not been previously breached may give easier access to the peritoneum and non-adherent viscera. Adhesions may be dense where there has been chronic infection and discerning the edges of the bowel wall may only be possible by palpation. Severe inflammation may cause fistulae to develop between adjacent structures. If this is not appreciated prior to separation of these structures, a small opening into the bowel as a result of a fistula may not be noticed at the time of surgery.

Intestine in a previously irradiated field is often severely affected, and adhesions formed following radiation injury may obliterate all tissue planes, with fusion of loops of bowel. Dissection must be very cautious when embarking on attempted adhesiolysis in these cases, as multiple perforations may occur and irradiated tissue heals poorly. Sutured perforations or anastomoses are at high risk of failure and subsequent leak of intestinal contents.

Malignant disease may cross and completely fuse adjacent visceral peritoneal surfaces covering the gastrointestinal tract, with possible subsequent fistula formation. Dissection along original tissue planes may not be possible without inevitable damage to the bowel and, in any case, has little oncological benefit. If en bloc resection is at all possible, then this should be performed. However, in many cases the extent of the disease precludes this surgical strategy. Remaining options include accepting inoperability, debulking of tumours or surgical bypass procedures. Outcomes from some malignancies, particularly ovarian, are improved by a reduction in tumour load by debulking.

Finger dissection is usually the safest way of lifting tumour off bowel surfaces. If it is not possible to resect a length of bowel perforated during debulking, dissection should err on the side of leaving residual disease. Attempts to suture perforations in the midst of malignant infiltration are unlikely to be successful, and are bound to fail if there is any degree of distal obstruction. This latter is, of course, a common problem with disseminated peritoneal disease.

Damage caused by dissection may be solely restricted to the serosa and not involve the full thickness of the bowel wall. The underlying submucosa and mucosa are usually able to maintain gastrointestinal integrity, but if subject to excessive distension, ischaemia or any diathermy, necrosis and subsequent perforation may ensue. Injury can occur even if the full thickness of the bowel wall is intact. Ischaemic injury may be caused by incorrect ligation and division of mesenteric blood vessels or by excessive attempts at haemostasis. Trauma to the mesentery may result in a mesenteric haematoma. The local pressure effect created can cause a segmental ischaemic injury. If tied too tightly, sutures used for anastomoses or repairs to intestinal defects can result in pressure necrosis, not only of tissue within the suture but also in adjacent bowel wall. Diathermy used at high power or for an excessive time can produce full-thickness tissue necrosis. A pernicious consequence of diathermy injury is that the damaged area will maintain gastrointestinal integrity for some time before the necrotic area sloughs and perforates. The injury may, therefore, go unnoticed at the time of surgery, only to present later with intra-abdominal sepsis.

Diathermy injury is a particular risk of laparoscopic surgery. Laparoscopic instruments may be in contact with the bowel outside of the field of view of the laparoscope. If diathermy current is initiated inadvertently an injury may not be seen to occur. Laparoscopic instruments, although insulated along most of their length, often have a short conducting area just proximal to the working area. This may come into accidental contact with the bowel when attention is concentrated on the working tip of the instrument.

Another type of injury is also associated with access, namely creation of a pneumoperitoneum prior to laparoscopy. It is common gynaecological practice to use a Veress needle to puncture the peritoneum and insufflate. Bowel puncture with this method is more likely if the viscera are prevented from being displaced by adhesions, or if the bowel is distended from obstruction. Other complications of Veress needle puncture are well described and include urological and vascular injury. An alternative to use of the Veress needle is the open or Hassan technique. The linea alba and peritoneum are incised under direct vision and a blunt-ended insufflating trocar is inserted. This method is recommended where adhesions are thought likely, but it has its hazards. The incision used for the open method is usually as small as possible to obtain an airtight seal around the trocar. This limits visibility, and bowel adherent beneath can be damaged by the attempts to gain access by blunt dissection. In cases of doubt, incisions for either method of laparoscopic access should be made at sites distant from previous incisions. The left upper quadrant is usually a favourable position.

Other injuries associated with laparoscopic surgery include not only the diathermy injuries already mentioned but also punctures caused by inaccurate positioning of instruments. Instruments left within laparoscopic trocars, but outside the field of view of the laparoscope, are particularly likely to result in injury. Also, the absence of stereoscopic vision reduces depth of field perception, and bowel positioned behind the surgical field may be damaged by excessive insertion of instruments. Slow and smooth movements of laparoscopic instruments are crucial to safe laparoscopic surgery. Instruments must not be manipulated unless within the field of view of the laparoscope, and should be removed completely if not in use. Inadvertent activation of diathermy should be guarded against constantly.

Unrecognized injury to the bowel is the greatest hazard and may occur when vision is limited both in laparoscopic and open surgery. Transvaginal procedures may result in trauma to loops of small bowel dropping into the pelvis, particularly if they are fixed following previous pelvic surgery. If injury is suspected, the bowel must be scrutinized, looking for eversion of mucosa and leak of gastrointestinal contents. Soft compression of the bowel either side of the site of injury, and pressurization of that segment, can eject luminal contents and confirm perforation. At the end of any extensive dissection it is always prudent to inspect the bowel methodically from proximal to distal, looking carefully for serosal tears and unrecognized perforations. This inspection should itself be gentle, as traumatized but still intact bowel can be torn in the process. This inspection should not just be limited to the small bowel, but should also include the colon. Again, there are specific hazards associated with this manoeuvre, namely splenic trauma and subsequent haemorrhage from retraction of the splenic flexure of the colon.

Serosal defects may be either left alone if minor, or sutured to provide some reinforcement. However, serosal sutures often pierce the mucosa and, if not placed satisfactorily, may be worse than leaving exposed submucosa. In cases where there are multiple or large serosal tears, the safest course is often to resect that segment of bowel. This is particularly important if there are multiple perforations. A succession of full-thickness repairs runs the risk of narrowing the gut lumen. This may cause proximal dilatation and 'cutting out' of the sutures. Colonic injury can rarely be safely repaired by simple closure of a perforation. The strategy with the least risk of serious complications, particularly when the bowel is unprepared, is to bring out the perforated section of colon as a stoma. Alternatively, colon may be resected and anastomosed along anatomical lines.

Specific operative techniques

Bowel resection and anastomosis

Although numerous techniques of equal efficacy and safety are described for intestinal anastomoses, resection of both small and large bowel must conform to certain common principles. It is important that the segment of bowel to be resected is selected carefully. For resection of small bowel, there is no lower limit to the length resected, but it should include adjacent areas of serosal damage. The remaining small bowel should be well over 100 cm long, as lengths less than this are not enough to provide adequate surface area for enteral nutrition alone. Ligation of small bowel mesenteric vessels requires only small haemostatic forceps and enclosure of as little tissue as possible with each ligature. If large amounts are ligated, this may occlude nearby vessels, affecting the blood supply of the bowel ends to be anastomosed. Dissection of the small bowel mesentery should not extend deep into the base of the mesentery, as damage to the main mesenteric vessels may occur. Resection and anastomosis near the ileocaecal valve should be avoided because it is difficult to preserve adequate mesentery for the last few centimetres proximal to the caecum.

Colonic resections are limited by vascular anatomical constraints. Arterial supply to the right and transverse colon is provided by the ileocolic, right colic and middle colic arteries, branches of the superior mesenteric artery. The left and sigmoid colon are supplied by ascending branches of the inferior mesenteric artery. There is an arterial anastomosis along the marginal artery between the two systems which passes around the splenic flexure of the colon. Resections usually require ligation of at least one main artery and removal of the length of colon supplied by that artery, resulting in the right, transverse, left and sigmoid colectomies. Resection of the distal sigmoid colon and upper rectum will involve ligation of the inferior mesenteric artery or its branches, and may also require mobilization of the splenic flexure.

There are two vital principles of constructing safe intestinal anastomoses: there should be a good blood supply and the bowel ends should not be under tension. Accurate anatomical preservation of mesenteric blood supply with adequate mobilization of the bowel allow adherence to these two principles. Anastomoses can be either hand-sewn or stapled, with many techniques described for tissue apposition. One simple technique is the inverting interrupted mattress suture (Fig 12.2). This has the advantage of being able to be used for any intestinal anastomosis. The first pass of the suture is all layers and is then reversed to take mucosa and submucosa only. If the knots are on the inside, the suture will automatically invert the edges of the anastomosis, preventing mucosal eversion. Also, with this technique any distension of the bowel should increase anastomotic apposition rather than distraction. Intestinal injury can also be repaired using this method, but it may not be suitable for single, very small defects. In these cases a simple two-layer interrupted closure is usually adequate. In small bowel injury it is occasionally useful to extend a perforation so that a more formal repair can be constructed. Serosal tears may be closed by one-layer closure, given the caveats described earlier.

Intestinal resections do not always allow subsequent anastomosis and restitution of the normal faecal stream. Pelvic disease may render the rectum inaccessible or bowel distal to the resection may be obstructed. Moreover, extensive disease often encases bowel and adjacent organs to such an extent that resection is not feasible and obstruction has either occurred or is incipient. The safety of primary repair of intestinal trauma, particularly to unprepared colon, cannot always be relied upon. When anastomosis is not possible or safe, diversion of the faecal stream

may be necessary. This may be achieved with either a defunctioning or an end intestinal stoma.

Obstructing lesions may be bypassed as long as careful examination of the distal bowel does not reveal other stenoses. Early peritoneal ovarian metastases may cause small bowel obstruction, and a single point stenosis is particularly suitable for either entero–enteral or entero–colic bypass. Extensive disease may produce many areas of narrowing, and a loop of bowel will need to be exteriorized as a defunctioning stoma. Defunctioning loop colostomies are the least technical to construct, but are only possible where the colon has a mesentery, namely the transverse and sigmoid colon. Through either right upper quadrant or left iliac fossa incisions, the rectus sheath is split to allow delivery of a loop of colon. The colon is supported by a 'bridge', usually of plastic, across the incision on top of the skin. The colon is then opened and sutured to the skin edges. The bridge can be removed safely after 5 days. Transverse colon may prolapse through a stoma, and attempts to prevent this include siting the stoma as close to the hepatic flexure as possible, thus anchoring the proximal limb.

Small bowel loop stomas should be as distal as possible, to reduce intestinal output. The right iliac fossa usually puts least tension on the delivered bowel. The proximal limb needs to be everted into a spout, so that, with a close-fitting stoma bag, small bowel contents pass without excoriating the skin. Similar principles apply to small bowel end stomas. End colostomies are delivered through the rectus sheath wherever the length of bowel allows, and a simple enterocutaneous suture will secure the stoma. It is important, particularly in obese patients, to deliver some colonic mesentery alongside the bowel, otherwise the stoma may subsequently retract.

End stomas are indicated following intestinal resections where subsequent anastomosis is not possible. In such circumstances the remaining distal bowel can either be closed and left within the abdomen, or itself brought out to the skin as a mucus fistula. Any closure of the distal limb will be at risk of dehiscence if the remaining bowel is obstructed, and in such cases construction of a mucus fistula is mandatory. Siting

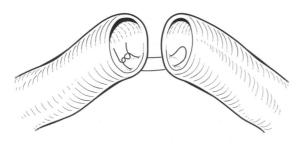

Fig. 12.2 Inverting interrupted mattress suture.

a mucus fistula will depend on the length of bowel and mesentery available. One of the most common indications arises when sigmoid colon is divided and remaining colon and rectum are obstructed in the pelvis. The mucus fistula may then be brought out to the lower end of a midline wound.

Intra-abdominal drains are rarely useful following elective gastrointestinal surgery. Leakage of gastrointestinal contents from an anastomotic failure rarely appear in a drain, and if they do it is usually a late sign. Suction drains left in situ may cause necrosis of bowel wall applied to the holes in the drain if the vacuum is not released. Drains may be useful if placed in the pelvis to reduce the likelihood of pelvic haematoma formation with subsequent abscess formation. Similarly, in emergency surgery, established infection may require continuing drainage.

Abdominal closure

The most common currently used technique for closing a midline incision is the mass muscle closure. This uses a continuous monofilament suture, often in two strands, taking the full thickness of the rectus sheath. Jenkins' rule states that the length of suture required should be three times the length of the incision, and each traverse of the sheath should be 1 cm apart and 1 cm deep lateral to the wound edges. Commencement at each end of the incision with two lengths of suture allows completion of the closure in the middle of the wound. This enables easy access for finishing the closure, with good visualization of any underlying bowel.

In cases with gross contamination of the peritoneal cavity with either pus or gastrointestinal contents, it is occasionally necessary to consider a further laparotomy after some days of stabilization. In these situations the abdomen may be left open either temporarily or permanently, as a laparostomy. There are numerous techniques for temporary coverage of the exposed viscera, and once granulation begins, the wound may heal by secondary intention. If possible, however, the abdomen should be closed within 5 days as a laparostomy may result in haemorrhage or fistula formation, and always leaves an incisional hernia. Less severe contamination, particularly in emergency cases, may have a high skin and subcutaneous wound infection rate. One strategy to reduce the risk of septic wound breakdown is to leave the skin wound open. Once the wound is clean, delayed primary closure may be undertaken. However, this usually requires a general anaesthetic, and in some cases the skin wound may not be closed at all but left to heal by secondary intention. If a subcutaneous monofilament suture is used for the skin, it can be left loose and, with subsequent traction on the ends, can close the wound, at least partially.

Postoperative management

The management of the postoperative patient in any operation involving the bowel is a matter of continual vigilance for the potential complications of intra-abdominal sepsis. The stable patient progresses steadily over a period of 2–5 days, with increasing mobility, reducing analgesic requirements and normal gastrointestinal function. The latter includes tolerating oral fluids and diet and normal bowel actions. Any deviation from this course should immediately raise concerns about the integrity of intestinal anastomoses or infected intra-abdominal collections (Fig. 12.3). Observation of vital signs are key to monitoring satisfactory postoperative progress.

Fig. 12.3 Indicators of sepsis following gastrointestinal surgery

- Increasing abdominal pain after initial improvement
- Persisting nausea and vomiting
- Persisting abdominal distension
- Inflammation of wound with or without purulent discharge
- Discharge of clear fluid from the wound, suggesting dehiscence
- Tachycardia (pulse rate >90)
- Tachypnoea (respiratory rate >20)
- Peripheral vasodilatation
- Pyrexia
- Neutrophil leucocytosis
- Rising urea and creatinine
- Hypotension
- Oliguria

Tachycardia, tachypnoea and pyrexia should not be ascribed to basal atelectasis or other extra-abdominal complications without careful assessment of the abdomen. Urine output needs to be very carefully monitored until the patient is tolerating oral fluids and is mobile.

Examination of the postoperative abdomen should assess the wound and any associated inflammation or discharge. Clear fluid without surrounding wound cellulitis may indicate an incipient wound dehiscence. Pain and tenderness inappropriate to the length and site of the wound may suggest underlying peritonitis. There are few investigations that can be relied upon to be abnormal in the face of intra-abdominal sepsis. A neutrophil leucocytosis, particularly rising from normal in the immediate postoperative period, is cause for concern, as is a rise in the C reactive protein. Abnormalities of electrolytes may reflect inappropriate intravenous fluid management but an occult collection can lead to such systemic sepsis that renal function is compromised. A reduction in peripheral oxygen saturation is also associated with systemic sepsis, and any suggestion of haemodynamic instability or inadequate oxygenation should be quantified by measurement of arterial blood gas and acid–base status. It should always be remembered that an arterial pH within the normal range only signifies that the patient is not *acidaemic*. Arterial bicarbonate and the base excess may well indicate *acidosis* in the presence of a low normal pH. Acidosis should always initiate an intensive search for a source of sepsis.

Imaging of the abdomen and pelvis becomes essential when complications of surgery are suspected. An erect chest X-ray may reveal pulmonary complications, but it is vital that such findings are only accepted as the cause of a deterioration if abdominal and pelvic complications are excluded. Free gas underneath a hemidiaphragm is only residual gas from a laparotomy or laparoscopy for a very short time, usually less than 24 hours, and if this is noted after this time, it must be pursued. A pleural effusion may result from subphrenic collections the other side of the diaphragm.

A plain supine abdominal X-ray may be useful. Very dilated loops of small bowel are more likely to be evidence of obstruction, perhaps from adherence to a septic collection, than 'an ileus'. The latter diagnosis should be treated with some scepticism, as small bowel motility does not cease after a laparotomy. Only gastric and colonic motility are reduced. An abdominal X-ray can demonstrate a large pelvic collection of widespread peritoneal fluid. Intra-abdominal collections are often identified by an abdominal or pelvic ultrasound scan and may be treated by guided percutaneous drainage. Computed tomography is even more sensitive for collections and is a useful investigation in the 'slow' patient in whom complications are suspected. As oral water-soluble contrast is used routinely, delineation of obstructed bowel is especially clear and, if proximal, a leak from a small bowel anastomosis may be demonstrated.

Importantly, however, if clinical deterioration occurs, and particularly if intra-abdominal sepsis is thought likely, re-operation should always be considered, even if imaging is either not immediately available or does not show an obvious abnormality. Early re-operation within 5 days following initial surgery is unlikely to encounter dense adhesions and carries a lower mortality risk than a delayed diagnosis of intra-abdominal sepsis due to faecal contamination.

Conclusion

The gastrointestinal tract presents many challenges in gynaecological and obstetric surgery and, if at all possible, the gut should be avoided. Morbidity and mortality associated with contamination of the peritoneal cavity by contents of the gut lumen are such that great care must be taken to preserve gastrointestinal integrity. Planned gastrointestinal resection carries increased risk compared to most gynaecological surgery but even this does not compare to the risks of unrecognized bowel injury.

FURTHER READING

Knaus W A, Draper E A, Wagner D P, Zimmerman J 1985 Prognosis in acute organ system failure. Annals of Surgery 202:685–693

Techniques from the urologists

Rick Popert

General comments

The incidence of urinary tract injury

The frequency of injury to the urinary tract, particularly the bladder and urethra, is difficult to appreciate from the literature: most are recognized and repaired at the time of the injury and go unreported. None the less, given the huge numbers of pelvic procedures carried out, the numbers of injuries are really quite small.

Graber et al (1964) noted 16 bladder injuries in over 800 hysterectomies, an incidence of less than 2%.[1] Of these, 11 were repaired at the time of the injury without further complication, whereas the five that were unrecognized all developed postoperative vesicovaginal fistula. Wharton (1956) reviewed over 16 000 major gynaecological procedures and noted only 83 bladder injuries, an incidence of about 0.5%.[2] In the 77 patients in whom the injury was recognized and corrected at the time of the surgery, complications did not occur; once again, it was the unrecognized injury in six patients that resulted in vesicovaginal fistula. It tends to be the more extensive pelvic dissections that are associated with the greatest number of bladder and ureteral injuries; however, the variety of procedures in which individual cases can occur covers the whole range of operations, from insertion of a Veress needle for establishing a pneumoperitoneum to a radical Wertheim's hysterectomy.

Injury to the urethra is rare, and most commonly in the past has been related to obstetric trauma. With the advent of modern obstetrics this has all but disappeared, except in Third World countries, where obstructed labour remains a significant problem. Iatrogenic injury to the urethra during vaginal or uterine surgery is unusual, and is most often associated with urethral diverticulectomy. It occurs in up to 5% of cases of simple diverticulectomy and in a much higher percentage of those that are acutely inflamed.

Ureteral injury is three to four times more common during abdominal than vaginal hysterectomy. The more extensive pathology requiring the abdominal approach may be a factor. The incidence of ureteric injury arising as a complication ranges from 0.5 to 1% of all major pelvic surgery.[3] However, the true incidence of injury may be higher. Although surprising, it is true that complete obstruction of a single ureter may be asymptomatic and may go unrecognized. Solomon et al (1960) reported ureteric injury with an incidence of 2.5% in 200 women undergoing major pelvic surgery, evaluated with postoperative intravenous urography.[4]

A high index of suspicion for potential injury is needed during any surgical procedure if it is to progress safely. If, as one proceeds during a procedure, one takes the time to look and ask oneself, 'Could I have injured the …?' and then, quite deliberately, check the anatomy and integrity of the 'at-risk structures', then a difficult operation is likely to progress safely. Any injury should be identified quickly and dealt with, with minimal complications. It may be a truism but, 'If you don't look, you cannot see' applies. Unfortunately, a number of urinary tract injuries will go unrecognized and are only discovered some days after the primary surgical procedure has been carried out. This produces understand-

able consternation to the surgeon, the staff and, not least, the patient. Although one would tend to assume that immediate treatment and repair of any injury is appropriate, this may well be the last thing one should do, until the exact nature, site and the extent of any injury has been determined and appropriate resuscitation has been given.

Instruments

No particularly unusual instruments are required to effect repair of the urinary tract, but there are some that are always useful to have around:

- DeBakey vascular forceps, short and long: atraumatic and ideal for handling periureteric tissues and the bladder mucosa.
- Lahey forceps: a right-angle forceps ideal for getting around or going under the ureter or vascular structures to receive or carry ties.
- Babcock or Allis forceps: for elevating the edge or apices of a viscus.
- Naunton Morgan needle holder: it opens with a box-like mechanism and works well in confined spaces, particularly the pelvis.
- A curved needle holder: often works better in the pelvis.
- Nylon tape: to 'sling' the ureter (I find nylon tape better than vascular slings). When elevated, the tape provides better traction for mobilization. When passing it under the ureter it should be wet.
- Ureteric catheters 6–10 French: these are always useful for running up the ureter, either in the opened bladder or through an ureterotomy.
- Infant feeding tubes: often in general, gynaecological and obstetric theatres ureteric catheters are not available, but infant feeding tubes come in a similar range of sizes and are a very good substitute.
- Catheters: a selection of silastic catheters are essential. If one has to place a suprapubic catheter while repairing a bladder injury, go big, 20 Fr. at least. If there is bleeding, the use of a three-way irrigating catheter is recommended.
- Methylene blue or gentian violet: distending the bladder with 400 mL of inked water will

help to confirm a leak or a repair, intravenous injection can help to identify an injured ureter.

Surgical exposure

Whenever, as a trainee, I had to call for assistance from a senior, invariably the very first thing done by the senior surgeon would be to increase the exposure. This would be by either adjusting the retraction or, most commonly, while adding to my embarrassment, simply making the incision bigger. If uncertain of one's ground, make sure one's exposure is adequate. A 24-cm wound will heal just as quickly as a 15-cm one; a bigger hole lets in more light and allows a better view. Sometimes simply tilting the table away from you, or towards you, will help. Putting the patient head down (Trendelenburg) and packing the bowel away from the operating site can make a big difference, especially by reducing pelvic venous engorgement.

Lighting

Rarely, as a trainee, did I see surgeons using a headlight. I have certainly found this to be a useful adjunct, particularly in the pelvis. Blood and the depth of the pelvis tend to dissipate the effect of the light. Fibreoptic flexible light sources are used daily in urological endoscopy, and it is a simple matter to get an assistant to hold one above the wound, but beware—they get hot and can burn. Cold light sources that can be attached to retractors are available.

Sutures

The rule is 'use whatever you like on the urinary tract, *as long as it is absorbable*'. I usually use 3/0 Monocryl® or Vicryl® as a stay suture and to close the bladder. For the ureter I will use 3/0 as a stay suture but 4/0 Vicryl® for any anastomosis or repair. Interrupted sutures should be applied to the ureter, but the bladder can often be closed with a single layer as a continuous suture. If in doubt, using a continuous suture to the mucosa and interrupted Lembert sutures to the bladder wall is always safe.

Urinary drainage and drains

Always make sure that adequate drainage of the bladder has been achieved with a decent-sized catheter (a suprapubic through the anterior wall of the bladder if the bladder has been repaired). A drain placed to the pelvis in the region of the repair will cover any temporary leak (not uncommon).

I tend to avoid using a suction drain to the urinary tract. I suspect this encourages urine to leak. A 20 Fr. Wallace or Robinson drain is satisfactory. A drain is mandatory if there has been a significant bladder or ureteric injury. There are plenty of times when I have considered not draining the pelvis, and on occasion I have regretted doing so, but I have never regretted leaving a drain in.

Causes and sites of injury

Bladder injury

The bladder is the most common site of iatrogenic injury in the course of pelvic surgery. The empty bladder is extremely difficult to damage and it should not be forgotten that the safest thing is to keep the bladder empty by catheterization during any pelvic procedure. The bladder usually moves easily away from the finger or scissors, because it is not a fixed pelvic structure except for where the urethra is attached to the pubis by the pubourethral ligaments. Anything that disturbs the normal anatomy will increase the risk of injury, such as chronic inflammation following previous surgery, malignancy and radiotherapy. The thinner the bladder wall, the more likely that damage may occur.

The loss of normal tissue planes following previous surgery or radiotherapy increases the risk of injury. Careless surgical dissection or problems dealing with bleeding increase this risk further. Injuries that occur during the course of either abdominal or vaginal hysterectomy are not always the result of a 'difficult or bloody pelvic dissection'. Indeed, the ones that disclose themselves late are often described in the operation note as having been 'routine'. The typical injury is located either on the trigone between the ureteral orifices or on the posterior bladder wall, just above the trigone. Such injury is most likely while attempting to mobilize the base of the bladder off the cervix, the upper vagina or the uterine fundus, or while closing the vaginal vault and catching the posterior wall of the bladder with the suture. The view may have been suboptimal because of unexpected profuse haemorrhage, making recognition of the surgical planes difficult.

Bladder neck and urethral injury

Other gynaecological procedures that may be associated with bladder injuries include surgery for incontinence, repair of transvaginal cystocoele or excision of a urethral diverticulum. Injury to the urethra itself is very rare and most commonly occurs in association with injury to the sphincter active area at the time of urethral diverticulectomy.

Obstetric bladder injuries, although rare, are well described, and not restricted to a prolonged second stage of labour in the Third World. They are most often associated with caesarean section and occasionally forceps deliveries. The usual cause of bladder injury in caesarean section is due to inadequate mobilization of the bladder reflection off the lower uterine segment. It may be stuck from scarring due to a previous section, or there may have been a failure to catheterize the bladder and unrecognized retention.

Ureteric injury

Ureteric injuries most often occur during the difficult (often bloody) hysterectomy or radical Wertheim's hysterectomy, where the risk equates to the extent of the disease and/or previous radiotherapy. The advent of laparoscopy and laser ablation of endometriosis and adhesions has been associated with an increased incidence of ureteric injury.

Fig. 13.1 summarizes the causes and sites of urinary tract injury.

Fig. 13.1 Causes and sites of injury
<ul><li>Hysterectomy<ul><li>base of bladder (dissection off the cervix)</li><li>ureters (relation to lateral fornices and the broad ligaments)</li></ul></li><li>Caesarean section<ul><li>anterior wall and base of bladder</li></ul></li><li>Colposuspension<ul><li>bladder (dissection of vaginal wall, placement of sutures)</li><li>ureters (stitch too far postero-laterally)</li></ul></li><li>Tubo-ovarian (including laparoscopy)<ul><li>uretic (lateral pelvic wall)</li><li>beware pelvic inflammatory disease (PID) and endometriosis</li></ul></li><li>Anterior colporrhaphy<ul><li>urethra (placement of plicating sutures)</li><li>failure to recognize urethral diverticulum</li></ul></li><li>Sling procedures<ul><li>dissection between urethra and anterior vaginal wall</li><li>urethral erosion</li></ul></li></ul>

Types of injury

When considering the causes and the subsequent management of urological injuries, it can be helpful to classify the types of injury that might occur. These may be described as either 'direct' or 'indirect' (Fig. 13.2). The type of injury may have a major impact upon how injury to a particular structure will present and how it is subsequently managed.

Direct injury (immediate)

It is not difficult to picture the scenario leading to a direct injury. This is simply the cutting, tearing, diathermizing or the placing of a suture around or through the ureter or bladder. This

Fig. 13.2 Types of injury
<ul><li>Direct and immediate<ul><li>cutting into a viscus</li><li>placement of a suture through or around it</li></ul></li><li>Indirect and delayed<ul><li>devascularization</li><li>stitch/ligature abscess</li><li>risks increased with radiotherapy/previous surgery</li></ul></li></ul>

is the group of injuries that is often recognized immediately, and consequently is the easiest to repair, with often an assured outcome. These are often unfortunate mishaps, and difficult to prevent when things have not gone smoothly during a particular procedure. They are recognized by careful attention to detail and a healthy suspicion of the potential for injury during even the simplest of procedures.

Indirect injury (delayed)

It is the indirect injury that tends to have a delayed presentation, the patient may be non-specifically unwell, and it may take some time for the extent of an injury to declare itself. These tend to be devascularization injuries, often due to injudicious dissection with the stripping of adventitia and the development of a stitch or ligature abscess. The risks of such a scenario developing are significantly greater in cases associated with previous radiotherapy and or previous surgery.

Management of urinary tract injury

Preventive measures

The key thought should be 'Care and attention to detail' (Fig. 13.3). The direct injury may not be preventable, but it is the attention to detail that allows one to recognize the injury immediately, and to repair it safely and securely. Always ensure that the bladder is adequately drained before starting a procedure. Insist on prophylactic antibiotics to include cover for the urinary tract, in case of injury. Gentamicin 3 mg/kg provides appropriate cover and is cheap to boot.

Fig. 13.3 Prevention of injury

- Care and attention to detail
- Preoperative intravenous urography (IVU)
  - difficult surgery
  - pelvicalyceal dilation on ultrasound
  - previous urological surgery
- Preoperative catheterization
  - to keep bladder empty
  - to prevent overdistension

Adequate preparation before commencing the pelvic or abdominal dissection is essential. This includes an adequate incision to get the job done and light to see by. If one encounters a problem during the dissection due to adhesions, fibrosis or scarring, then take things more carefully. Reassess the situation regularly as one proceeds, take time to identify the anatomy, make judicious use of slings round structures as they are identified. Go back and check on what has been done, especially 'at-risk' structures. If unhappy or uncertain, do not be afraid to ask for help.

Pelvic haemostasis

It is worth making some comments on haemostasis as it applies to the urinary tract. If bleeding is encountered, try to deal with it as you proceed, don't lose control of the situation. Panicking and blindly under-running a bleeding area close to the cervix, the lateral fornices or deep within the pelvis, is fraught with danger. It is extremely easy to catch the ureter, which runs under the uterine artery (a branch of the superior vesical pedicle). Remember 'water flows under the bridge' and the only place in which it is possible to palpate a ureteric calculus is through the lateral fornix. If one is losing control of the situation, the priority is the patient. Stop trying to under-run bleeding areas, accept that the situation is getting out of control and do something about it. Advise the anaesthetist of the problem, make sure the patient is in the Trendelenburg position (head down) and prepare to control the bleeding by packing and pressure. Ask for blood, including fresh frozen plasma.

This achieves four things:

1. It lets the anaesthetist know that you are aware of a problem but that you remain in control of the situation.
2. It gives you time to take stock of the situation and plan your next move, remembering that in the urinary tract the key to safety is the anatomy.
3. You can still find the ureter at the pelvic brim in the intersigmoid recess between the sigmoid mesentery and the iliac artery. This is a reliable constant.

4. Identify the ureter throughout its length and control the bleeding.

Once vision has been restored, the retroperitoneum should be opened at the pelvic brim and the ureter identified. Sling the ureter with a nylon tape, elevate it and you can dissect over the anterior surface of the ureter to the superior vesical pedicle. This is easily ligated and divided medial and lateral to the ureter (the pedicle comprises 2–3 segments). Once this is done, one can easily identify the ureter throughout its course as it approaches the bladder and set about controlling the bleeding, secure in the knowledge that the ureter is safe.

Avoiding injury to the bladder

All pelvic surgeons will injure the bladder at one time or another; however, as long as the injury is recognized and repaired, it heals well. The site of injury often determines the probability of postoperative complications. The urinary bladder is an extraperitoneal musculomembranous sac that functions primarily as a urinary storage reservoir. The bladder is relatively resistant to injury when collapsed, so the first line of defence is drainage by a urethral catheter. This should be done in all cases prior to caesarean section, vaginal or transabdominal surgery.

Retropubic dissection in the face of previous pelvic surgery is hazardous and it is better sometimes to open the bladder at the dome or anteriorly (where it is most easily repaired) to aid dissection from the symphysis rather than risk a large, ragged accidental laceration. Carelessness during dissection of the thin-walled bladder or in relation to control of bleeding may result in lacerations, which are difficult to repair.

Injury to the bladder base tends to be more significant (it is less easily recognized). This injury can occur in vaginal hysterectomy, while attempting to enter the anterior cul-de-sac, during low transverse caesarean sections and during abdominal hysterectomy, while separating the bladder from the cervix or when closing the vaginal cuff. The bladder tends to be opened during blunt dissection. Careful *sharp dissection*

with counter traction on the bladder is the key to preventing a bladder injury.

Identifying a bladder injury

The sickening realization that one has entered the bladder inadvertently is often heralded by the presence of unexpected wetness in the wound (Fig. 13.4). Filling the bladder with dilute methylene blue is often unnecessary, as the situation can often be confirmed by careful observation and the simple distension of the bladder with water from a bladder syringe. The problem with methylene blue is that, unless very dilute, it stains everything and so it can be more difficult to identify the mucosa from the bladder wall during a repair. To define the extent of the injury, it may be necessary to cystoscope or simply open the anterior wall of the bladder and catheterize the ureters directly. This ensures they have not been compromised and protects them during a repair.

Opening the bladder

There are occasions when it is better to open the bladder primarily to either confirm or prevent an injury occurring. The advantage is that one gets to choose the site and it is consequently easier to repair. It is best to open a moderately distended bladder and so, before any operation, make sure there is easy access to the catheter. It is best to distend the bladder with 200 mL of water. Not saline, because it interferes with diathermy function and it is less bloody to open a bladder with diathermy than with a scalpel or scissors.

Fig. 13.4 Recognizing perioperative injury
• Could I have damaged the urinary tract? — urine in the operative field — blood in the catheter bag — check the integrity of the bladder and the ureters • In doubt? — open the bladder dome — ureteric injury excluded by catheterization — methylene blue via catheter or intravenously

First, the anterior and lateral bladder wall should be mobilized by blunt dissection. It can be helpful to free up the peritoneal reflection off the vault. Choosing the site for the cystotomy is fairly obvious, it tends to present itself.

The cystotomy should be transverse and low enough to provide easy access to the ureteric orifices without being so deep as to make vision poor or access difficult. Having chosen the site for the transverse cystotomy place two full-thickness 2/0 Vicryl® stay sutures through the antero-lateral margins on either side, and two full-thickness stay sutures above and below the intended line of incision. The bladder should be elevated with the stays and, using a diathermy probe, an incision made. It is often surprising how thick the wall of the bladder is. One often finds that the stay sutures are not full thickness; if so, they should be replaced as one proceeds. Once the bladder has been entered, there is a rush of water and urine into the wound, so be ready with the sucker. Lift the edges with the stay sutures or Babcock forceps and extend the cystotomy under direct vision (Fig. 13.5).

It may be necessary to extend an injury to the bladder in order to more easily define the margins for closure. This is most easily achieved by applying the same principles, using stay sutures to elevate the edges.

Repairing a bladder injury

A bladder injury is usually easily corrected if identified at the time of surgery (Fig. 13.6). The bladder with its excellent blood supply heals quickly, provided the mucosal edges are re-approximated and continuous, unobstructed urinary drainage is maintained.

Once the extent of the injury has been defined, the margins of the repair can be determined. It is often better to consciously extend the injury so that these margins can be better

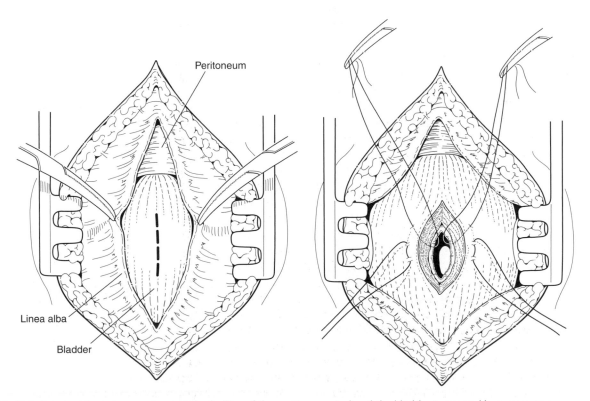

Peritoneum

Linea alba

Bladder

Fig. 13.5 Suprapubic cystomy — the muscles bellies of the recti are parted and the bladder is opened between stay sutures using diathermy (fill the bladder with water not saline). Resite the stay sutures and extend the incision as required.

Fig. 13.6 Repair of bladder injury

- Puncture injury
  — drain and suprapubic catheter (SPC; minimum 16 Fr.)
- Larger hole
  — define the extent of the injury
  — OPEN THE BLADDER, check the ureters
  — place stays in the margins (N, S, E and W)
  — insert the SPC through the anterior wall
  — close in two layers WITHOUT TENSION
  — omental interposition
  — drain the site of repair

defined and a tension-free repair effected. I believe that in all cases of bladder injury or large cystotomy it is safest to bring a Foley suprapubic catheter (SPC) out through the anterior wall of the bladder. This should be placed before the bladder is closed and should be combined with a urethral catheter for 48 hours or so. This prevents the occasional vesical leak resulting from a difficult repair or the blocking of a solitary

urethral catheter. With a decent suprapubic catheter, control is assured. It is also more comfortable for the patient, particularly if they have to go home with a catheter in situ. The catheter should stay for 7–10 days and can then be clamped and removed if there are no significant residuals.

Intra-operative injury is best repaired in two layers, using a 2/0 or 3/0 *absorbable* suture (Figs 13.7, 13.8 and 13.9). The cystotomy is best closed with a running full-thickness suture. The second layer, if necessary, may be either a running or interrupted suture placed in an inverting manner. Do not use non-absorbable sutures.

Posterior bladder wall or trigonal injury

If there is injury to the posterior bladder wall or the trigone, then it is essential to confirm patency of the ureters. Closing the bladder from without makes it difficult to see the ureteric orifices and therefore puts them at risk. If one is concerned,

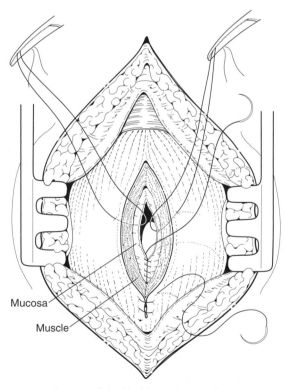

Mucosa

Muscle

Fig. 13.7 Closure Of the bladder — the muscle and inner layer are closed as a continuous layer with an absorbable suture.

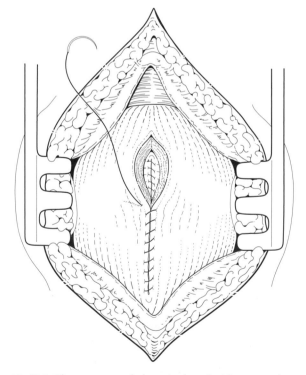

Fig. 13.8 The outer muscle layer is closed with a second layer as either a continuous in interrupted suture. A suprapubic foley catheter should be brought out through the closure or, more safely, through a separate stab before the bladder is closed.

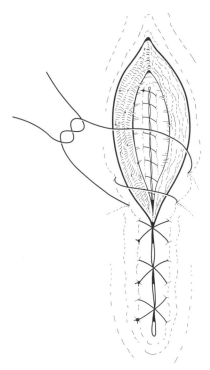

Fig. 13.9 The very thin-walled bladder may best be closed by interrupted absorbable sutures. This is particularly useful in closing the posterior wall, base and trigone of the bladder. Ensure drainage is adequate and check repair with a cystogram at 2–3 weeks.

it is much safer to acknowledge the risk and avoid potential injury by opening the bladder anteriorly, catheterizing the ureters and then repairing the posterior wall or trigone. In this instance there seems to be much less give in the bladder wall, and I tend to use interrupted sutures. I have no problems with leaving the knots on the inside of the bladder, as long as absorbable sutures have been used.

If omentum is available, this should always be mobilized and tacked to the site of repair and interposed between any suture lines, for instance vaginal closure. This minimizes the risk of subsequent fistulation.

The adequacy of the repair should be checked by bladder distension, and any identified leaks closed with interrupted figure-of-eight sutures. Before closing the incision, a drain should be placed into the perivesical space. I avoid suction drains because I feel they tend to encourage urine to leak through the repair. Urine is so good at

finding its way out that to actively encourage a leak seems illogical. The drain is removed once drainage is less than 25 mL in 24 hours.

Managing a urinary leak

Occasionally a prolonged urinary leak may occur which causes concern. If there is a question as to whether or not this is urine, then the easiest way to confirm is to send a sample in a U&E bottle. Don't confuse the laboratory by asking for an estimation of the urea, simply send it as a serum sample. If the level of urea and creatinine is equivalent to that of serum, then the drainage is *not* urine and one can be reassured. If the urea and creatinine is sky high, then simply leave the drain, make sure the catheters have not blocked by flushing them gently with 25 mL saline, if necessary change the urethral catheter for a larger one—up to 22 Fr.—and wait for things to dry up over the next few days.

As long as the leak is controlled, there are unlikely to be any significant metabolic problems. However, if a urinary leak persists, despite adequate bladder drainage, then one should be concerned that there may have been an unrecognized ureteric injury. If a cystogram confirms a bladder leak, then continue to sit tight and consider bilateral nephrostomies, which may encourage the situation to dry up. If there is no evidence for a bladder leak, then an intravenous urogram is indicated to exclude a ureteric injury. In the presence of a ureteric injury, there is often a delayed nephrogram on the side of the affected ureter, and there may be extravasation of urine.

Figures 13.10 and 13.11 summarize management of the stable and unstable patient, respectively.

Fig. 13.10 Managing the stable patient

- Read the operation notes, catheterize
- Urgent ultrasound or IVU
  — upper tract dilation
  — delayed nephrogram, extravasation of urine
- Cystogram
- Percutaneous nephrostomy (delayed antegrade)
- Cystoscopy, retrograde study and stenting
- EXPLAIN AND REASSURE
- EXPLORE AND REPAIR

Fig. 13.11 Managing the unstable patient

- Moribund with Gram-negative septicaemia
  — urgent resuscitation and diagnosis
  — intensive support and percutaneous nephrostomy
- EXPLAIN AND REASSURE
- EXPLORE AND REPAIR
  — to drain the pelvis of extravasated urine
  — to remove occlusive sutures or ligatures
  — to establish good urinary and wound drainage
- BILATERAL INTUBATED URETEROSTOMY

Urethral injury

The urethra should never be dissected without a catheter in situ, which facilitates immediate recognition of injury. This should be closed with 3/0 or 4/0 absorbable suture. The sutures should be placed interrupted, horizontally and include a second layer if possible to separate the primary repair from the vaginal suture line. If there is any doubt at all about the soundness of the repair, then a Martius fat pad should be harvested from the labia majora and used to support the repair, with the vaginal wall being closed loosely over it with interrupted sutures.

Ureteric injury

'The venal injury is to the ureter, but the mortal sin is failing to recognize it.' The complication of unrecognized ureteric injury can be devastating and its successful management provides a considerable challenge.[5]

Urologists are keenly aware of the anatomy of the ureters and rarely do they injure the ureter inadvertently. It would not be expected that a relatively inexperienced, or even an experienced, gynaecological surgeon should attempt repair of ureteric injury without seeking experienced and specialist help. Urologists are always very happy to be called upon to advise, and would far rather exclude or deal with a ureteric injury primarily, rather than manage the surgical nightmare as a consequence of delayed recognition of a significant ureteric injury.

It is probably beyond the expectation of junior trainees to attempt more complex ureteric repair and reconstruction, but they should be able to carry out an intubated ureterotomy, a cystotomy to enable catheterization of the ureters, repair a bladder laceration and place a large suprapubic catheter. Although a discussion of the finer points of ureteric repair and reconstruction are beyond the remit of this chapter, some discussion is worthwhile, if only to illustrate some of the general principles of urological surgery as it applies to gynaecological injury of the urinary tract.

Avoiding injury to the ureters

The ureter is injured most frequently during radical hysterectomy, especially in previously irradiated patients. However, since radical hysterectomies are carried out less commonly now, most injuries occur during simple hysterectomy. The presence of benign and malignant pelvic tumours, pelvic inflammatory disease, postradiation fibrosis and endometriosis add to the difficulty of any procedure and increase the risk of ureteric injury.

Prevention of ureteric injury depends upon several principles. Preoperative knowledge of the course of the ureters is essential in cases where known pelvic pathology may distort the anatomical position of the ureters. Intravenous urography should be carried out preoperatively before cases of severe procidentia, large adnexal tumours, large fibroids, particularly when intraligamentous, severe pelvic inflammatory disease, endometriosis, and where there has been previous pelvic surgery, particularly in association with radiotherapy.

Familiarity with the danger points where ureteral injury commonly occurs is important. Most injuries occur in the distal segment of the ureter, where it lies in close approximation to the uterine artery, uterosacral ligaments or the vaginal cuff. Other sites for potential injury are near the infundibulo-pelvic ligament and the lateral pelvic sidewall near the broad ligament. Often the event leading to the injury is excessive bleeding, and therefore if this has occurred, once control has been obtained then it is appropriate to examine all these areas and to mobilize the ureter throughout its length to reassure oneself that it is intact.

Another principle is the intra-operative identification of the ureters and their course. If there is no significant gross pelvic pathology, inflammatory disease or endometriosis, the ureters may be easily visible through the thin posterior parietal peritoneum, and there should be little danger of injury. The ureter can often be identified through the broad ligament by pinching the ligament between finger and thumb and rolling the ureter to identify it. Alternatively, if the pelvic pathology makes this difficult, or there is excessive bleeding, it is better to go back to basic anatomy and identify the ureter throughout its length.

The ureter may be identified at the pelvic brim in relation to the common iliac vessels, as described previously. If this proves difficult, then the ureter may be approached laterally by a manoeuvre which facilitates the ligation of the uterine artery while ensuring that the ureter is protected. This is done by entering the retroperitoneum behind the round ligament, opening the loose areolar tissue on the lateral pelvic wall between the peritoneum and the division of the common iliac artery into its external and internal branches. Divide the adventitia overlying the origin of the internal iliac and follow it until its division into the obliterated umbilical, superior vesical and uterine artery. This last branch is ligated and divided. The ureter can be easily identified attached to the under surface of the pelvic peritoneum, where it is reflected medially. The main blood supply to the uterus is thus controlled with little danger to the ureter, which can be safeguarded throughout its pelvic course.

Finally, preoperative ureteric catheterization can be considered. It will probably be necessary to liaise with urological colleagues about this, but it is useful to insert ureteric catheters cystoscopically prior to pelvic surgery, particularly if one is expecting distorted anatomy. The ureteric catheters should be at least 6 Fr. to facilitate palpation. Alternatively if, during surgery, one is having difficulty identifying the ureters, or one suspects a ureteric injury, then it is best to open the bladder anteriorly and pass catheters up each ureter. To aid identification of the ureteric orifices, the patient should be taken out of the usual Trendelenburg position, (which pools the urine in the renal pelves) and be given a bolus of frusemide and 10 mL of indigo carmine or methylene blue intravenously. A brisk diuresis of blue urine ensues, which will identify any ureteral leak above the bladder, as well as the ureteric orifices. If it is necessary to leave the ureteric catheters, then these should be brought out though a puncture cystotomy in the anterolateral bladder wall on each side, and out through the anterior abdominal wall (Fig. 13.12).

Intra-operative management of ureteric injury

The treatment of ureteral injury secondary to pelvic surgery depends upon a number of factors: when the injury is recognized (intra-operative or postoperative), the condition of the patient, the extent and the location of the injury and the status of the opposite renal unit. Injuries recognized intra-operatively include ligation, crushing, transection and avulsion. The number one priority is the patient. If a ureteric or bladder

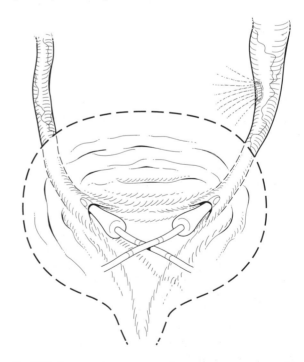

Fig. 13.12 Retrograde ureterography or catheterisation of the ureters following is a cystotomy may be helpful in identifying the site of injury and planning an approach to repair of the injury.

injury is recognized, then even the most experienced should not be too proud to call for help, even if it takes 2 hours for a urologist to get to the theatre (there are still many hospitals that have no in-house urological service). Often, the event that led to the injury is excessive pelvic bleeding and it is the management of the bleeding or a bowel injury that is most important. If the condition of the patient is unstable, then management of the ureteric injury can be deferred until the situation has been stabilized and the patient is safe.

If the situation is so dire that it is necessary to pack the pelvis, then no effort should be made to deal with the ureteric injury, other than doing an intubated ureterotomy above the brim of the pelvis.

Intubated ureterostomy

As a surgical procedure this is a life saver (Fig. 13.13). It reliably diverts the urine and can

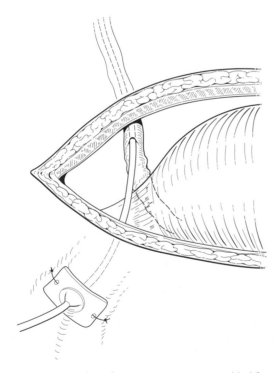

Fig. 13.13 The intubated ureterostomy is a veritable lifesaver because it provides a reliable method of achieving urinary diversion. It may be all that required when combined with the drainage of pelvic collections and haematoma in the sick and unstable patient.

salvage the worst of situations. All that is required is an 8 or 10 Fr. infant feeding tube, which is passed up to the renal pelvis through a 0.5–1 cm vertical ureterotomy above the ligated ureter, or through the proximal end of the transected or avulsed ureter. The distal end of the ureteric catheter is exteriorized through an abdominal stab wound and sutured to the skin. The ureterotomy, or the open end of the ureter is closed around the catheter with a 3/0 absorbable suture, the ends left long to secure the tube.

The pelvis should be drained and a large bladder catheter placed.

Simple nephrectomy

Occasionally, for the stable patient who has a normal contralateral kidney but has terminal cancer, or when the involved ureter is draining an already compromised poorly functioning kidney, then a simple nephrectomy may be the ideal procedure. Maximal benefit with minimal complications should be the intention in these cases. Intentional proximal ligation of the ureter above the injury should not be considered because of the risk of fistula formation and sepsis. The Pfannenstiel incision can be extended, hockey-stick fashion, into the flank to allow the nephrectomy to be done.

Repair of ureter (middle third)

In general, the best time to repair an injury is immediately. All ligation injuries above the pelvic brim should probably be treated by excision of the ligated segment and a spatulated anastomosis over a splinting ureteric stent (Fig. 13.14). Above the pelvic brim it is easy to mobilize the ureter, simply by running one's finger up behind the ureter, lifting it off psoas above and below the level of the injury. The ureter can often be made to overlap by 2 cm, ensuring a tension-free repair. I use interrupted 4/0 absorbable sutures. Once the back wall has been completed, a J-J stent can be passed over a guidewire into the bladder (fill it with dilute methylene blue and blue saline emanates from the side holes when the stent reaches the bladder), and the other end negotiated into the

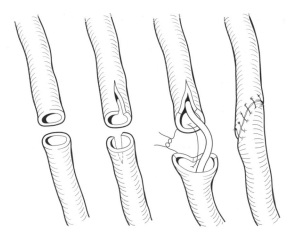

Fig. 13.14 If the ureter is accidentally severed or crushed then excision and primary repair may be easily effected in the middle and upper third but with great difficulty in the lower third. The keys are a spatulated anastomosis, under no tension with splintage and adequate drainage.

renal pelvis (the guidewire can be run in through one of the stent side holes) (Fig. 13.15). The stent can be removed 2 weeks later using a flexible cystoscope.

Repair of ureter (lower third)

Unfortunately, most ureteric injuries occur below the pelvic brim. In these cases the blood supply to the lower third of the ureter has often been compromised and it is inappropriate to consider re-anastomosing the ureter. If the ureter is intact and has been freed of any encircling sutures and a J-J stent can be positioned successfully, then the option of conservative management could be

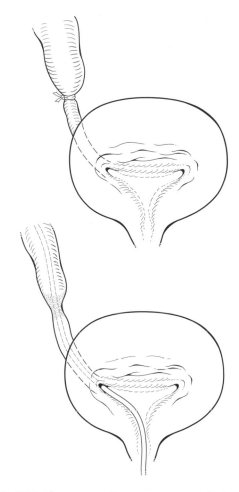

Fig. 13.16 The conservative manangement of a lower third ureteric injury can be consdered if the injury is identified early, and ligatures removed and the ureter is stented successfully. The stent should remain in place for a minimum of 6 weeks.

considered, although the site of injury should still be drained (Fig. 13.16).

If there is any doubt, then a re-implantation of the ureter will be necessary. The psoas hitch procedure, the Boari flap and a transuretero-ureterostomy are useful urological operative techniques for re-establishing continuity between the ureter and the bladder (Fig. 13.15). Of the three, the most versatile, and the one associated with least complications, is the psoas hitch procedure (Fig. 13.17). The psoas hitch is a means of extending the bladder's dome or lateral wall superiorly and anchoring the bladder to the

Fig. 13.15 Repair of ureteric injury

- Upper- and middle-third injuries
  - excise and mobilize the damaged ureter
  - spatulate the two ends
  - overlap at least 1 cm each (no tension)
  - interrupted 3/0 or 4/0 Vicryl®
  - omental wrap to repair with drain
- Lower-third injuries (difficult)
  - more likely to present late, so more stuck
  - less room for mobilization
  - consider psoas hitch or Boari flap reconstruction
  - transuretero-ureterostomy

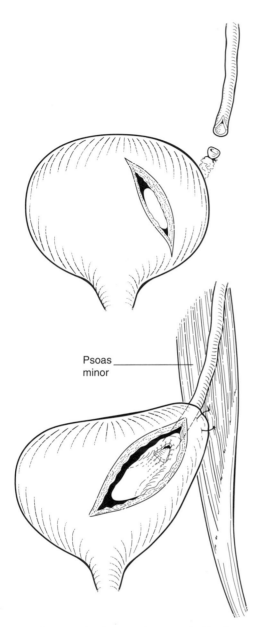

Psoas
minor

Fig. 13.17 The psoas hitch procedure is probably the most versatile of reconstructive procedure for injury of uterer's lower third. The bladder is excised in the transverse axis and hitched to the psoas minor tendon thus taking the tension off the uretervesical anastomosis that should be stented. The bladder should be drained with both urethral and suprapubic catheters.

surface of the psoas muscle, thereby bridging the gap between the ureter and bladder. It is not the place of this chapter to describe in detail the technique of a psoas hitch, suffice to say it is one

of the most adaptable methods of reconstructing injuries to the lower third of the ureter. By the combination of a psoas hitch and lowering the kidney by renal dissection and nephropexy, tension-free re-implantation of even short proximal ureters can be achieved. In cases where there is pelvic inflammatory disease, in the previously irradiated pelvis, or in delayed repair where there is significant fibrosis, the ureter may need to be stented for up to 3 months.

Management of delayed presentation of ureteric injury

Most ureteral injuries are recognized postoperatively. Often the patients will be non-specifically unwell with signs and symptoms, which are rather vague, and may be disguised because of wound pain. There may be a history of postoperative ileus, pyrexia, flank pain, excessive vaginal drainage, a pelvic collection and oliguria. A ureteric injury will usually declare itself in one of three ways:

1. External leakage of urine via the drain or the wound.
2. Internal leakage of urine with reduced urine output, a pelvic collection or urinary peritonitis.
3. Signs of ureteric obstruction with constitutional symptoms, reduced urinary output and loin pain.

An intravenous urogram (IVU) will confirm the diagnosis 90% of the time. In this situation the patient will require aggressive treatment of any associated infection, resuscitation and consideration given to inserting a nephrostomy. This should be carried out without delay to divert the urine and preserve renal function on the affected side. An antegrade nephrostogram (with antibiotic cover) may be carried out after 72 hours, and it is not unreasonable for an attempt to be made to pass a stent into the bladder by an experienced interventional radiologist. There should be no hesitation in proceeding to explore and repair or reconstruct once the patient has been stabilized (Fig. 13.18). In the long run, a problem rapidly identified and corrected will often be viewed as an unfortunate but acceptable

Fig. 13.18 The principles of surgical management

- Provide adequate antibiotic cover
  — gentamacin 3–5 mg/kg
  — broad-spectrum cover
- Sutures must be ABSORBABLE
- Suture lines must be TENSION FREE
- Omentum to WRAP AND SUPPORT REPAIR
- Drain the bladder with a SUPRAPUBIC
- Drain the pelvis (non-suction)
- MAKE SURE DRAINAGE IS ADEQUATE

complication, whereas a failure to recognize a problem, compounded by a delay or suboptimal management, tends to lead to a protracted, and possibly unsatisfactory, recovery in an unhappy patient.

Delayed presentation of a ureteric injury longer than 3 or 4 weeks usually presents with flank pain, infection, fever or profuse vaginal discharge (ureterovaginal fistula). An IVU is usually diagnostic but a cystoscopy and retrograde ureterogram will confirm, and are useful to exclude a vesicovaginal fistula. Sepsis many months later may be the only sign of ureteric damage.

Classic surgical teaching would advocate that injuries discovered early, within days of the primary surgery, be repaired immediately, those discovered later should have treatment delayed for 3 to 6 months. It is presumed that delayed repair is easier and more successful in the absence of haematoma, inflammation and oedema. In my experience, allowing continued delay makes the surgery more difficult. The ureters and bladder tend to become fixed and scarred. By all means, divert the urine with a nephrostomy and attempt an antegrade stenting once sepsis has been controlled. If successful, fine, but if not, then early aggressive treatment of ureteral injuries has much to recommend it. Even in the presence of frank pelvic infection, which may be a contra-indication to primary repair or reconstruction, there is merit in carrying out a laparotomy and drainage of a pelvic collection, combined with establishing adequate control of urinary drainage.

Occasionally, if there is significant loss of ureteral length, or there is an irradiated, inflamed

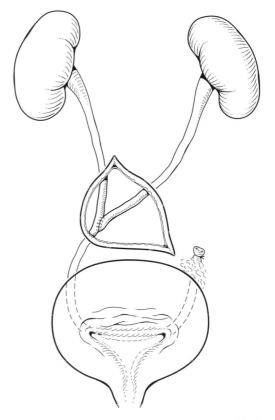

Fig. 13.19 Trans uretero-ureterstomy may be a useful alternative in the severely-damaged ureter. There should be no tension, a gentle curve and the anastomoses that should be wide stented and drained. The contralateral ureter must be normal – it may be put at risk.

ureter, or one side of the pelvis is filled with cancer, which precludes reimplantation, then a transuretero-ureterostomy may be the only option (Fig. 13.19). In this procedure the ureter is transected above the problem, mobilized and swung across to be joined end to side to the contralateral ureter, with a spatulated anastomosis. The contralateral urinary drainage must be normal, otherwise the procedure may result in further problems.

The use of omentum in repairing the urinary tract

The omentum may be interposed between two layers of healing tissues and can be mobilized

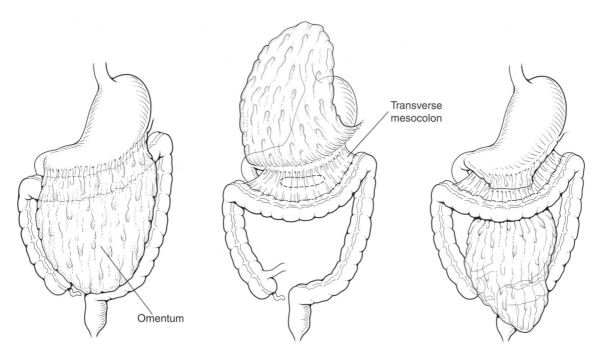

Transverse mesocolon

Omentum

Fig. 13.20 The omentum is a wonderful source of support for any bladder or ureteric repair. Omental interposition should always be used to separate suture lines, particularly between the posterior wall of the bladder and the anterior vaginal wall. Te greater omentum is detached from the transverse colon along the avascular plane and led through a hole in the mesocolon.

if necessary and used to cover the whole urinary tract, including the perineum. It can be used to fill dead spaces, to prevent the development of fibrosis around the ureter in cases involving endometriosis, and to provide neovascularization where required (Fig. 13.20).

Often sufficient omental length can be achieved by fully mobilizing along the avascular plane between the left omentum and the left transverse colon. The omentum can be swung to wrap around a ureteric repair and will usually reach to support the distal ureter above a psoas hitch re-implant. If greater mobilization is required to interpose between the posterior bladder wall and the vagina, then full mobilization of the omentum will be required, but it is essential that the blood supply is preserved. The omentum derives its blood supply from the left and right gastroepiploic vessels, which form the gastroepiploic arcade that courses alongside the greater curve of the stomach. Again starting from the left-hand side, the left gastroepiploic

artery is divided and then the short gastrics are divided favouring the stomach side of the gastroepiploic arch, preserving the gastroepiploic arcade derived primarily from the right gastroepiploic artery extending to its origin from the gastroduodenal artery.

Although formal dissection of the omentum is not easy, if reasonable care is taken to avoid haematomas and the procedure is not rushed, it is an extremely important source of protection for any repair. It is often not as difficult as it would seem, particularly if there has been some delay in repair, because a portion is often lying close by, ready to be mobilized and put to good use.

Concluding remarks

No surgical procedure can be without any risk. It is an awareness of the potential for injury and the steps necessary to avoid such injury that separate the experienced surgeon from the novice. If injury does occur and is recognized immediately, it can invariably be repaired without complication if basic surgical principles are adhered to. It is often more difficult to manage the injury that discloses itself late, and to manage these injuries well requires the greatest experience. It is far preferable to recognize and admit there is a problem, organize prompt resuscitation with appropriate investigation and early intervention. Don't forget to culture the urine. If the patient has no catheter, then catheterize with at least an 18 Fr. catheter.

If help is needed, call for it early, don't place the patient in a side room and wait until after the weekend. Radiologists are on call to provide clinical support—use them. Consult with the on-call urologist early, before the investigations have been completed, and let the urologist know the results as soon as they are available. Ideally, once the patient has been seen, she should be transferred to the urology ward as soon as possible. I think it is the most distressing thing in the world for a patient to be placed in a situation where there is uncertainty. The degree of uncertainty is accentuated in a ward where the nursing and medical staff may be unclear themselves. Far better that the patient be managed within the appropriate specialty where the day-to-day management of such problems is viewed as routine rather than with trepidation.

REFERENCES

1. Graber E A, O'Rourke J J, McElrath T 1964 Iatrogenic bladder injury during hysterectomy. Obstetrics and Gynecology 23:267–273
2. Wharton L R 1956 Methods of preventing injury to the ureters and bladder during gynaecological operations. Annals of Surgery 143:752–763
3. Mattingly R F 1977 Operative injuries of the ureter. In: Telinde R W (ed) Operative gynecology. Lippincott, Philadelphia, p 293
4. Solomon E, Levin E J, Bauman J et al 1960 A pyelographic study of ureteric injuries sustained during hysterectomy for benign conditions. Surgery, Gynecology and Obstetrics 111:41
5. Higgins C C 1967 Ureteral injuries during surgery. Journal of the American Medical Association 199:118

FURTHER READING

Mundy A 1983 Injuries of the lower urinary tract. Surgery 1:67–70
Mundy A 1983 Injuries of the upper urinary tract. Surgery 1:96–98

Techniques from the vascular surgeons

Peter Taylor and David Gerrard

Introduction

One of the most feared events in the practice of obstetrics and gynaecology is the occurrence of torrential haemorrhage which appears suddenly, with no obvious or treatable cause and which is catastrophic enough to threaten the patient's life. This chapter will attempt to identify the common causes and discuss a logical way of controlling the bleeding and treating such rare events until help arrives. Cases from the authors' experience, which exemplify the major points, will be discussed.[1]

Common causes of bleeding

When patients who are pregnant present with torrential abdominal bleeding, the term often applied is abdominal apoplexy. This does not attempt to specify a cause, indeed this is often not identified until the bleeding is brought under control. The second clinical scenario in obstetrics where massive bleeding may occur is after birth, when uncontrollable uterine bleeding may be encountered. In gynaecological practice uncontrollable pelvic bleeding may occur due to inadvertent injury of major arteries and/or veins in the pelvis. Sometimes this happens during the insertion of instruments to perform laparoscopy or during operations to remove lymph nodes from the iliac arteries and veins during Wertheim's hysterectomy. Very rarely, these vessels may be injured during inadvertent perforation of the uterus during endoscopic procedures.

Immediate action on the discovery of haemorrhage

The first action is not to panic. Inform the anaesthetist that there is bleeding so that blood can be crossmatched, and fresh frozen plasma and platelets ordered. Group O, rhesus negative blood may be used if necessary. Make sure there is good exposure by lengthening the wound, or by making a different incision (e.g. a midline laparotomy). Ensure that the lighting is good and that there are enough assistants to assist with retraction and to operate two suckers, which are essential if bleeding is profuse. Call early for senior help if you are a junior, and for vascular help if you are not experienced in vascular surgery. Remove all the blood from the abdomen using a combination of large swabs and suckers. Use the largest packs available to control bleeding. Keep the pressure on the swabs until help arrives. Start from the pelvic brim and work down, securing all bleeding vessels on the way with 4/0 or 5/0 monofilament sutures. The use of clamps is to be avoided unless major arteries are involved. Clamps may injure and tear fragile pelvic vessels and large veins lying beneath the visible bleeding vessel. Likewise, diathermy is to be avoided, as it rarely controls venous bleeding. It may work temporarily, but in scenarios of massive haemorrhage, the bleeding from the diathermy site usually starts up again when mean arterial pressure returns towards normal, and when coagulation may become deranged. If all the major bleeding points have been secured, but the patient is still bleeding in the form of an ooze which collects in the pelvis, use large packs to tamponade the bleeding in the pelvis and abdomen, and look again in 24 hours.

While it is preferable to avoid ureteric injury, control of life-threatening haemorrhage is clearly the priority and injury to a ureter can be resolved later. The most important part of emergency treatment for haemorrhage is to stop the bleeding in order to preserve life.

The patient must be sent to the intensive care unit. Any haematological abnormalities should be corrected with transfusion of platelets and clotting factors. The use of warming blankets such as the Bair Hugger® are very effective in correcting hypothermia. Low body temperature can affect the blood's ability to clot. A core temperature below 31°C will prevent natural haemostasis. Early second-look laparotomy should be avoided, as opening the abdomen may reduce the patient's core temperature further and prevent the correction of coagulation abnormalities. There are two exceptions to this. One is further severe haemorrhage, which suggests that packing may be inadequate or that a major blood vessel is still bleeding. The other is the development of abdominal compartment syndrome.

Raised intra-abdominal pressure may produce complex physiological derangement, leading to multi-organ failure.[2] At pressures below 10 mmHg, cardiac output is maintained but hepatic arterial blood flow is reduced. Decreased cardiac output, renal impairment and hypoxia may occur with higher pressures, and anuria is frequently caused by intra-abdominal pressures greater than 40 mmHg. A decrease in visceral perfusion leads to tissue hypoxia, acidosis and the generation of oxygen free radicals from bacterial translocation. Cerebral perfusion pressure may be decreased secondary to elevation of thoracic airway pressure. These adverse events are superimposed on the underlying cause, and ongoing haemorrhage and hypovolaemia are likely to exacerbate the problem. However, patients are usually able to tolerate raised intra-abdominal pressure for 24 hours, during which time the majority of bleeding has nearly always stopped. Relief of intra-abdominal pressure invariably reverses the adverse physiological processes discussed above. If there are residual bleeding points, these are easily identified and can be secured with 5/0 polypropylene sutures. It is important to ensure that all haematological abnormalities are corrected with transfusion of blood, platelets and fresh frozen plasma. Rarely, if there is further unacceptable bleeding which cannot be controlled, the abdomen can be re-packed and a further inspection made in another 24 hours.

If the bleeding is torrential and the cause cannot be found, the abdomen should be packed and arteriography performed with a view to embolization. This technique avoids the potential

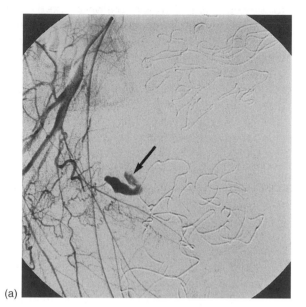
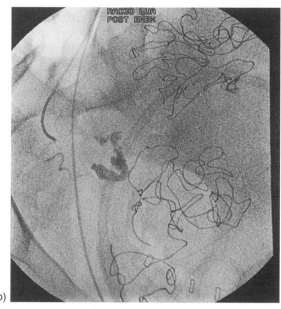

Fig. 14.1 Angiograms demonstrating pelvic bleeding (arrow) followed by successful coil embolization of the feeding artery. Note the presence of abdominal packs.

complications of further surgery, which include significant failure rates for internal iliac artery ligation, ureteric injury and loss of fertility. Transcatheter pelvic arterial embolization is usually performed in the X-ray department, as excellent radiographic equipment is required. The patient should therefore be relatively stable so that transfer can be performed safely. The majority of X-ray departments can now accept ventilated patients, so that transfer of patients direct from theatre or the intensive care unit can be carried out. The aim is to identify the source of the bleeding and selectively embolize the vessel, usually with coils (Fig. 14.1).[3] If successful, the pelvic circulation can be preserved, resulting in the possibility of the patient having further pregnancies.[4]

Case report 1: Gynaecology

A 36-year-old nurse was undergoing a Wertheim's hysterectomy when unexpected torrential venous and arterial bleeding started from the pelvic side walls during clearance of the lymph nodes from the iliac vessels. The situation rapidly became critical and the patient became hypotensive and tachycardic. Twenty units of blood were used before vascular surgical help

was called for. Packs were used to remove a large quantity of blood from the abdomen and pelvis, and the pelvis was packed with swabs. The bleeding was controlled with pressure on the swabs, and the anaesthetist was able to catch up on the blood loss and order more units of blood, together with fresh frozen plasma and platelets. Blood samples were sent for full blood count, a clotting screen (prothrombin time and activated partial thromboplastin time) and for crossmatch of more units of blood. Starting from the top, all bleeding points were secured with polypropylene sutures, using finger pressure to control the vessels.

The patient was transfused a total of 45 units of blood. On removal of the packs at 24 hours, two minor bleeding points were under-run, and no further packs were required. The patient had a foot drop which was thought to be secondary to spinal cord ischaemia as a result of hypotension. The patient succumbed to metastatic ovarian cancer 4 years later.

Obstetric causes of haemorrhage

Abdominal apoplexy with massive bleeding, occurring in patients who are pregnant, is usually secondary to rupture of a visceral or renal

207

aneurysm. The most common site is the splenic artery, followed by the renal artery. Less common sites are the hepatic, superior mesenteric, gastro-duodenal and gastroepiploic arteries. A midline incision ensures access to all areas of the abdomen, and is (theoretically) associated with the least blood loss. Two suckers are used to remove blood from the abdomen, especially from the subphrenic spaces, as blood will continually flow from these spaces, contaminating the field, which then confuses the search for the source of the bleeding. Large packs are used in each quadrant of the abdomen after the blood has been removed. The anaesthetist is then able to catch up with the blood loss and order replacement packed cells, platelets and fresh frozen plasma. The packs are removed sequentially. The general, and then the specific, area of blood loss can then be identified. Usually, rupture of the aneurysm has taken place. Once the aneurysm sac is opened, the feeding vessels can be identified and oversewn with polypropylene sutures. There is usually both antegrade and retrograde flow into the aneurysm sac, both of which need to be secured. If the bleeding is still uncontrolled and not identifiable, and the anaesthetist cannot keep up with the blood loss, then all intra-abdominal bleeding can be controlled with a clamp on the aorta above the coeliac axis. The stomach is pulled to the patient's left with the right hand, and the lesser omentum can be broken through easily with a finger. This opens the lesser sac, and the aorta can be felt on the spine, separated by the crus of the diaphragm. Pressure can be applied with a blunt instrument on to the spine to control the bleeding, or the crus can be dissected, often with blunt dissection, and the aorta occluded with a vascular clamp. If the bleeding is found to come from the pelvis, then the infrarenal aorta can be controlled. This is found by reflecting the small bowel on to the right side of the anterior abdominal wall. The aorta can be easily palpated in the midline, as long as the patient has a blood pressure above 60–70 mmHg. The posterior peritoneum is then opened and the aorta can be dissected directly posteriorly. The sides of the aorta can be freed from the surrounding tissue and a vascular clamp applied. These two territories may not be familiar to obstetricians and gynaecologists, and they may have more confidence in finding the distal aorta by following the iliac arteries up from the pelvis and clamping the aorta just above the origin of the common iliac arteries.

Patience is important when trying to identify difficult bleeding points. Sometimes, blood pressure is low and the bleeding minimal when the site is first inspected, so be prepared to go back to areas that were thought to be secure, especially if blood is contaminating the packs left in that area. As mentioned previously, in pelvic bleeding it is important that the internal iliac arteries are not ligated. This rarely makes any difference to the bleeding, as there is a rich anastomosis between the external and internal iliac arteries, so that the bleeding point is rarely controlled. There is also very good cross flow from one side of the pelvis to the other. These arteries may also be a useful conduit for interventional radiologists to embolize bleeding points when surgery has failed to control them. If they have been ligated, then a useful and effective means of control cannot be used.

Visceral aneurysms

These are usually saccular and less than 2 cm in diameter. They occur most frequently in the splenic artery (60%), followed by the hepatic artery (20%). The rest occur infrequently in the superior mesenteric artery, the coeliac axis, the arteries to the stomach and pancreas, and are least frequent in the arteries to the small bowel and colon.[5] The risk of rupture of a splenic aneurysm has been estimated to be about 2%. However, rupture is associated with pregnancy, and has a high maternal and fetal mortality of 70% and 75–90%, respectively.[6,7] Any aneurysm more than 2 cm should therefore be treated in women of childbearing age. This previously involved surgery, with either under-running of the vessel and/or splenectomy, but endoluminal techniques have now become available, and aneurysms can be thrombosed with the use of coils and/or stent grafts.[8] Initially, rupture of a splenic aneurysm may give back pain associated with shock, as blood fills the lesser sac. Continued bleeding may cause blood to exit through the lesser foramen and run down the right paracolic gutter, so giving rise to right iliac fossa pain. The signs of shock rapidly ensue.

Renal aneurysms occur in about 0.1–0.3% of the population, and are associated with hypertension. There is an increased risk of rupture in pregnancy, but the mortality is lower compared to splenic aneurysm rupture, with a 50% maternal mortality and a 50–80% risk of fetal death.[9,10] The choice of repair may be arterial reconstruction with either synthetic or vein grafts, embolization for intraparenchymal aneurysms, or sometimes the only option in the emergency situation is nephrectomy. New endovascular techniques are becoming available, such as exclusion of the aneurysm with stent grafts.[11]

Case report 2: Abdominal apoplexy

A 45-year-old woman developed severe abdominal pain which radiated up to both shoulders. She was brought in to Accident and Emergency collapsed, with an unrecordable blood pressure. She was effectively resuscitated and ultrasound performed in the department showed fluid in the peritoneal cavity. She was transferred to theatre for emergency laparotomy. A full-length midline incision was made and all blood removed from the abdominal cavity, which was then packed. No blood was observed when packs were removed from the lower abdomen, but there was constant blood arising from packs left around the stomach. Eventually, the blood was found to be coming from the greater curvature of the stomach, and on close inspection, the gastroepiploic artery was found to have parted, and was actively bleeding from both ends. These were oversewn, and the patient made an uneventful recovery.

Case report 3: Obstetrics

A woman with one child gave birth to twins, but unfortunately had placenta accreta. The twins were in a parlous state, and were transferred to the neonatal intensive care unit. As much of the placenta was removed as possible, and the patient was transferred back to the ward. She suffered a cardiac arrest due to severe haemorrhage, and was taken to theatre, where a hysterectomy was performed. Unfortunately, she continued to bleed and both internal iliac arteries were ligated. She was transferred to the intensive care unit, and after a total of 70 units of blood, her diaphragm became splinted and ventilation compromised. The platelet count and clotting screen were near normal following transfusion of relevant blood products. At laparotomy, all the blood was removed from the abdomen and the pelvis packed. There was bleeding from every surface that had been dissected. She required a further 20 units of blood, taking her total to 90 units. Volunteers were requested, and three nurses gave one unit each of fresh O negative whole blood, which was then transfused directly into the patient. This was safe in this particular patient as there could have been very few of her own antibodies left in circulation. The effect of fresh whole blood was immediate, with a marked decrease in bleeding. The pelvis was packed, and the packs were removed 24 hours later when no further bleeding points were encountered. The patient underwent reconstructive surgery to one of her ureters. She also developed weakness of hip flexion, such that for the first 3 months, she was confined to a wheelchair. The neurological problems were attributed to spinal cord ischaemia secondary to hypotension. After 3 months, she and her twins had all made a full recovery.

Important points

Patients who have major haemorrhage following childbirth are usually young and fit. They are able to compensate well for the loss in blood volume as they have good venomotor tone, and the only physical sign may be a tachycardia. When the blood pressure falls, it may be followed quickly by a cardiac arrest. Luckily, such patients will respond to rapid transfusion, and despite the situation being seemingly hopeless, can make a complete recovery.

Always inspect the posterior wall of any vessel injured during insertion of instruments at laparoscopy. The vessel, especially a vein, may have suffered a through and through injury, and although the front wall is successfully repaired, the patient may still die of haemorrhage from the back wall.

Pack the abdomen and pelvis with the biggest packs you can find, and liaise with the anaesthetist to order blood, platelets and fresh frozen plasma. Allow enough time to stabilize the blood pressure before any attempts are made to secure the bleeding points.

Call for help early on, either more senior help from your specialty, or from vascular surgeons or general surgeons who can deal with blood vessel trauma.

Make sure you have good exposure, good lighting and enough assistants to help retract and to use two suckers.

Start from the top and work down. Stop the bleeding with finger pressure, and overrun the bleeding points. Avoid the use of diathermy and clamps.

If in doubt, pack the abdomen and pelvis. Closure of the abdomen may be difficult under these circumstances but is always possible. A continuous mass closure using number 1 nylon or polydioxanone suture should be used. The method of skin closure is less important. Drains should not be used as this will defeat the object of packing, which is to tamponade the bleeding vessels. The patient should be returned to the operating theatre in 24 hours, when the clotting screen and platelets are in the normal range.

Consider arteriography and embolization of persistent uncontrollable haemorrhage. The main cause of postpartum haemorrhage is an atonic uterus with retained placental fragments. A recent series of selective uterine embolization resulted in either the cessation or dramatic reduction of bleeding.[12] No major complications were encountered and normal menstruation resumed in all women who retained their uterus.

REFERENCES

1. Houghton A D, Taylor P R 1996 Iatrogenic life-threatening massive pelvic haemorrhage – report of four cases and guidelines for management. Journal of Obstetrics and Gynaecology 16:422–423
2. Schein M, Rucinski J, Wise L 1996 The abdominal compartment syndrome in the critically ill patient. Current Opinion in Critical Care 2:287–294
3. Vedantham S, Goodwin S C, McLucas B et al 1997 Uterine artery embolisation: An underused method of controlling pelvic haemorrhage. American Journal of Obstetrics and Gynecology 176:938–948
4. Murao H, Kinjo K, Uemura S et al 1998 The subsequent pregnancy outcome to transcatheter angiographic embolization and internal iliac artery ligation for obstetrical hemorrhage. Acta Obstetrica et Gynaecologica Japonica 50:351–354
5. Panayiotopoulos Y P, Assadourian R, Taylor P R 1996 Aneurysms of the visceral and renal arteries. Annals of the Royal College of Surgeons of England 78:412–419
6. Barrett J M, Van Hooydonk J E, Boehm F H 1982 Pregnancy related rupture of arterial aneurysms. Obstetrical and Gynaecological Survey 37:557–566
7. Caillouette J C, Merchant E B 1993 Ruptured splenic artery aneurysm in pregnancy. Twelfth reported case with maternal and fetal survival. American Journal of Obstetrics and Gynecology 168:1810–1813
8. Reidy J F, Rowe P H, Ellis F G 1990 Splenic artery aneurysm embolisation – the preferred technique to surgery. Clinical Radiology 41:281–282
9. Cohen J R, Shamash F S 1987 Ruptured renal artery aneurysms during pregnancy. Journal of Vascular Surgery 6:51–59
10. Robroek A, Van Dick H A, Roex A J M 1994 Rupture of renal artery aneurysm during pregnancy. European Journal of Vascular Surgery 8:375–376
11. Bui B T, Oliva V L, Leclerc G et al 1995 Renal artery aneurysm. Treatment by percutaneous placement of a graft stent. Radiology 195:181–182
12. Pelage J-P, Le Dref O, Jacob D et al 1999 Selective arterial embolization of uterine arteries in the management of intractable post-partum hemorrhage. Acta Obstetrica et Gynaecologica Scandinavica 78:698–703

Techniques from the plastic surgeons

John Pereira and Derek Mercer

Introduction

The term 'plastic' surgery originates from the Greek term *plasticos*, meaning to mould. Plastic surgeons operate in conjunction with many specialties, covering a multitude of pathologies and anatomical sites. There are no magical secrets to the work of plastic surgeons, the principles of meticulous planning, dissection with attention to neurovascular supply, gentle tissue handling, haemostasis, asepsis and wound closure without excess tension can be applied by all surgeons to ensure success. What follows is a brief account of areas where the principles of plastic surgery can be applied to obstetric and gynaecological practice to avoid common problems, as well as information on other areas of overlap and co-operation between the two specialties, a knowledge of which will benefit the reader, encourage joint management and ultimately improve patient care.

Incisions and wound closure

Frequently, surgeons are judged by the scar that they leave. It is a constant reminder to patients that they have had an operation, and is responsible for a steady stream of referrals to the plastic surgical clinic. Frequently attention to detail *before* the first incision will avoid subsequent problems.

Surgical scars are a permanent mark of our day-to-day work. The acceptability of a scar depends on many factors. We have all encountered patients with terrible scars that we would feel could be improved, only to be told proudly 'See this? Mr X did this when he saved my life!'

Similarly, we have seen beautifully healed scars which patients find unacceptable, causing them to shop around various surgeons in an attempt to achieve 'perfection'. Somewhere between these extremes lie most of our patients. It is our duty as surgeons to understand wound healing and factors that influence it, so as to maximize the aesthetic result and minimize complications for our patients.

Wound healing

Wound healing is typically described as a three-phase process, comprising an *inflammatory* phase, a *fibroplastic* phase and a *maturation* phase. In truth, these phases merge in a dynamic sequence of events that ends in a soundly healed wound, without undue delay or problems for the patient (or surgeon).

The *inflammatory phase* is initiated at the time of wounding. Initial vasoconstriction is followed by vasodilatation, resulting in the formation of a platelet coagulum within the wound. Capillaries and venules become leaky in response to histamine, and leucocytes and serum enter the wound. Polymorphonuclear leucocytes perform initial wound débridement and are themselves phagocytosed by mononuclear leucocytes, which become the predominating cells beyond 48 hours.

The *fibroplastic phase* begins on day 2 or 3, lasts for up to 4 weeks, and is heralded by the appearance of fibroblasts in the wound. Fibroblasts are responsible for the production of fibrillar collagen and 'ground substance', the background chemical components in which collagen fibrils assemble to re-establish tissue structure and strength. The end of this phase is characterized by a reduction in fibroblasts and ground substance, and an abundance of relatively poorly organized type 3 collagen.

The *maturation* phase occurs from around 2 to 4 weeks. Synthesis and breakdown of collagen is increased in a co-ordinated fashion, resulting in no net loss or gain of scar mass. The quantity of type 3 (healing) collagen reduces, and that of type 1 (usual) collagen increases, as does the organization and cross-linking of the collagen fibres. At 60 days the wound should reach its maximum strength, around 80% that of unwounded skin. Maturation continues, with organization and a gradual reduction in scar vascularity, seen clinically as the colour change from red/pink early on, to pale and flat by 6–18 months.

While all this is going on, keratinocytes, deprived of contact inhibition, mobilize from adjacent cells and basement membrane, and migrate across the wound surface. Once a confluent layer has been formed, contact inhibition is again established, as are the normal ordered layers of the epidermis.

Congenital and acquired factors may influence wound healing, and any preoperative appraisal should include an evaluation of these factors. While it is inappropriate to list exhaustively the various conditions and their effects on healing, it would be incomplete to neglect various factors from a good history, these may include:

- previous personal or family history of bad scarring;
- connective tissue disorders such as cutis laxa, pseudo-xanthoma elasticum or Ehlers–Danlos syndrome;
- local wound factors, such as previous radiotherapy, multiple previous scars or infections;
- severe anaemia, hypoproteinaemia, uraemia or jaundice;
- poor diet, resulting in vitamin (A, C, E) or zinc deficiency;
- heavy smoking;
- diabetes mellitus;
- chemotherapy, steroids and immunosuppressant drugs;
- cachexia or obesity.

Incisions and wound closure

Half the battle is to identify the factors that put a patient at risk of poor healing; the other half is to counsel patients about the risks of bad scars. Medico-legal actions are easily avoided by truthful explanation and accurate documentation about the possibilities of a poor scar or delayed wound healing. Pointing out the historical factors that increase a patient's risk of a poor outcome at the outset of treatment allows the patient to understand that the blame for poor scars may well not lie with the surgeon. Having said that, there are some fundamental principles that may improve the outcome of wound closure:

- careful planning in 'Langer's lines';
- gentle tissue handling;
- accurate vertical-sided incisions;
- predictive and reactive meticulous haemostasis;
- appropriate wound drainage;
- correct selection of suture material;
- closure in layers, reducing tension on the cuticular suture;
- external support of the wound;
- prevention of wound infection with prophylactic antibiotics if appropriate and suitable dressings;
- avoidance of excessive stress on the wound until maximum strength has been achieved (60 days).

While all surgeons may have different preferences, a reasonable closure technique for the lower abdomen may include 0 nylon for the rectus sheath (mass closure of posterior and anterior sheath), 2/0 polydioxanone for Scarpa's fascia, 3/0 Monocryl® interrupted buried knot subcuticular, and 3/0 Monocryl® running intradermal suture to close the skin. This closure in layers achieves two objectives. First, it prevents the scar in the skin from adhering to the rectus sheath (a common complaint from unhappy patients), and secondly it distributes tension away from the final skin stitch, thus reducing the problem of scar stretch and hypertrophy (see later). Recent studies in weight reduction and body contour surgery have confirmed the structural strength and importance of the superficial fascial system (SFS/Scarpa's fascia in the abdomen). Two points should be clarified here; first, mass closure techniques *must not* include large bites of the rectus muscles, as this will cause tissue ischaemia and necrosis, leading ultimately to wound infection and failure. Secondly, if an absorbable suture is substituted for nylon in this layer, it should be a slowly absorbing material such as PDS®. More rapidly absorbed stitch material will result in hernia formation.

Bad scars

When a patient complains of a bad scar, it is important to establish exactly the nature of the complaint. Clearly, incisional hernia and keloid require different approaches to management, but as we have alluded to earlier, the patient's perceptions and expectations are not always clear or realistic. Only by carefully taking a history and performing a thorough examination can the problem be fully understood. Common complaints are of thick, itchy scars (hypertrophic or keloid), stretched scars (poor collagen or poor closure), or contour irregularities (tethering, hernia). Occasionally, scars may cause pain due to neuroma formation, or functional difficulties due to constriction and contracture.

The exact pathogenesis of abnormal scars is not fully understood. Keloids and hypertrophic scars are due to an abnormality of collagen homeostasis within the scar, a process normally regulated by growth factors and cytokines. For some reason (genetic, environmental or surgical) there is a derailment of the normal control mechanisms, resulting in poor scars.

Hypertrophic scars are characteristically raised above the level of the surrounding skin, red/pink in colour and may itch. They stay within the boundary of the scar, may occur at any site or age, but often occur in the young in scars that are under undue tension (around joints for example). There is an equal sex ratio, and the natural history is for the scar to improve with time. There is some evidence that treatment with silicone gel sheet and pressure may speed up the process. Resistant scars, and those where a predisposing factor such as infection, de-hiscence, delayed wound healing or undue tension can be identified, may respond to surgical revision, correcting the predisposing cause.

Keloid scars (Fig. 15.1), on the other hand, are more aggressive, and characterized by extension of scar tissue beyond the boundaries of the original incision. Keloids are more common in coloured skins, females, and may show familial tendencies. They can commence several months after the original insult, and rarely improve with time. Most commonly they occur on the anterior chest, earlobes and face, but in those with a racial

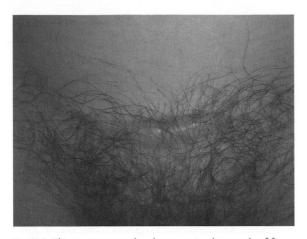

Fig. 15.1 This section scar has been excised on each of four sections. Every time, a thick, itchy, keloid scar has resulted. Clearly, further excision is not indicated, a trial of steroid injections would be an appropriate step forward.

or genetic predisposition, abdominal and perineal scars can be affected. Unlike hypertrophic scars, keloids rarely improve with time, and are unpredictable in their response to therapies. Again, patient expectations need to be managed, and a sensible treatment plan established with the patient. This may involve steroid injections (triamcinolone acetate 10 mg/mL or 40 mg/mL) into the scar at 6-weekly intervals to try and soften and flatten the scar, as well as reduce itch. Care must be taken to keep the steroid within the scar, as extravasation is complicated by local skin and fat atrophy, as well as pigmentation changes. Frequently, steroids achieve sufficient improvement in symptoms to avoid surgery, and they remain the mainstay of management for most sufferers. Repeat injections may be indicated if symptoms relapse. Steroids will not cure a keloid. They may reduce it in size, make it soft and less irritable, and this will often suffice. Surgical excision alone, whether intralesional or complete, is often rewarded with rapid and aggressive recurrence. It is therefore reserved for non-responders to steroids, and often combined with steroids or radiotherapy in the postoperative period. Even with combination therapies, relapse rates range from 50 to 100%.

Stretched scars reflect poor wound support or poor collagen synthesis. From the above description of healing, it can be seen that collagen is turned over during the maturation phase, and scars reach 80% of normal strength by 60 days. Excessive tension during this period, or poor collagen synthesis due to increasing age, for example, can result in stretched, depressed scars. Often patients find these scars acceptable, as the colour fades rapidly and they are not typically itchy or uncomfortable. Revision requires surgical refashioning with layered closure and long-term wound support.

Contour deformity is probably the most common complaint seen in lower abdominal scars. Failure to close wounds in layers results in tethering of skin to the underlying rectus sheath. Tissue above tends to overhang this tethered scar in an unsightly fashion, fungal and bacterial infections may occur under this overhang. Treatment for this problem usually requires management of infection and scar revision. While meticulous closure may improve cosmesis of the transverse lower abdominal incision, there remains the problem of the obese patient with an excessive lower abdominal apron. This group of patients are at high risk of wound complications, and present a difficult access problem for the gynaecological surgeon. A combined approach of initial 'access apronectomy', gynaecological intervention, and subsequent plastic closure can be used to great effect in these cases.

Scar revision

There are many techniques for scar revision. In the majority, simple scar excision, mobilization of good-quality adjacent tissue, and closure in layers will improve the local situation. In general, old scars should be excised, allowing fresh, healthy tissues to be re-opposed. Obstetricians are privileged in this respect, as 9 months of biological tissue expansion should render a wound that is never closed under tension despite scar excision! When scars are tethered to fascia, excision can be difficult without causing potential weakness and risk of herniation. A useful approach here is to *incise* around the original scar and de-epithelialize it, leaving the scar tissue on the fascia. Mobilization of local tissue and closure *over* the old scar is then undertaken in a standard layered manner.

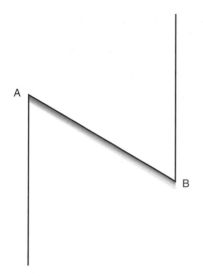

Fig. 15.2 Z-plasty involves the creation of two equal triangular flaps that transpose and close. The total resultant length A–B is greater after transposition. The incisions should all be of equal length, and the angles between scar and incision around 60°.

Although rarely indicated in simple scars on the abdomen, Z-plasty (Fig. 15.2), Y–V-plasty and W-plasty are revision techniques that have a place in treating contracted scars in the perineum. These techniques attempt to lengthen and break up tight straight-line scars or release scar webs that can occur after poorly planned incisions in this area. This is achieved by transposition or advancement of skin flaps into the wound, and is best performed by a trained reconstructive surgeon.

Reconstructive surgery in obstetrics and gynaecology

Gynaecological oncology

The management of gynaecological malignancy presents a challenge for both the oncologist and reconstructive surgeon. When considering surgery as a treatment modality, many factors must be taken into account. It is convenient to think of these as the 'Ps'.

The first P is the *pathology*. Accurate tissue diagnosis, radiological evaluation and staging, and examination under anaesthesia (EUA) are mandatory in order to understand the disease status and resection/reconstruction required. It is easy to underestimate the extent of resection required in recurrent disease, postirradiation skin and invasive disease within a pre-invasive field change. Incisional biopsies at the time of EUA are very helpful here. Only with this information can the surgeon, oncologist and patient discuss treatment options accurately.

Having accurately diagnosed the pathology, the *purpose* of planned treatment must be established; this may be curative or palliative. While it may seem unkind to perform major surgery for palliative reasons, we have treated numerous patients with postirradiation recurrences, who have been socially crippled by pain, odour and discharge, with excellent results. While long-term cure may not be possible, quality of life is restored for a variable period of time.

Patient wishes and *performance status* are the next two areas to consider. This is particularly important in gynaecological reconstruction, where the complexity of operation increases with functional demands. For example, it is relatively straightforward to reconstruct the perineum after exenteration, but a further level of complexity is added if vaginal reconstruction is required. Clearly, not all patients will request vaginal reconstruction, and a simpler technique will be available here. Moreover, not all patients are fit for major ablative and reconstructive surgery, and full preoperative assessment with the help of the anaesthetic department and physician is a prerequisite in the elderly.

Previous treatment and *postoperative adjuvant therapy* are the next two areas to consider. Old scars may compromise reconstructive options. Stomas and catheters may complicate the design and mobilization of flaps. Irradiation renders wound healing less efficient, and makes tissues stiff and poorly suited for reconstructive use. Moreover, if postoperative therapy is scheduled, the reconstructive surgeon has a deadline for complete wound healing, to allow for commencement of the adjuvant chemo- or radiotherapy.

Only after all the above factors have been carefully weighed up can the details of the *planned procedure* be finalized. When planning reconstruction, a good reconstructive surgeon will not only have a plan, but a fall-back position in case of operative difficulties with the first option, and, almost always, a further option up one's sleeve for dealing with flap failure or recurrence of disease at a later date. This philosophy dates back to Harold Gillies, one of the fathers of modern reconstructive surgery. He stated, 'Have a plan, and a pattern for the plan. Have a plan and a lifeboat!'

Reconstructive options

When approaching reconstruction, it is conventional to look at solutions to a problem in a logical progression of simple to complex options. This approach is often described as the 'reconstructive ladder'. The most simple end of the spectrum, the lowest 'rung' of the ladder, is to leave the defect to heal by secondary intention; the top rung is the use of composite free tissue transfer; and, in between, the rungs include direct closure, skin grafting, local and distant cutaneous or myocutaneous flaps. Although the complexity of surgery increases as the ladder is ascended, this does not mean that it is not appropriate to jump straight to a more complex option rather than rigidly sticking to a stepwise progression of reconstructive options. Each option has its advantages and disadvantages in terms of outcome versus complexity and donor site morbidity, and the surgeon must weigh up the pros and cons of each. With increasing familiarity and reliability, the 'ladder' becomes more of a 'toolbox', to be dipped into as required.

The perineum is a complex three-dimensional area, combining the functions of micturition, defaecation and sexual function. Comfort, flexibility and durability are essential to allow normal sitting and locomotion. All these factors must be taken into account when planning surgery. Fortunately, it has a rich blood supply upon which to base reconstructive techniques.

Defects that require reconstruction tend to fall into one of the following categories:

- abdominal wall (secondary tumours)
- vulval defects (partial and complete)
- vaginal defects (partial and complete)
- pelvic floor resurfacing after exenteration.

These will be dealt with in sequence, and the pros and cons of options discussed.

Abdominal wall reconstruction

Defects of the abdominal wall are usually encountered after direct tumour extension, secondary tumours, or implantation of tumour at the time of earlier resection. Occasionally, necrotizing fasciitis can produce full-thickness defects. Reconstruction of the structural layers of the abdominal wall requires the use of synthetic mesh or fascia lata for the muscle/fascial layers, and cover with vascularized skin. This is best achieved by using the vertical rectus abdominus myocutaneous flap (VRAM) with mesh, or the tensor fascia lata flap (TFL) from the lateral leg, bringing with it a vascularized layer of fascia lata. Figures 15.3 and 15.4 show an ovarian secondary in the abdominal wall widely

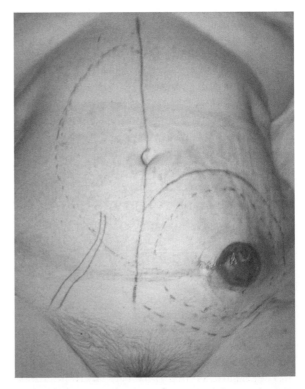

Fig. 15.3 Tumour implantation from an ovarian carcinoma.

supply. Myocutaneous flaps based on the rectus abdominus muscles and gracilis muscles also have a role in large defects. Again, the exact choice will depend upon the experience and preference of the surgeon, previous incisions, and size and geography of the defect. Figures 15.5 and 15.6 show a fungating vulval lesion with lymphadenopathy in both groins, treated by excision, bilateral groin dissection, a right hemi-transverse rectus abdominus myocutaneous flap (TRAM) to the mons, and bilateral buttock crease cutaneous transposition flaps to the posterior

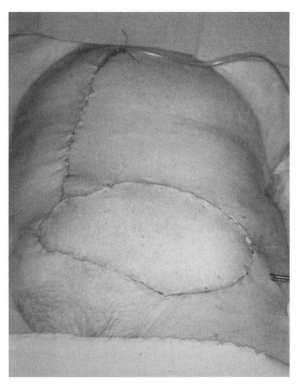

Fig. 15.4 Reconstruction with a right vertical rectus abdominus myocutaneous (VRAM) island flap over a double layer of synthetic mesh.

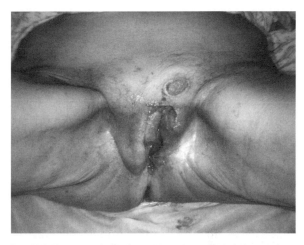

Fig. 15.5 Fungating vulval carcinoma, irradiated skin and bilateral lymphadenopathy, a challenging surgical terrain.

resected and reconstructed using a VRAM flap. The flap has been islanded and is transposed to cover a mesh placed in the lower abdominal wall defect. The flap is based on the deep inferior epigastric vessels, which supply the rectus muscle and its overlying skin. Donor site morbidity includes abdominal scars as shown, abdominal weakness, and risk of herniation. The advantages are that the flap is extremely reliable, quick and easy to raise, and can be mobilized without extra preparation or movement of the patient. Typically the patient mobilizes after 48 hours, and is rehabilitated as for an abdominal hernia repair.

Vulval defects

Vulval defects may be partial or complete. Options for reconstruction include healing by secondary intention (small defects that have not been irradiated), direct closure, and local cutaneous flaps based on the perineal blood

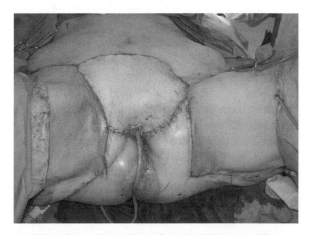

Fig. 15.6 After excision, three flaps have been used for resurfacing: bilateral gluteal fold flaps for the vulva and a hemi-transverse rectus abdominus myocutaneous flap for the mons pubis.

vulva. This was followed up by external-beam radiotherapy, and good palliation of symptoms was achieved.

Vaginal reconstruction

Reconstruction of a functioning vagina is a great surgical challenge, whether for congenital absence, or after tumour ablation. The quantity and sensitivity of remaining introital tissue is an important contributor to the patient's sexual pleasure. The reconstructive goal is to create a stable, durable vaginal tube of adequate dimension for intercourse, with acceptable donor scars and morbidity.

Tubularized skin graft for neovaginal reconstruction was introduced by McIndoe in 1938. It is still commonly used, especially in vaginal agenesis. A new vaginal pocket is created between the rectum and the bladder and this space is resurfaced with split-thickness skin grafts harvested from the lateral thigh, or a full-thickness graft from the groin. The skin graft is draped over an appropriately sized plastic vaginal mould, inserted into the pocket, and retained by suturing the labia together. The mould is removed after 3 weeks for graft inspection, and if all is well, replaced again for a further month. Thereafter, a slightly smaller insert is kept in situ for 6–12 months to prevent graft contracture. Regular dilation or intercourse is essential to maintain an open introitus. Stenosis is less common when full-thickness grafts are used. It is reported that, with time, the new vagina assumes some mucosal characteristics and may become sexually responsive. Using skin graft for vaginal reconstruction after resection for cancer can be successful only if the bladder and rectum remain in place to support the grafts, and there has been no prior irradiation to the field. Where there is no vascularized support for a graft, this must be imported, or flaps of tissue with their own blood supply employed. In procedures that require supralevator resection, or that preserve anterior or posterior vaginal cuffs, extensive dissection for myocutaneous flaps may itself disrupt normal unaffected structures and contribute to additional morbidity. In these cases neovaginal reconstruction using an omental flap with split-thickness skin graft lining can avoid these difficulties while providing adequate pelvic fill and functional restoration. The omentum, which has an excellent blood supply, is mobilized and pedicled on the left gastroepiploic artery, passed into the pelvis along the left paracolic gutter, and lined with a skin graft on a stent as described above. This method is technically simple, safe and reliable.

In those cases where skin grafts are unsuitable, local flaps of skin from the adjacent perineum can be raised bilaterally on the rich perineal blood supply, sutured together to create a tube and transposed into the defect. Recently, this technique has become increasingly popular, the flaps are quick to raise, reliable, and have the advantage of also being sensate. A stent is not required long-term, and stenosis is less of a problem than with skin grafts.

The last cutaneous reconstructions are based away from the perineum, and rely upon a muscle and its blood supply to maintain an island of skin that is tubed to form the vagina. Two main options are available here. From above, passed down through the pelvis, the VRAM flap, as mentioned before, can be tubularized into a vagina. From below, islands of skin carried on the gracilis muscle can be raised bilaterally and passed up to form a tube. Both options have the disadvantage of scars remote from the perineum, but produce good results in expert hands.

The final technique for vaginoplasty involves a pedicled large bowel flap, islanded, closed at its deep end and transposed into the pelvis. This technique has the advantage of a self-lubricating mucosal surface, and fewer cutaneous scars. Endoscopically assisted techniques are now evolving which further enhance cosmesis. The disadvantage is that a bowel repair is required, with its attending risks, and stenosis at the bowel/cutaneous junction can be a problem.

The exact technique of vaginoplasty will be selected by the reconstructive surgeon after analysis of the 'Ps' mentioned above.

Exenteration

The final need for reconstruction of the perineum is that of resurfacing following removal of all pelvic function, with creation of a urinary diversion, colostomy and excision of the vagina. These defects can sometimes be closed primarily, but in the face of previous irradiation it is often advisable to import healthy tissue and excise the radiotherapized areas, which will heal slowly if at all. Again, the mainstay flaps for this are the VRAM from above, and the gracilis from below. The muscle element of the flap is used where possible to fill dead space low in the pelvis and provide a plug in the pelvic floor. Although the VRAM is a bulkier flap and is more reliable than the gracilis, its harvest may compromise positioning of the urinary diversion and colostomy, and careful planning with the stoma nurse and resecting surgeon is essential.

Other conditions

Cutaneous endometriosis

Extrapelvic endometriosis is fortunately uncommon, but should be suspected in women with subcutaneous masses, which give cyclical symptoms of pain and swelling, and with cutaneous lesions that bleed or discharge at menstruation. The common sites for presentation are in the umbilicus, laparotomy, section, and laparoscopy scars, and in the perineum. Cutaneous lesions are usually small and complete surgical excision has a high cure rate. For lesions that are large, subcutaneous or recurrent, preoperative hormonal therapy with danazol or leuprolide is recommended by some to reduce the size of the lesions, and possibly the risk of further recurrence.

Female genital repair, refashioning and enhancement

In recent years there have been an increasing number of procedures requested and performed for functional and aesthetic problems of the vulva and vagina. The 'designer vagina' is one of the latest cosmetic enhancements offered by some aesthetic clinics. Procedures range from reductions of excessively redundant labia majora and minora (which become sore at intercourse, interfere with urinary stream, or simply look unnatural) to liposculpture of the mons, fat and filler injections to the labia, and vaginal tightening or hymen reconstruction. As with all 'aesthetic' procedures, the patients should be carefully counselled and screened for psychological disorders before surgery is undertaken. A clear understanding of the patient's functional and aesthetic requirements is a prerequisite for success. Incisions must be designed to avoid scar contractures and potential discomfort and clearly consideration to sensory nerve supply is all-important. It remains to be seen if this is a growing market or a passing fashion!

Necrotizing fasciitis

Finally, no chapter on gynaecology and plastic surgery would be complete without a mention of necrotizing fasciitis (NF). This is an aggressive bacterial infection (often group A β-haemolytic streptococci) of the superficial fascia and subcutaneous tissues. Overall mortality remains around 20%. Although the condition is uncommon, early recognition is essential for effective management. In the perineum NF can occur spontaneously or after surgery, Bartholin's abscess (Fig. 15.7), episiotomy, septic abortion or pudendal anaesthetic blocks. Usual predisposing factors include diabetes, renal disease, malignancy, malnutrition, intravenous drug abuse, alcoholism, immunosuppresion and morbid obesity.

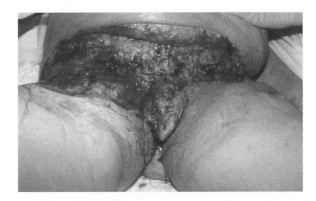

Fig. 15.7 Necrotizing fasciitis following a Bartholin's abscess in a diabetic. This shows the typical extent of excision required to control the infection. Further inspection should be undertaken daily until no further necrotic tissue remains.

Presentation is often insidious, but the characteristic feature is a rapidly spreading skin discoloration, with severe pain, disproportionate to the local signs. The patient may quickly become toxic with pyrexia, tachycardia, tachypnoea and hypotension. Multi-organ failure is common. Early diagnosis is the key here; fluid resuscitation and oxygen therapy are instituted while theatre and ITU facilities are alerted. It should be remembered that the area of NF is always significantly larger than the extent of the visibly involved skin. Bold and radical surgical débridement is life saving. Large excisional defects are reconstructed with skin graft once the patient is stable. Early plastic surgical assistance in these cases has been shown to reduce mortality and morbidity. *Always suspect the diagnosis when pain is disproportionate to local signs*—one day you will find it and save your patient's life.

ACKNOWLEDGEMENT

The author wish to thank Mr. Naguib El-Mottardi, Locum Consultant Plastic Surgeon St. Thomas' Hospital, for help in preparing the text and photographs.

FURTHER READING

Cormack G, Lamberty G 1994 The arterial anatomy of skin flaps, 2nd edn. Chuchill Livingstone, Edinburgh

Genitourinary repair and reconstruction. Selected Readings in Plastic Surgery 8(40). Baylor University Press, Dallas, Texas

Lockwood T E 1991 The superficial fascial system of the trunk and extremities: a new concept. Plastic and Reconstructive Surgery 87(6):1009–1018

McCraw J, Massey F, Shanklin K, Horton C 1967 Vaginal reconstruction with gracilis myocutaneous flaps. Plastic and Reconstructive Surgery 58:176–183

Martello J, Vasconez H 1995 Vulvar and vaginal reconstruction after surgical treatment for gynaecological cancer. Clinics in Plastic Surgery 22(1):129–140

Monstrey S, Blondeel P, Van Landuyt K et al 2001 The versatility of the pudendal thigh fasciocutaneous flap used as an island flap. Plastic and Reconstructive Surgery 107:719–725

Mustoe T A et al 2002 Guidelines on scar management. Plastic and Reconstructive Surgery 110(2):560–571

Sadove R, Horton C 1988 Utilizing full-thickness skin grafts for vaginal reconstruction. Clinics in Plastic Surgery 15(3):443–448

Tobin G, Pursell S, Day T 1990 Refinements in vaginal reconstruction using rectus abdominus flaps. Clinics in Plastic Surgery 17(4):705–712

Wee J, Joseph V T 1989 A new technique of vaginal reconstruction using neurovascular pudendal-thigh flaps: A preliminary report. Plastic and Reconstructive Surgery 83:701–709

Woods J, Alter G, Meland B, Prodratz K 1992 Experience with vaginal reconstruction utilising the modified Singapore flap. Plastic and Reconstructive Surgery 90:270–274

Wound Healing, wound closure, abnormal scars. Selected Readings in Plastic Surgery 9(3). Baylor University Press, Dallas, Texas

Yii N, Niranjan N 1996 Lotus petal flaps in vulvo-vaginal reconstruction. British Journal of Plastic Surgery 49:547–554

Appendix:
A guide to instruments commonly used in obstetric and gynaecological surgery

Darryl Maxwell

The diversity of instruments developed by manufacturers to aid surgeons is extensive. Instrument catalogues are impressively large telephone directory size publications in which the Obstetrics and Gynaecology sections occupy substantial space. The range of instruments selected for discussion in this review is not comprehensive and covers only a small portion of available choice. Those included reflect personal experience and what is considered to be available for use in operating theatres throughout the UK. Any individual surgeon wishing to learn more, or to borrow ideas from another speciality, is strongly advised to consult available catalogues or communicate directly with the manufacturers.

Dissecting forceps (also called thumb forceps)

As the name suggests, these types of forceps are used to handle tissue during dissection and suturing. These forceps grip when compressed between thumb and fingers, allowing quick pick up and release movements during dextrous pelvic dissection or to grasp the needle during suture placement. They are either of light or heavy construction with or without teeth at the tips. The approximating teeth help to grasp tissue or the suturing needle. Choice depends on the intended purpose, and one of each sort is generally found on each instrument set. Serrated inserts are often added to the inside of the arms of toothed forceps to facilitate tissue handling. The non-toothed variety is preferred for handling peritoneum and more delicate tissue such as bowel.

Common examples are:

- **Bonney forceps:** toothed and non-toothed. The needle forceps have 1 × 2 tenaculum teeth at the end, plus fine sharply defined serrations in the inserts to provide non-slip surfaces with which to grasp the tissue and suture needles.

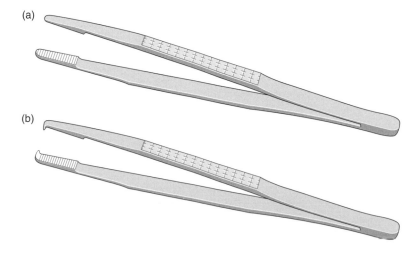

Fig. A.1 Bonney dissecting forceps:
(a) serrated;
(b) 1/2 teeth.

● **McIndoes:** not as heavy as Bonney's forceps, with a single 'stop' inside the handles.

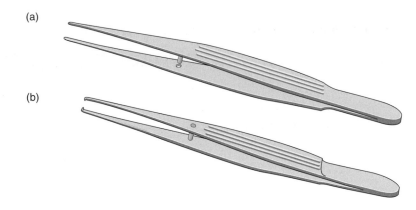

Fig. A.2 McIndoe dissecting forceps:
(a) serrated;
(b) 1/2 teeth.

● **Gillies:** an even lighter variety with two 'stops' inside the handles.

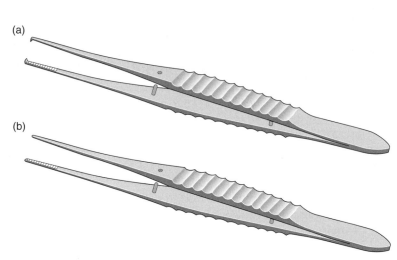

Fig. A.3 Gillies dissecting forceps:
(a) 1/2 teeth;
(b) serrated.

- **DeBakey forceps:** a wide range of light atraumatic general-purpose tissue/vascular forceps. The angled type is quite useful for handling periureteric tissues and bladder mucosa.

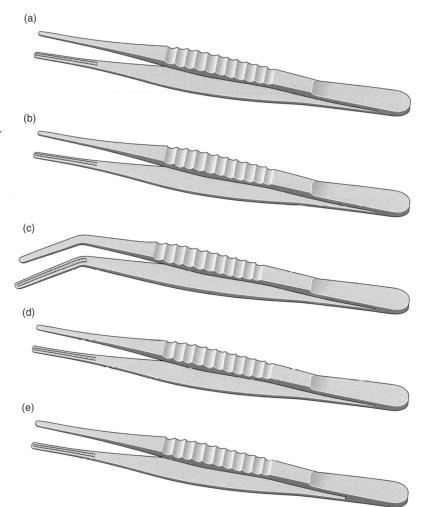

Fig. A.4 DeBakey dissecting forceps:
(a) atraumatic, 1.5 mm jaw;
(b) atraumatic, 2 mm jaw;
(c) atraumatic, angled, 2 mm jaw;
(d) atraumatic, 2.4 mm jaw;
(e) atraumatic, 2.7 mm jaw.

Tissue forceps

These forceps have apposing tips and are hinged in the middle with a ratchet lock at the handle. The blade shape and surface configuration is specific to the intended use (see illustrations). Opposing surfaces may have fine serrations and/or small interlocking teeth. They are most suitable for static tissue holding during area dissection around the secured tissue.

Common examples are:

- **Lanes:** suitable for grasping large blocks of tissue destined to be removed as a specimen.

  Fig. A.5 Lanes tissue forceps, 1/2 teeth, fenestrated.

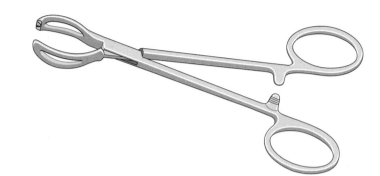

- **Littlewood:** a gentler forceps for handling tissue that is to remain.

  Fig. A.6 Littlewood tissue forceps, 2/3 teeth.

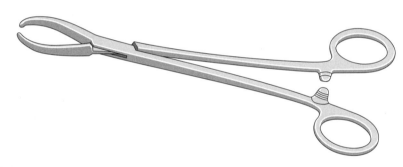

- **Allis:** have a series of approximating teeth at the end. Can be short or long.

  Fig. A.7 Allis tissue forceps.

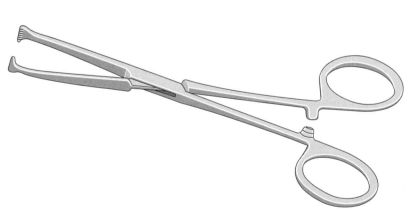

- **Babcock:** such forceps have flat apposing surfaces with fine parallel cross serrations. The blades have a ring-like shape and are designed to handle bowel that can 'bulge' into the curvature of the blades and so be held securely. Available in varying jaw widths, they are used almost exclusively to handle bowel in elevating the edge or apices of a viscus.

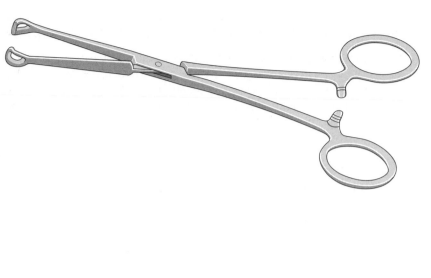

Fig. A.8 Babcock tissue forceps, serrated jaws.

- **Duval:** these have a triangular 'bite' that is wide and non-crushing.

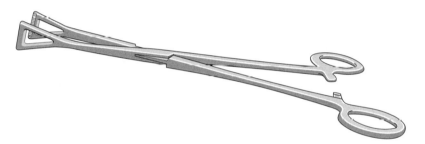

Fig. A.9 Duval tissue forceps, serrated.

Haemostatic forceps (also called artery forceps or hemostats)

Light instruments with spring handles and generally quite small, delicate tips with transverse serrations along the jaws, they are used to isolate bleeding points or small vascular pedicles. There are numerous types and they can be curved or straight, longer or shorter, according to intended use and the individual surgeon's preference. The immense variety of size, shape, length and design has made these a very utilitarian instrument.

Common examples are:

- **Mosquito forceps:** the simplest, lightest example.

  Fig. A.10 Mosquito Micro haemostatic forceps, straight and curved.

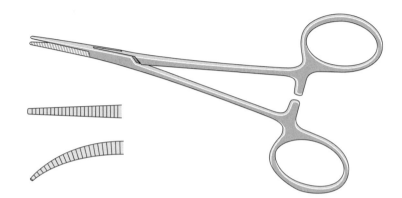

- **Mosquito Halstead**

  Fig. A.11 Mosquito Halstead haemostatic forceps:
  (a) straight serrated jaws;
  (b) straight, 1/2 teeth.

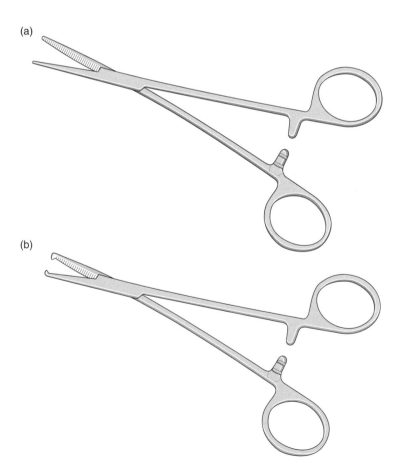

(a)

(b)

- **Spencer Wells:** a slightly heavier version, which can be curved or straight.

  Fig. A.12 Spencer Wells haemostatic forceps, straight and curved, serrated jaws.

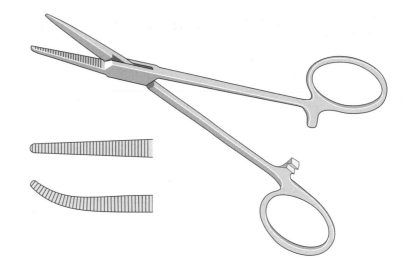

- **Kocher's:** heavier with approximating tenaculum teeth at the tip. Can be curved or straight and many different sizes. Used by some as a clamp at hysterectomy, the editor does not consider them suitable for that purpose.

  Fig. A.13 Kocher haemostatic forceps, straight and curved, 1/2 teeth.

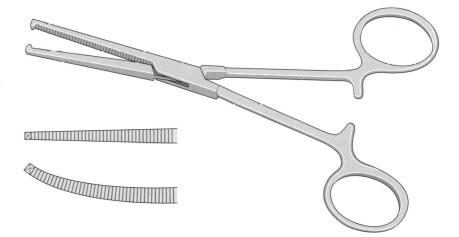

- **Oschner's forceps:** similar to Kocher's.

  Fig. A.14 Oscher haemostatic forceps, straight and curved, 1/2 teeth.

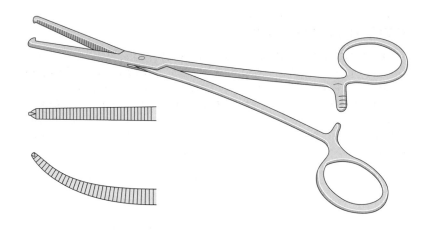

- **Lahey forceps:** these are right-angled forceps, ideal for getting around or going under the ureter or vascular structures to receive or carry ties. They were designed originally for gall bladder and thoracic work.

  Fig. A.15 Lahey haemostatic forceps, curved, longitudinal serrations.

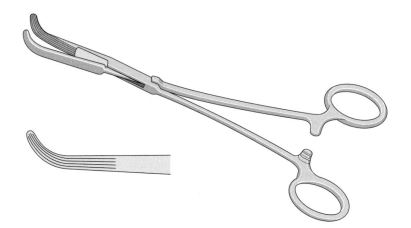

Hysterectomy clamps

When removing the uterus, a key requirement is the repeated clamping of discrete pedicles of tissue for subsequent mobilization and ligature. Because the enclosed tissue is often very vascular (particularly the recently gravid uterus), clamps need to have a robust ratchet lock in the handle combined with secure jaw closure that prevents tissue escaping from the jaws while at the same time minimizing tissue trauma. Serrations along the inside of the jaws aid in securing tissue, while interlocking tenaculum teeth, approximately at the distal tip of the jaw, prevent lateral play. Generally there are three types of serrations:

1. serrated (serrations which run transversely across the jaw);

2. longitudinal serrations (which run the length of the jaw);

3. cross-serrations (a criss-cross pattern—not very commonly used).

As a general rule, longitudinal serrations are preferred.

Many types are available. Clamps in common use are:

- **Bonney:** these are angled clamps with cross-serrations and 1 × 2 teeth at the tip.

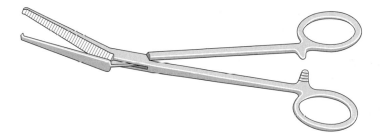

  Fig. A.16 Hysterectomy clamps: Bonney, angled on flat, 1/2 teeth.

- **Gwilliam:** longitudinal serrations with 1 × 2 teeth at the tip. Curved or straight variations are available.

  Fig. A.17 Gwilliam hysterectomy clamps:
  (a) straight, longitudinal serrations, 1/2 teeth;
  (b) curved on flat, longitudinal serrations, 1/2 teeth.

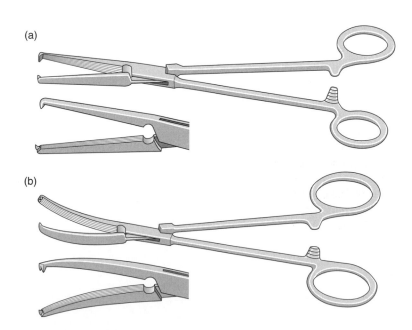

(a)

(b)

- **Heaney:** there are several varieties but these are generally only available with an angled serration. A characteristic feature is the presence of a wide single or double 'cross'-tooth along the jaws to improve apposition. They do not have longitudinal serrations, as these cannot be machined due to the presence of the cross-teeth.

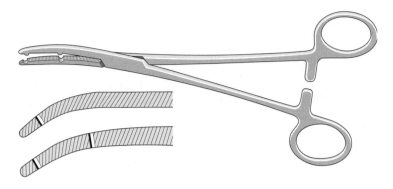
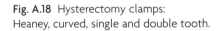

Fig. A.18 Hysterectomy clamps: Heaney, curved, single and double tooth.

- **Maingot:** a straight or curved clamp with a tongue-and-groove jaw with 1 × 2 teeth.

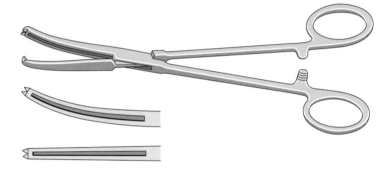

Fig. A.19 Hysterectomy clamps: Maingot, curved on flat and straight, 1/2 teeth

- **Zeppelin:** these are designed specifically for use at hysterectomy, coming in a variety of sizes and curves. They are more delicate, lightweight instruments, designed specifically to minimize tissue trauma and to allow for maximum vision in the operating field. A specific range for vaginal hysterectomy has also been introduced. Zeppelin clamps have achieved widespread acceptance since their introduction.

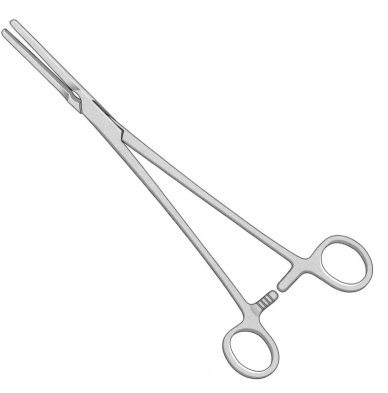

Fig. A.20 Zeppelin hysterectomy clamp.

- **Chelsea angle clamps:**
these are available in angled
and straight versions. They are
similar to Bonney hysterectomy
clamps but slighter longer with
shorter, more robust jaws.

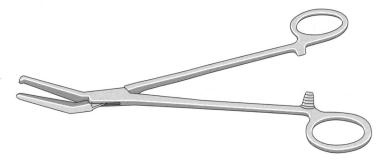

Fig. A.21 Hysterectomy clamps:
Chelsea angle clamp.

- Other clamps favoured by some are Howkin's and the McCullough's.
The special feature of the latter is that they have large finger apertures
in the handles (bows)—apparently McCullough had big thumbs!
Both are featured in catalogues infrequently and may be difficult to
obtain.

Fig. A.22 Howkin's
hysterectomy clamp

Other lighter clamps
sometimes adopted for
use at hysterectomy are:

- **Moynihan cholecystectomy:**
these have relatively short,
heavy curved jaws,
transverse serrations and
no teeth.

Fig. A.23 Hysterectomy
clamps: Moynihan
colecystectomy forceps,
curved on flat, box joint.

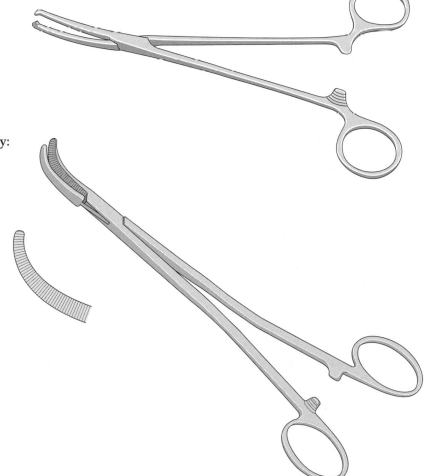

- **Lahey cholecystectomy:**
these have relatively small,
curved jaws, longitudinal
serrations and no teeth
(see Fig. A.15).

Abdominal retractors

Hand-held retractors

- **Langenbeck:** a very common hand retractor, available with small, medium and large blades.

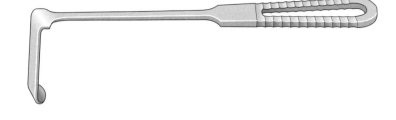

Fig. A.24 Hand-held retractors: Langenbeck, single ended.

- **Morris:** also very common, larger blades, available double ended.

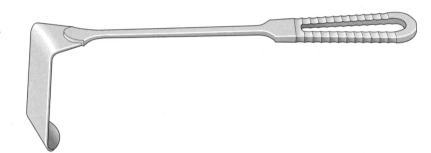

Fig. A.25 Hand-held retractors: Morris, single ended.

- **Doyen:** commonly used at caesarean section, it comes with blades of three different sizes.

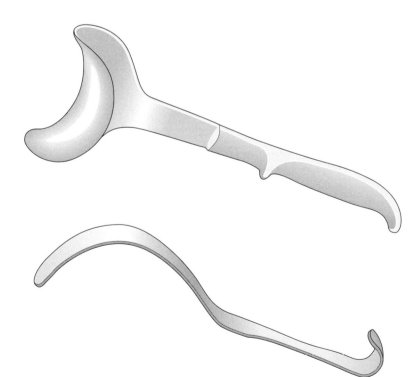

Fig. A.26 Hand-held retractors: Doyen.

- **Deaver:** a general surgical bowel retractor available in different lengths or widths.

Fig. A.27 Hand-held retractors: Deaver abdominal.

- **De Lee:** a useful general-purpose retractor.

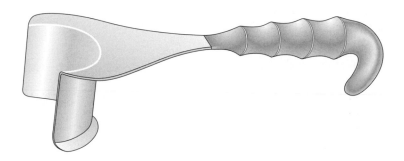

Fig. A.28 Hand-held retractors: De Lee universal retractor.

Self-retaining retractors

- **Balfour:** a very common retractor for O and G use. This is a spreading retractor with central and lateral blades. There are alternative sizes to every component, the many permutations allowing adaptation for specific operative needs.

  Fig. A.29 Self-retaining retractors: Balfour, fenetrated end blades.

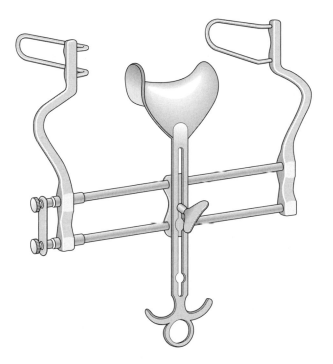

- **Gosset:** a two-bladed spreading retractor, available in short and large sizes.

  Fig. A.30 Self-retaining retractors: Gosset, two blades.

- **Turner Warwick:** a versatile ring retractor with numerous different adjustable components. Much loved (or hated) by those who have used it.

  Fig. A.31 Self-retaining retractors: Turner Warwick adult retractor set.

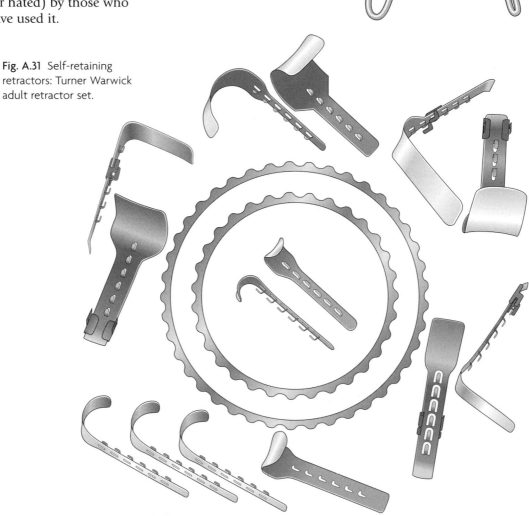

Operating scissors

Scissors for operating in the pelvis fulfil two different surgical needs. Scissors with powerful blades and long handles give leverage when dealing with scar tissue or cleavage dissection of the 'separate-and-cut' type. The more finely constructed variety is designed for accurate delicate dissection and separation of filmy adhesions, possibly involving peritoneum, Fallopian tubes or bowel. One of each type is normally available on most laparotomy sets. Surgical scissors can be straight, curved or angled, but generally have chamfered ends; sharp pointed scissors are rarely used in pelvic surgery.

Typical examples are:

- **Mayo:** a wide range is available.

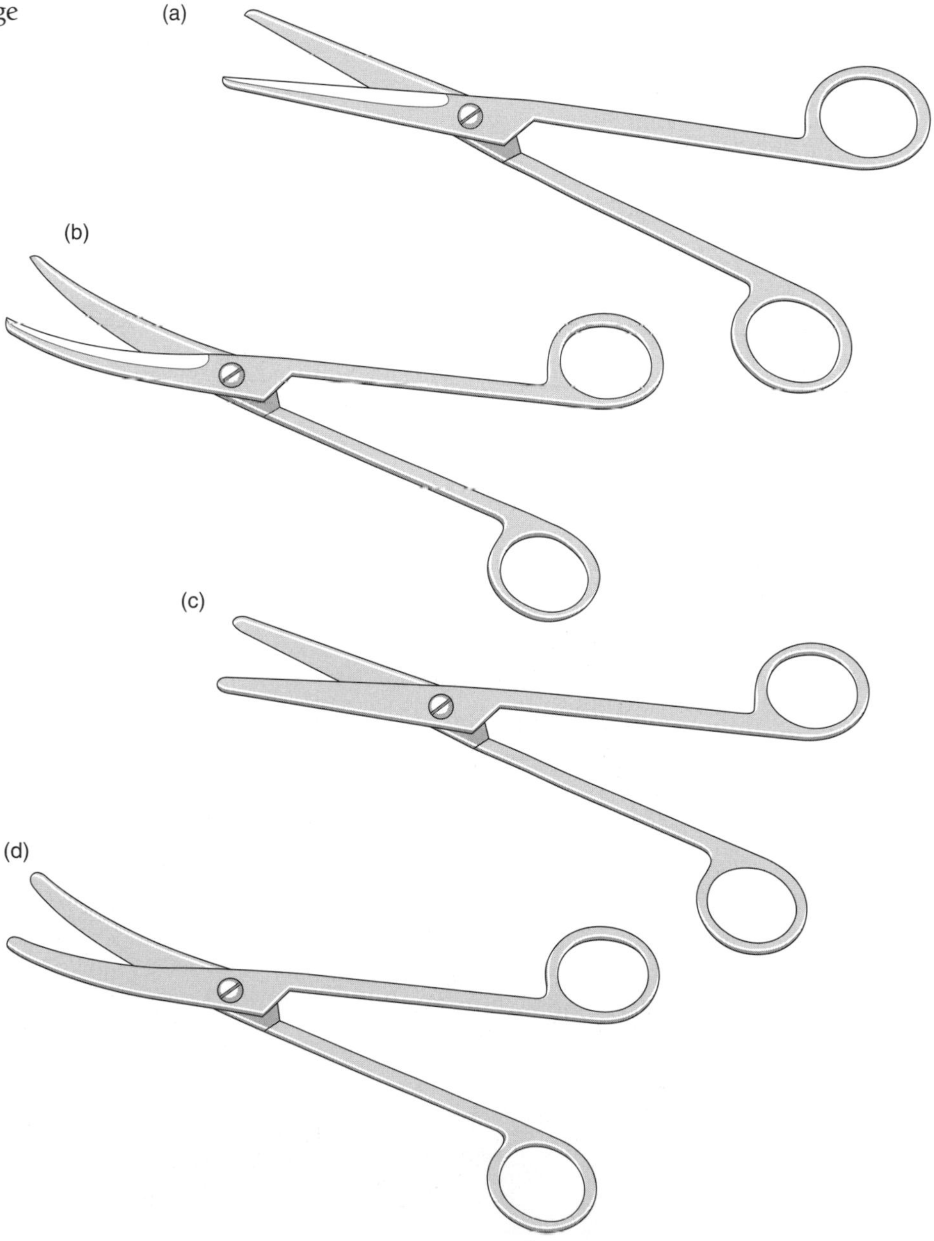

Fig. A.32 Mayo operating scissors:
(a) straight, bevelled blades;
(b) curved, bevelled blades;
(c) straight, round blades;
(d) curved, round blades.

(a)

(b)

(c)

(d)

- **Metzenbaum:** a wide range is available, with the lighter scissors being particularly good for fine dissection.

Fig. A.33 Metzenbaum operating scissors:

(a) straight, blunt/blunt;

(b) curved, blunt/blunt;

(c) fine, straight, blunt/blunt;

(d) fine, straight, sharp/sharp;

(e) fine, curved, blunt/blunt;

(f) fine, curved, sharp/sharp.

- **McIndoe:** similar to the 180 mm curved, blunt Metzenbaum scissor (Fig. A.33b) (not the other sizes).

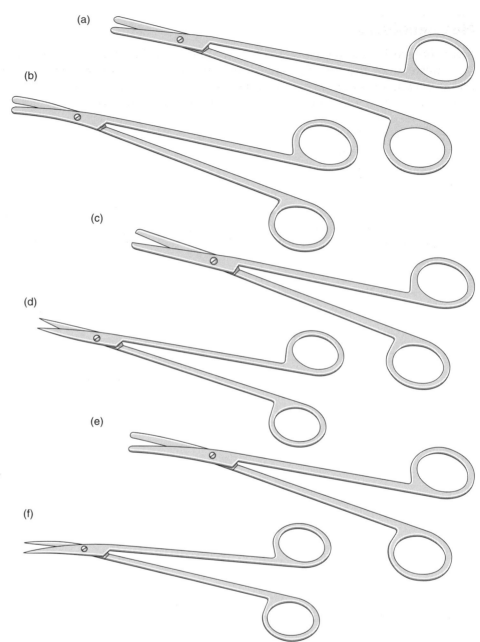

(a)

(b)

(c)

(d)

(e)

(f)

Needleholders

Needleholders have short, serrated jaws to hold the needle securely and a smooth locking mechanism at the handle. The type with tungsten carbide (TC) inserts inside the jaws achieves maximum grip on suture needles. Needleholders can be straight or curved, and long-handled varieties are available. The curved and/or long needleholders may facilitate access to deeper confined spaces in the pelvis.

Common examples are:

- **Mayo:** these come in the widest range of sizes.

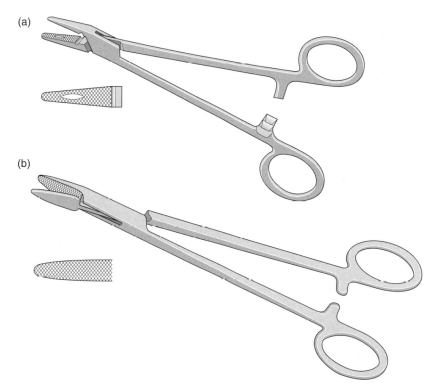

Fig. A.34 Mayo needleholders:
(a) light pattern, serrated jaws;
(b) wide, serrated jaws.

- **DeBakey's:** widely available.

Fig. A.35 DeBakey needleholders.

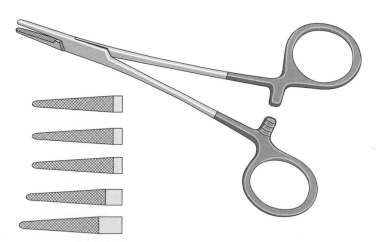

- **Thomson—Walker:**
  the cranked shanks allow
  an S-curve with a normal
  straight jaw.

  Fig. A.36 Thomson—Walker
  needleholders, serrated jaws.

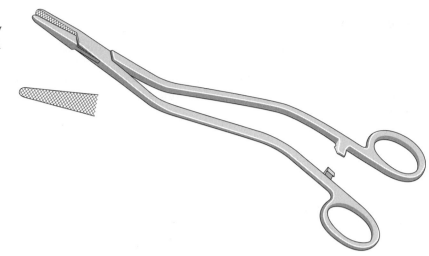

- **Naunton Morgan:**
  opens with a box-like
  compound action suited
  for work in confined
  spaces, e.g. the pelvis.

  Fig. A.37 Naunton Morgan
  needleholders, compound action,
  serrated jaws.

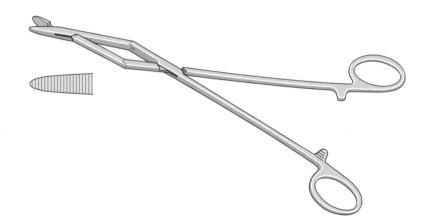

Index

239

241